LIVING WITH VISION PROBLEMS

The Sourcebook for Blindness and Vision Impairment

Jill Sardegna; Susan Shelly;
Allan Richard Rutzen, M.D.;
Scott M. Steidl, M.D., D.M.A.

Checkmark Books®

An imprint of Facts On File, Inc.

Living with Vision Problems: The Sourcebook for Blindness and Vision Impairment

Checkmark Books
An imprint of Facts On File, Inc.
132 West 31st Street
New York NY 10001

Library of Congress Cataloging-in-Publication Data

Living with vision problems: the sourcebook for blindness and vision impairment /
Jill Sardegna . . . [et al.].
       p. cm.
  Includes bibliographical references and index.
  ISBN 0-8160-4281-0 (pb.: alk. paper)
    1. Vision disorders—Popular works. 2. Blindness—Popular works.
    I. Sardegna, Jill.
  RE51 .L585 2002
  617.7′12—dc21   2001058102

Checkmark Books are available at special discounts when purchased in bulk quantities for businesses, associations, institutions, or sales promotions. Please call our Special Sales Department in New York at (212) 967-8800 or (800) 322-8755.

You can find Facts On File on the World Wide Web at http://www.factsonfile.com

Text design by Evelyn Horowitz
Cover design by Cathy Rincon

Printed in the United States of America

MP FOF 10 9 8 7 6 5 4 3 2 1

This book is printed on acid-free paper.

CONTENTS

PREFACE

Sight is one of human beings' most precious gifts, and yet one of the most taken for granted. Most of us routinely go about our daily business, relying on our sight to get around, complete our work, recognize friends and family, read, and generally make our lives easier and more enjoyable.

Too often, only when we develop problems with our eyes or eyesight do we appreciate what a miracle the sense of sight is—or was.

Living with Vision Problems is an easy-to-use sourcebook on the subject of blindness and issues that relate to blindness. It addresses topics as far ranging as the mechanics of the eye to traditional biases and prejudices against blind people. It seeks to help readers achieve a better understanding of how the eyes work, and of the problems that can occur with the eyes and with vision. It also addresses laws affecting blind or visually impaired individuals, procedures and medicines used to treat vision problems, and diseases and disorders that can affect the eyes and their sight.

The major issues of vision impairment are discussed chapter by chapter. An extensive section of easily-referenced A to Z entries follows, and detailed appendixes provide all the information needed to find additional resources or organizations that serve your particular needs.

Living with Vision Problems is designed to be a functional tool for a consumer or patient looking for information relating to the eyes. The book is not intended to be used as a diagnostic tool, but it will be useful in providing readers with information that can be used to make informed decisions in conjunction with their doctors. However, it is no substitute for the care and supervision of trained medical professionals.

A great deal has changed regarding blindness and vision problems in recent years, leaving the public hungry for information on new technologies and treatments such as keratotomy, LASIK surgery, and progressive addition lenses; newly recognized potential causes of vision damage such as automobile air bags and shaken baby syndrome; and new options for the blind such as Braille music, the Employment Assistance Referral Network, and guide horses. Recent years have also brought some important milestones such as the World Blind Sailing Championship and the Mount Everest expedition of Eric Weihenmayer, who became the first blind person to climb the legendary peak.

All of it is covered here and all information included in this book is a current and up-to-date as possible in a field governed by rapid medical advances and regularly changing statistics. *Living with Vision Problems* will be the perfect guide for you and your family when facing blindness or other vision disorders, but be sure to consult your physician before making decisions or commencing treatment.

—Susan Shelly
Shillington, Pennsylvania

—Allan Rutzen, M.D., and Scott Steidl, M.D.
University of Maryland School of Medicine

ACKNOWLEDGMENTS

Professional people working with all aspects of blindness and vision impairment generously gave of their time and talents to advise, counsel and inform us. We would like to acknowledge their contributions and offer our appreciation to Roger R. Cackler, County of Santa Clara Social Services, Dr. Peter D'Alena, Richard E. Dietl, The President's Committee on Employment of People with Disabilities, Juliet Esterly, Council of Rehabilitation Specialists, Dr. Deborah Gilden, Smith-Kettlewell Institute of Visual Sciences, Jessie A. Goehner, National Industries for the Blind, Joseph J. Hennessey, Western Blind Rehabilitation Center, E. K. Hudson, National Association for Parents of the Visually Impaired, Michelle Laboda, American Academy of Ophthalmology, Diane Lipton and Pam Stenberg, Disability Rights, Education, and Defense Fund, Joe Jackson, Media Access Office, Michael Larsen and Elizabeth Pomada, Sally Mangold, California State University, San Francisco, Marc Mauer, National Federation of the Blind, George McNally, United Cerebral Palsy, Michaelann R. Meehan, RP Foundation Fighting Blindness, Tom Moore, Eye Bank Association of America, Mary Ellen Mulholland and Dr. Sandra Timmerman, American Foundation for the Blind, Dr. Harry Murphy and Neil Scott, California State University, Northridge, Diane B. Piastro, Carol Ranalli, James C. Riley, California State Department of Rehabilitation, Arnay Rosenblat, National Multiple Sclerosis Society, Victoria Sheffield, Helen Keller International, Sandy Smith and Kenneth Stuckey, Perkins School for the Blind, Michael A. Thoennes, Foundation for the Junior Blind, Todd Turiff, National Society to Prevent Blindness, Heidi Williams, Vivian Younger, our friends at ABLEDATA, M.C. Migel Memorial Library and Information Center and National Rehabilitation Information Center. Our special thanks to our editors, Nicholas Bakalar, Kate Kelly, Sarah Fogarty, and James Chambers.

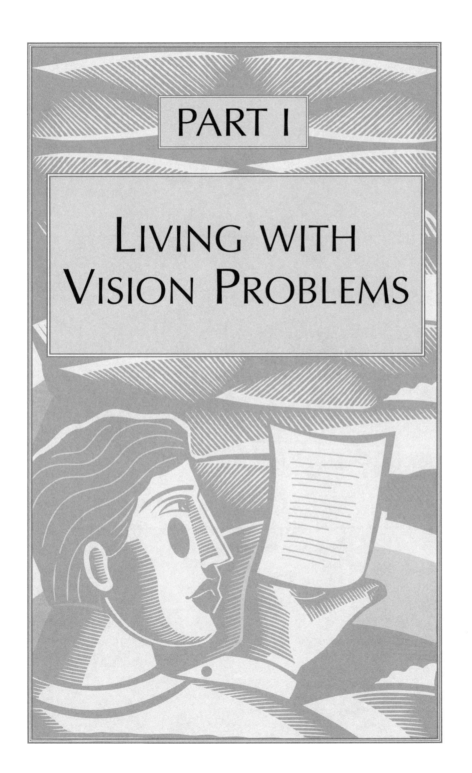

PART I

LIVING WITH VISION PROBLEMS

NOTE

The diagram of the eye that appears below will be useful in clarifying matters of anatomy and structure, and will be essential in understanding many of the entries throughout the book.

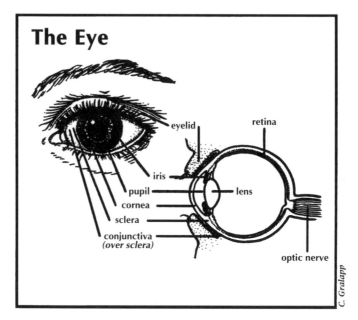

Cross section of the eye. Reprinted by permission of the American Academy of Ophthalmology.

CHAPTER 1

WHAT IS A VISION PROBLEM, AND WHAT IS BLINDNESS?

Many of us already are experiencing some sort of vision problems, and many more of us will have problems at some time within our lives. Some of us, unfortunately, will experience blindness.

There are an estimated 775,800 blind people in the United States today, and more than another 2 million who are visually impaired. Experts say we can expect to see a significant increase in vision problems and blindness as the nation's 76 million baby boomers age. In fact, it is estimated that there will be twice as many visually impaired people by the year 2030 as there are today, due primarily to age-related eye disease.

The good news is that doctors and researchers are learning more and more about the causes and treatment of eye disease. They are optimistic that eye care will continue to advance, and new and better treatments will be found for the most common and destructive eye diseases.

In this chapter, we will examine the definitions of blindness and vision impairment and how the two conditions are different. What exactly does it mean to be visually impaired? Or to be blind? We will also learn about different types of vision impairment and a little about eye anatomy and how a healthy eye works.

WHAT IS A VISION PROBLEM?

There are many kinds of vision problems, ranging from mild to very severe. A vision problem is any condition that affects your sight. Vision problems can be caused by disease or through injury to the eye. Sometimes the problem is with the eye itself, sometimes it is initiated in the part of the brain that receives messages for sight.

A few examples of the many, many kinds of vision problems include

- Nearsightedness
- Farsightedness
- Astigmatism
- Retinal detachment
- Color blindness
- Night blindness
- Cataracts
- Conjunctivitis

3

- Glaucoma
- Strabismus
- Macular degeneration

Obviously, the degree of vision problems varies greatly. Generally, however, vision problems are classed within three categories: visual impairment, low vision, and total blindness. Definitions of each of these categories have been developed and are based on the ability of the affected person to perform different kinds of daily tasks.
Here is a look at what each of these categories involve:

- *Visual Impairment.* The degree of visual impairment ranges greatly, but it always affects a person's ability to learn, or to perform normal daily tasks. Visual impairment can be improved with glasses or contact lenses, but can't be brought back to normal levels through those means.
- *Low vision.* A person with low vision is impeded in his or her ability to learn, or to perform normal, daily tasks. He/she is, however, still able to use available sight to obtain useful information about his/her surroundings. A New York City–based group called Low Vision Associates estimates that one of every six Americans suffers from low vision. A person with low vision can be legally blind and yet still have some sight. Generally, low vision is described as vision that's poor enough to prevent a person from reading a newspaper while wearing his or her regular glasses.
- *Blindness.* A person is blind when he/she has a complete absence of vision, or no perception of light.

Vision problems can prevent people from being able to drive, read, or just successfully navigate life in their own homes. Imagine not being able to see a clock on a table near your bed or turn your oven thermometer to the proper setting. Vision problems are extremely common and cause varying degrees of impairment. You will learn much more about many types of vision problems in the rest of this book. Following is an overview of blindness—the most severe type of vision problem.

WHAT IS BLINDNESS?

Legal blindness is a phrase that refers to a specific level of visual acuity. Visual acuity is a measure of vision clarity. Legal blindness is defined as having best-corrected visual acuity of 20/200 or worse in the better eye. A person with a field of vision not exceeding 20 degrees also is considered to be legally blind.

That definition, however, does not really tell us much about what it's like to be blind. Let us take a closer look at the legal definition of blindness and try to gain some perspective on what it means to be blind. Exactly what is 20/200 vision, anyway?

A person with 20/200 vision would have to be only 20 feet away from an object to see what a person with normal, or 20/20 vision, could see from 200 feet. Imagine trying to watch your child or grandchild perform in a school play or run down a soccer field with 20/200 vision.

Legal blindness also includes those people with good-quality vision but only a small visual field. This is what some call "tunnel vision." It can include people whose field of vision is 20 degrees or less. A person with a normal field of vision can see 180 degrees, with vision extending to either side. A 20-degree field of vision is extremely narrow. A person with a very narrow field of vision, however, may be able to see normally the things within that field.

We should remember that 20/200 vision or a 20-degree field is maximum vision for a person who is legally blind. Blindness extends from 20/200 down to a total loss of sight.

In complete blindness, there is no perception of light. This does not necessarily mean, however, that a person who is completely blind sees darkness. A person who is totally without sight offered an excellent explanation of complete blindness on an Internet site. He said that people with no vision don't see darkness—they see nothing.

Recognizing that it is difficult to separate those two concepts, this blind person offered the following explanation. "Darkness is what you see when you're blindfolded," he wrote. "Totally blind people have no sight at all. They don't see darkness, they see nothing. The same kind of nothing that a sighted person would see if he tried to look around using the palm of his hand as an organ of sight."

Think of the large E on the eye chart at your doctor's office. A person with 20/200 vision can see that letter from no farther than 20 feet away from the chart. A person with normal vision can see it from 200 feet back.

RECOGNIZING AND DIAGNOSING VISION PROBLEMS

You would think that vision problems would be easy to recognize when they occur. Sometimes they are. If you suddenly experience double vision, for instance, that is a clear indication that you are having a vision problem. Often, however, vision problems are not so obvious, making them more difficult to recognize.

Children with vision problems often do not recognize them, because they may not know what normal vision is. A child who has always had a problem has no way of knowing that he/she doesn't see the way other people do. A parent or teacher often will recognize a child's vision problem before he/she is aware of it. The adult will notice that the problem interferes with learning or conducting normal daily tasks.

Some common vision problems and their symptoms are listed below:

- Blurred vision when looking at objects that are far away (may indicate nearsightedness, also called myopia)
- Blurred vision when looking at objects that are close up (may indicate farsightedness, also called hyperopia)
- Trouble telling the difference between red and green while in dim light (may indicate color blindness)
- Trouble seeing objects in dim light (may indicate night blindness)
- Horizontal or vertical lines that appear blurry or irregular (may indicate astigmatism)

If you have any of the symptoms listed above, you should contact your eye doctor for an appointment. If you have any of the symptoms listed below, you should contact your doctor and tell him or her that you need an appointment as soon as possible.

- Flashing light sensations or floaters in your eyes that weren't there previously
- Sudden onset of light sensitivity
- A gradual loss of vision over days or weeks
- Extremely red eyes that do not include vision loss or extreme pain

And, if you have any of the following symptoms, don't wait. Get to your eye doctor or to an emergency room as quickly as possible.

- Sudden loss of vision
- Sudden onset of double vision
- Eye pain or changes in vision following eye surgery
- Any kind of trauma to the eye, including getting punched, snagged on a fishhook, poked with a branch, etc.
- Chemicals in the eye
- Any severe discomfort or pain in your eye

Only a doctor will be able to properly diagnose and treat a vision problem. In some emergency situations, quick treatment is essential to avoiding permanent eye damage or to minimizing damage.

THE ANATOMY OF A HEALTHY EYE

The eye is a complex and amazing sensory organ. In humans, the eyes generally are more developed than any of the other sensory organ. More brain power is used for the functions of eyesight than for any of the other senses of smell, touch, taste, or hearing.

Our eyes send constant bits of information to the optic nerve in our brains, where the information is processed, resulting in sight. Most of us take this ongoing near miracle for granted, not realizing what an intricate and amazing process it is.

In a healthy eye, many different parts work together to produce good vision. The illustration on page 2 shows the different parts of a healthy eye.

A normal eye is about the size of a Ping-Pong ball, and rests in a bony socket called the orbit. The orbit protects the eye and also contains muscles and nerves that enable the eyes and eyelids to move. Also found within the orbit are blood vessels and the lacrimal, or tear, gland. The outside of the eye is protected by the eyelid and eyelashes, which serve as filters to protect the eye from dust and other particles.

Below is a list and brief definition of the major parts of the eye:

- Cornea—the clear outer portion of the eyeball that transmits and focuses light into the eye
- Iris—the colored, circular part of the eye that helps regulate the amount of light that enters the eye. It controls the size of the pupil
- Lens—the transparent disc-shaped structure inside the eye that focuses light rays onto the retina
- Optic Nerve—the very important nerve that carries messages from the eye to the brain. The optic nerve carries the impulses formed by the retina to the brain, which interprets them as images and allows sight
- Pupil—the dark center in the middle of the iris that determines how much light is let into the eye. The pupil changes size to accommodate the amount of available light
- Retina—the inner layer of the eye that contains cells that are sensitive to light. The retina senses light and creates impulses that are sent through the optic nerve to the brain
- Macula—a small area in the retina that contains special cells that are very sensitive to light. The macula permits us to see fine details clearly
- Vitreous—the clear, gelatin-like material that fills the middle of the eye.

HOW A HEALTHY EYE WORKS

How do all these parts of the eye work together to transfer messages to the brain and allow us to see? How do we distinguish light from dark, and determine distances, colors, and sizes? How, exactly, does vision occur?

Briefly, what happens is that light reflects off an object and travels to the eye. It gets refracted, or bent, by the cornea and lens, and focuses into an image on the retina. But, as you know, the process of sight is not confined to just the eye. The retina is very important because it processes and sends visual messages through the optic nerve—a cluster of more than a million nerve fibers—to the brain.

The image that gets focused on the retina is upside down and reversed. It is not until the image gets to the brain that it gets turned around to produce the image that we actually see.

Light and Darkness

A healthy eye naturally adjusts to light and darkness. The pupil, which is an opening in the iris, changes in size to control the amount of light entering the eye. It becomes smaller in bright light because the eye doesn't require much light under those conditions. In dim light or darkness, however, the pupil gets bigger to allow in as much light as possible.

Distant and Near

To change its focus from objects that are far away to those that are close, the eye performs what is called accommodation. This means that the muscles around the eye adjust the shape of the lens to focus on something that is either far away or close. The lens becomes thicker when focusing on objects that are close and thinner for those that are far away.

Determining Color and Detail

The eye contains rods and cones, which are types of specialized light-sensitive cells located in the retina. They line the back of the eye and work together to help a healthy eye to see well. Cones provide color vision and help the eye to see fine detail. They function best in bright light. Rods function best in dim light and are important in night vision. They also help with side, or peripheral, vision.

The workings of a healthy eye are intricate and complicated, involving many parts of the eye as well as the brain. The brief descriptions here offer only a very general understanding of how the eye works and how vision occurs. A listing of other books and resources to help you learn more is located in the back of this book.

CHAPTER 2

WHAT CAUSES VISION PROBLEMS?

Problems with vision can result from a number of things. Many people develop vision problems as a natural result of aging—others are born with them.

Systemic diseases such as diabetes, hypertension, or thyroid disease, can cause vision problems. And, of course, some vision problems result from accidents during which there is trauma to the eye. In this chapter, we'll examine some of the problems caused by each of these factors.

AGE-RELATED VISION PROBLEMS

Problems with eyesight become increasingly prevalent as we age. In fact, vision impairment is rated as the third most common disability among older people.

By the time we reach our mid-40s, many of us will require reading glasses. This is due to a condition called presbyopia, which is a very common refractive error. Corrective lenses also are used to correct other refractive errors, including myopia (nearsightedness), hyperopia (farsightedness), and astigmatism (a condition which is typically associated with an uneven surface of the cornea).

Some people who have these conditions when they are young may notice that the problems get worse as they get older. This is due to constant changes in the eyes as we age.

Other eye-related problems sometimes occur due to changes in the muscles that hold the eye in place and allow it to move or in the skin around the eye.

The most serious age-related vision problems, however, are cataracts, glaucoma, and macular degeneration.

Cataracts

Cataracts are extremely common, and they are the leading cause of blindness worldwide. It's estimated that nearly 20 million people throughout the world have severe loss of vision because of cataracts, about 40,000 in the United States. In areas of the world with good health care, cataracts are not considered to be terribly serious because surgery usually can restore lost sight. Many parts of the world, however, do not have the funds or technology necessary for correcting eyesight lost to cataracts.

A cataract is a cloudiness or opacity that develops within the lens of the eye. There are different kinds of cataracts, but the most predominant type is the nuclear sclerotic cataract. It is called this because it occurs in the nucleus, or center, of the lens. As the lens of an eye ages, the center of it becomes larger, and the protein structure starts to change. The clear lens becomes yellowish and, after a period of time, can become increasingly brown. This interferes with the eye's ability to see objects at a distance. Many people who have cataracts have trouble driving at night, and they find they need brighter light in order to see properly. Very bright light, however, may also cause glare.

Cataracts are a natural result of aging, and everyone who lives long enough will develop cataracts to some degree. Occasionally, a baby is born with a cataract, either because it is an inherited condition or the result of a viral infection, such as German measles, contracted during pregnancy. Cataracts that develop during childhood usually are due to eye injury or are the result of a disease elsewhere in the body. They also can be caused by abnormal growth of the eye's lens.

> It's estimated that about 5,000 people in the United States go blind each year due to cataracts, despite the excellent medical help available. This is blamed on ignorance, fear, or refusal to undergo surgery.

Glaucoma

The optic nerve is a bundle of nerve fibers that carries visual messages from the eye to the brain. Glaucoma is a condition in which the optic nerve is damaged. Damage to these nerve fibers can cause blind spots, and total blindness if the disease is not treated and the optic nerve becomes completely destroyed.

More than 1 million Americans are fortunate to have had their glaucoma diagnosed early. The disease can then be treated, and vision loss possibly prevented. According to the American Academy of Ophthalmology, however, about 80,000 people in the United States are blind due to glaucoma, and another million are at risk for blindness because they are unaware of their glaucoma. Glaucoma is one of the leading causes of preventable blindness, and the single most common cause of blindness among African Americans.

Glaucoma often is called the silent thief of sight because its lack of symptoms makes it such an insidious disease. It can cause severe damage to the optic nerve, leading to irreversible vision loss, before a victim is even aware of having the disease.

The most common type of glaucoma is open-angle glaucoma. It occurs when pressure within the eye, called intraocular pressure, builds up and causes damage to the optic nerve. Intraocular pressure builds up when aqueous humor, the clear liquid within the eye, is prevented from draining properly. In a healthy eye, the liquid drains off and replenishes itself. If it can't drain, it backs up and causes pressure within the eye to increase.

The other basic form of the disease, closed-angle glaucoma, also is caused by a problem with the drainage of the aqueous humor. The blockage in closed-angle glaucoma occurs when the area into which the fluid drains is physically blocked. This type of glaucoma also is called narrow-angle glaucoma or angle-closure glaucoma.

Glaucoma is a puzzling disease. Some people who have elevated eye pressure, also called ocular hypertension, never experience damage to their optic nerve. And, there are some people with normal intraocular pressure who suffer damage to their optic nerve, regardless. That condition is an unusual kind of glaucoma called normotensive glaucoma, or normal-pressure glaucoma.

Blind spots can occur gradually, usually starting in the peripheral vision. By the time a person suffering from glaucoma notices the spots, the damage to the nerve has already been done.

One type of glaucoma—acute closed-angle glaucoma—comes on suddenly and has noticeable symptoms. Intraocular pressure rises rapidly, often causing acute eye pain. This condition is an emergency and should be treated immediately. The eye may become red and painful, and the patient may experience nausea. Other symptoms can include

- Blurred vision
- Appearance of haloes or rainbows around lights
- Headache

Glaucoma is more prevalent in African Americans than in Caucasians. In rare cases, children develop glaucoma, beginning in infancy, childhood, or adolescence. Congenital glaucoma usually appears shortly after birth but sometimes later in the first year of life. Congenital glaucoma often has noticeable symptoms, such as tearing, cloudiness of the cornea, and sensitivity to light.

Macular Degeneration

The third, and most common, of the big-three eye diseases that are linked to aging is age-related macular degeneration (ARMD). More than 13 million people in the United States show some signs of this disease, and it is considered the leading cause of vision loss in people ages 60 or older.

Macular degeneration affects the retina, the light-sensitive lining at the back of the eye that sends visual messages through the optic nerve to the brain. Specifically, it affects the macula, which is a small portion of the retina. The macula is necessary for seeing objects directly in front of you. Often, people with macular degeneration will lose this vision while retaining peripheral vision. Without central vision, reading, driving, and many other activities become extremely difficult, if not impossible.

There are two main types of the disease: dry and wet. In dry ARMD, also called the atrophic form, the cells in the retina become damaged. As these cells deteriorate, they release a substance that builds up, eventually forming deposits called drusen. While it is thought that most adult eyes contain some drusen, the deposits typically become more pronounced over time in people with age-related macular degeneration. Eventually, they cause changes to the cells of the retina, which causes further degeneration, and vision is affected.

Severe loss of vision occurs more quickly with the wet form of ARMD than with the dry form. With the wet form, also called the exudative form, abnormal blood vessels grow beneath the retina, resulting in bleeding and fluid leakage. In these cases, vision can suddenly become blurred or distorted. The abnormal blood vessels can cause severe scarring of the macula. When this occurs, vision can become extremely impaired. It is terribly unfortunate that some people develop both forms of ARMD, sometimes in the same eye.

> The wet form of ARMD affects only about 10 percent of all people who have the disease, but it is responsible for about 80 percent of the severe vision loss attributed to ARMD.

CONGENITAL VISION PROBLEMS

When a baby is born with severe vision problems, or is born blind, one of the following causes usually is responsible:

- An infection before birth
- An inherited disease
- A physical injury around the time of birth
- Too little oxygen reaching the brain before or during birth

Sometimes the damage that causes a child to be born with vision loss is in the eye itself, and sometimes it is to the part of the brain that receives and processes visual messages.

Some congenital vision problems include cataracts and glaucoma. Some childhood vision problems—that is, those that typically occur during childhood, but are not congenital—include strabismus and amblyopia.

Cataracts

As mentioned earlier in this chapter, babies occasionally will be born with cataracts—clouding of the lens of the eye. The cloudy lens prevents light from reaching the retina fully and causes vision to be blurred or hazy. The degree of visual impairment caused by cataracts varies, depending on how much of the lens is covered.

Glaucoma

Glaucoma, a condition in which the optic nerve is damaged, is another disease occasionally present at birth. Total blindness can occur if the disease is not treated and the optic nerve becomes completely destroyed. Congenital glaucoma usually appears shortly after birth and often has noticeable symptoms, such as tearing, cloudiness of the cornea, and sensitivity to light.

Strabismus and Amblyopia

It's estimated that about 4 percent of all children in the United States have strabismus, and 2 to 3 percent have amblyopia. Strabismus is an imbalance of the eye muscles that prevents the eyes from aligning properly so that they can both focus on the same object at the same time. When the muscle imbalance causes one eye to turn in toward the nose, the condition is commonly called crossed eyes. When it causes one eye to turn out toward the ear, it's commonly called wall eye.

Commonly called lazy eye, amblyopia often is the result of strabismus that has gone untreated. A child who has strabismus will eventually learn to focus on the vision produced by the stronger of his or her eyes and ignore the vision produced by the weaker, or lazy, eye. This causes the vision in the weaker eye to not develop fully and can result in reduced sight in that eye. Amblyopia also can be caused by a condition such as ptosis, which is a drooping of the eyelid.

DISEASE-RELATED VISION PROBLEMS

Eye problems sometimes don't begin in the eye at all, but are the result of a systemic disease that affects the entire body, including the eyes. Many people experience vision problems as a result of diseases such as diabetes, hypertension, carotid artery disease, or thyroid disease. Diabetes, which affects from 4 to 6 million Americans, can be particularly devastating.

Diabetes and Vision Problems

For various reasons, diabetes continues to be a major health problem in the United States. While this disease affects the entire body, the eyes seem to be particularly susceptible to the damage it causes. Historically, most people with diabetes have experienced some sort of eye problem during their lifetime as a result of the disease.

Diabetes affects the eyes in several potentially devastating ways. It can destroy optic nerve fibers, causing optic atrophy; increase the likelihood of cataracts and glaucoma; and affect the eye muscles, iris, and lens of the eye. The retina is the most commonly affected portion of the eye.

Diabetic retinopathy is a condition in which blood vessels in the retina are damaged, causing them to leak fluid or to bleed. This causes the retina to swell and form deposits called exudates. Most diabetic retinopathy does not begin for about 10 years after the diabetes has been diagnosed. A person who has had diabetes for a long time is at greater risk for diabetic retinopathy than someone who's been recently diagnosed.

Someone in the early stages of retinopathy may not notice any changes in vision. This makes the condition especially dangerous, because it can continue to advance without the person even knowing that he or she has it. The early form of diabetic retinopathy is called nonproliferative, or background, retinopathy.

Sometimes fluid collects in the macula, the central part of the retina. The macula allows us to see fine details. This type of fluid collection is called macular edema, and, if it occurs, reading and other tasks might be affected.

If the condition worsens, it's called proliferative retinopathy. At this stage, small new blood vessels grow on the surface of the retina. If the tiny vessels break and bleed, as they often do, it can cause serious vision problems. Blood from the vessels can leak into the vitreous, which is the clear, jelly-like substance in the center of the eye. Blood in the vitreous prevents light from passing through the eye to the retina, causing vision to be decreased.

The new vessels also can cause scar tissue to develop, which can make the retina pull away from the back of the eye. This is called retinal detachment, and can lead to blindness if not treated.

There are treatments for diabetic retinopathy, and, although it's considered a serious problem, it usually can be controlled when treated early.

Hypertension and Vision Problems

Hypertension, or high blood pressure, can affect the entire body, including the eyes. Over a period of time, hypertension can cause tiny arteries in the retina to become blocked, obstructing the flow of blood. The retina needs oxygen and nutrients from the blood in order to function properly; it becomes damaged when blood flow is diminished. The most severe eye problems caused by hypertension include retinal hemorrhages and retinal edema from the damaged arteries in the retina.

Carotid Artery Disease and Vision Problems

The carotid arteries, those that carry blood upward to the head, are extremely important to the eyes. One of the branches of the carotid artery is the ophthalmic artery. It is the main source of blood to the eyes. If the artery (there is one on each side, supplying blood to each eye) becomes clogged and blood is unable to pass to the eye, tissue becomes diseased and may lose function.

The most common problem affecting the carotid artery is atherosclerosis, which is when the artery becomes clogged and hardened. This often prevents blood from properly passing through the artery to the retina and the brain. In addition to eye problems, atherosclerosis can result in a stroke, if blockage becomes severe.

Thyroid Disease and Vision Problems

Disorders of the thyroid gland, which is located in the neck, also can cause problems in the eyes.

When the thyroid gland becomes diseased, the body creates antibodies. Antibodies are intended to fight off infection and disease, but in some cases, including thyroid disease, they attack normal tissue. For some reason, the eyes are particularly vulnerable to some of these antibodies, and damage can result.

Symptoms of thyroid eye disease are bulging eyes, problems with double vision, and damage to the optic nerve. Progression of this disease can be slow or aggressive, and eye problems can remain for years after the thyroid condition has been brought under control.

VISION PROBLEMS CAUSED BY ACCIDENTS

Thousands of accidents occur every day that result in eye injuries. Cleaning solutions splash into the eyes. An object flies out from under a running lawn mower and strikes the eye. A child pokes herself in the eye with a pointed object. Another child is hit in the eye with a pellet or BB. A teenager is blinded when fireworks explode in his face.

Most accidents involving the eyes are preventable. We will discuss prevention to a much greater extent in the next chapter.

If an injury to the eye does occur, it is extremely important to get prompt medical treatment. The eye is easily damaged, and delaying treatment can cause permanent eye damage and loss of vision.

CHAPTER 3

CAN YOU PREVENT VISION PROBLEMS?

You learned in the last chapter that vision problems can result from many different things. Some are preventable, others are not.

Eye problems caused by systemic diseases such as diabetes, for instance, may not be preventable but can be better controlled by proper management. Eye problems caused by hypertension can be greatly lessened by controlling the hypertension.

If there are any indications of genetic defects in your family, be sure you tell your doctor to allow for informed family planning. Congenital eye problems *may be* difficult to prevent, although good prenatal care can help prepare parents for what lies ahead. Congenital eye disease due to genetic conditions can sometimes be managed through nutrition, avoidance of certain foods, and taking particular supplements.

For the average person, probably the single most important thing you can do to prevent vision problems is to have regular eye examinations. This allows for early detection and treatment of some eye diseases. Everyone, including children, should have their eyes examined every few years, unless there are reasons to have them checked more frequently. Those over age 40 should get an eye exam every two years. Remember that some serious eye diseases, such as glaucoma, have no early symptoms and can only be detected during an examination.

UNDERSTANDING AN EYE EXAM

Routine eye exams can be conducted by an ophthalmologist or an optometrist. Technicians may assist in parts of the exam.

Ophthalmologists are medical doctors who specialize in the treatment of eye disorders. They can perform eye surgery, prescribe corrective lenses, and prescribe drugs. Because ophthalmologists are physicians, as well as being experts on eyes and eye care, they can be expected to have an understanding of the systemic illnesses that can effect your eyes.

Optometrists are trained and licensed to test vision, and they can prescribe corrective lenses. They cannot, however, perform surgery. They normally limit their practices to nonmedical treatment of eye problems. State laws vary in the extent to which they allow optometrists to prescribe medications.

Opticians are professionals who are trained to fit glasses and contact lenses, as prescribed by an ophthalmologist or optometrist.

When you have your eyes examined, the ophthalmologist or optometrist will test them in various ways. He/She will test the acuity of your vision by having you read the letters on an eye chart. Poor reading of the eye chart indicates a problem. Normally, the problem would be an incorrect prescription for glasses (usually for nearsightedness or farsightedness), but it could indicate a more serious problem, such as glaucoma.

The ophthalmologist or optometrist also will check the retina of each eye with an instrument called an ophthalmoscope. This allows the examiner to discover any disorders, such as retinal detachment, and also would reveal signs of a systemic problem, such as diabetes or hypertension. Normally, the pupils will be dilated before the retinal exam to give the examiner a better view. This is done by administering dilating drops into each eye and waiting for a short period of time (usually 15 to 30 minutes) for the drops to take effect. The balance of the muscles that control your eyes will be checked, in addition to an examination of the pupils. The doctor will check the shape and symmetry of your pupils, and examine how they react to light.

A test to measure intraocular pressure also will be conducted. This is most commonly done by using an instrument called an applanation tonometer. The test may require putting a local anesthetic and a dye in the eye.

An instrument called a slit lamp will be used to examine the cornea, lens, and other parts of the eye. A slit lamp illuminates and magnifies the eye, making it possible for the examiner to detect problems in the early stages.

The ophthalmologist or optometrist also may conduct tests to measure your visual field, eye coordination, and color vision. If there is indication of a problem with your eyes, further tests or procedures may be done.

If you are 65 years or older, consider having an eye exam every year, or at least every other year. Your risk of developing a problem such as cataracts, glaucoma, or macular degeneration increases as you get older, and early detection is crucial.

EYE EXAMS FOR CHILDREN

Vision screenings—and eye exams when necessary—are very important for children, and yet it's estimated that fewer than 20 percent of children are adequately screened. Screenings for children are so important because, often, youngsters don't recognize their own vision problems. They assume that the way they see is normal. It's estimated that vision problems affect one in 20 preschoolers and one in four school-age children.

A vision screening is intended to identify possible problems so they can be checked by an eye care professional. It doesn't take the place of a professional exam, but merely indicates when an exam is necessary. Remember that vision disorders that are undetected and untreated can result in a variety of problems, including permanent vision loss.

If your child is not being screened for vision in school or by his or her pediatrician, think about scheduling an appointment for an eye exam or check your local directory for an agency near you that may perform vision screenings. While eye examinations are extremely important, they aren't the only thing you can do to prevent vision problems.

According to Prevent Blindness America, a national volunteer eye health and safety organization, whose website www.prevent-blindness.org offers much good information, an eye screening should include the following three steps:

1. The screener should look at the child's eye for any visible signs of problems, such as watering eyes or swollen eyelids. He or she also should look for other signs, such as excessive rubbing of the eyes or squinting.
2. The screen should test for distance acuity and ability to focus through use of an approved eye chart.
3. Children through age nine should be given a test called stereopsis to make sure their eyes are working together properly. If they are not, the child is at risk of amblyopia (lazy eye).

EYE SAFETY

Most states require drivers and passengers to wear seat belts. Many require children to wear helmets when they ride bicycles. And yet, there are few regulations, outside of the workplace, to protect our eyes and our children's eyes.

There are thousands of eye injuries each year, and most of them are preventable. While eye safety in the workplace has improved due to increased regulations, a growing number of eye injuries are being sustained in the home, according to Prevent Blindness America.

Preventing Eye Injuries in the Home

Despite all our good intentions, most of us tend to get a little careless in our consideration of potential dangers to small children. We leave things lying around that we should not. Awareness is the first step in preventing serious problems from occurring. Prevent Blindness

America offers the following guidelines as ways to prevent eye (and other) injuries.

Preventing Eye Injuries

- Use safety gates at the top and bottom of stairs
- Provide lights and handrails to improve safety on stairs
- Pad or cushion sharp corners and edges of furnishing and home fixtures
- Install cabinet and drawer locks in kitchens and bathrooms
- Leave personal-use items (cosmetics, toiletry products), kitchen utensils, and desk supplies where they are not easily accessible to children
- Use occupant restraints, such as infant and child safety seats, booster seats, safety belts, and shoulder harnesses in cars
- Avoid toys with sharp or rigid points, shafts, spikes, rods, and dangerous edges
- Keep toys intended for older children away from younger children
- Use guards on all power equipment
- Keep paints, pesticides, fertilizers, and similar products properly stored in a secure area
- Avoid flying toys and projectile-firing toys; these pose a danger to all children, particularly those under five years old
- Beware of items in playgrounds and play areas that pose potential eye hazards
- Keep your tools in good condition
- Keep BB guns away from kids
- Inspect and remove debris from lawns before mowing
- Wear chemical safety goggles when using hazardous solvents and detergents
- Read and follow all manufacturer instructions and warning labels
- Do not mix cleaning agents
- Know that regular eyeglasses do not always provide enough protection when using power tools or other potentially dangerous tools
- Wear safety glasses or dust goggles to protect against flying particles, and chemical goggles to guard against exposure to fertilizers and pesticides

Preventing Eye Injuries at Work

At work, eye protection should be used whenever necessary. A recent survey by the Bureau of Labor Statistics revealed that three out of every five workers who suffered an eye injury were not wearing any protection. Proper eye protection should always be worn if there is any chance of flying objects, chemicals, harmful radiation, or other hazards. Even people who are just passing through such an area should wear eye protection.

Eye injuries in the workplace cost more than $467 million each year, according to the Bureau of Labor Statistics. Indirect costs, such as legal fees, judgments, and training replacement workers, increase that amount even more.

All new employees should be educated about eye safety and given the proper safety equipment, and everyone should be required to wear eye protection whenever applicable.

Preventing Eye Injuries at Play

About 40,000 people are treated in hospital emergency rooms each year for eye injuries sustained while participating in sports. And, it is reasoned, because many people are treated by trainers or in outpatient clinics, the actual number of eye injuries probably is two or three times that.

Eye injuries occur most often while playing basketball, baseball, and racket sports. Some problems that can result from sports injuries include the following:

- Fracture of the eye socket
- Scratches on the cornea
- Traumatic cataract
- Inflamed iris
- Blood spilling into the eye's anterior chamber
- Swollen retina

It is recommended that sports eyeguards be used while playing these and other sports. Sports eye guards are available at sports specialty or optical stores. Make sure that they fit properly and are comfortable. And, make sure that you wear them if, for example, you are at risk for eye trauma, if you have had a previous retinal detachment, or if you have high myopia. Your eye doctor can tell you if you are at high risk for sports-related injury.

Be especially careful when participating in sports or activities that involve shooting. Never allow a child or youth to use any kind of gun, sling shot, bow and arrow, etc. without proper supervision.

Preventing Eye Damage from Ultraviolet Radiation

There is increasing evidence that long-term exposure to ultraviolet (UV) radiation can cause serious damage to the eyes. Researchers think that it may contribute to the development of serious eye disorders, including cataracts and macular degeneration.

It is recommended that to protect the eyes from UV radiation, you wear both approved sunglasses and a wide-brimmed hat or cap. While the glasses will absorb the UV rays, the hat will prevent them from entering the eyes around the glasses. Make sure that the lenses you wear absorb 99 to 100 percent of both UV-A and UV-B rays. Not all sunglasses are effective at protecting your eyes. Kids' eyes need protection from UV rays too. Make sure they have appropriate eyewear and hats when spending extended time in the sun in both the winter and summer.

FIRST AID FOR EYE INJURIES

If an eye injury does occur, it is important to get it checked by a professional. In some emergencies, such as battery acid splashing into the eyes, or a fishhook becoming lodged in the eye, it is obvious that professional care is necessary. The need for care, however, isn't always so evident.

Many of us have had a black eye or two, and it is very likely were not treated for the condition. A black eye, however, may indicate internal damage to the eye and should be checked. If you get hit in or around the eye, you may apply a cool compress without pressure. This may ease pain and swelling.

If your eye or eyelid is cut or punctured, follow the steps listed below.

- Get medical help immediately
- Do not apply pressure until a professional sees the injury
- Do not try to wash out or pull out an object stuck in the eye
- Avoid touching the eye area to minimize the chance of infection

If you get a corrosive chemical or fluid in your eye, follow the steps listed below.

- Quickly wash out the eye by holding the opened eye under a gentle flow of running water
- Be sure to keep your head tilted toward the injured side so the chemical doesn't run into the other eye
- Hold your eye open with your fingers to allow the water to run over it
- Flush the eye for 10 minutes, cover it with a clean pad, and seek medical attention immediately

If you get a foreign object in your eye, follow the steps listed below.

- Lift the upper eyelid outward and down over the lower lid
- Allow your eye to tear to wash the object out, or use an eye wash
- See a doctor if you cannot remove the particle
- Avoid rubbing your eye

CHAPTER 4

HOW TO TREAT
VISION PROBLEMS

Many advances in the treatment of vision problems have occurred over the past few years, and many more are under way as professionals continue to better understand the eye and improve their methods of treating the problems that affect it. Researchers and doctors are working hard to improve existing treatments and find new treatments for age-related diseases such as macular degeneration, cataracts, and glaucoma. This research is extremely important as the United States's 76 million baby boomers age and the number of people suffering from vision problems increases. There also have been significant breakthroughs in treatments for children's eye problems and in the area of genetics.

Treatment for vision problems ranges from simple eye drops to precise, high-tech laser surgery. This chapter looks at some available treatments and how they are used. It also looks in the future of eye care and the advances that may lie ahead.

MEDICAL TREATMENTS

Medical treatments for eye problems fall into four basic categories:

- Topical eye drops
- Oral medications
- Intravenous medications
- Injections into or around the eye

While eye drops are known as topical drugs, oral and intravenous medications are called systemic drugs. Medical treatments are used in ophthalmology to treat eye diseases and disorders, to prepare the eyes for examination or surgery, to treat or prevent inflammation, and to diagnose disease or disorders.

Eye drops, or topical drugs, may be used to dilate the pupil of the eye. These are called mydriatics and are found in two basic forms: as sympathomimetics and as parasympatholytics. They are most commonly used during eye examinations to allow a physician to see into the eye.

Eye drops also come in antibiotic form and are used to treat ocular infections. Infections of the eye are treated according to whether the infecting agent is bacterial, fungal, viral, or protozoal. Different kinds of antibiotic drops would be used for each of those categories.

Another type of eye drop is of the anti-inflammatory variety. These may be used to treat allergies or to reduce swelling in the eye caused by an injury, surgery, infection, or uveitis, which is an inflammation of the uveal tract of the eye. Anti-inflammatory drugs are nearly always used following surgery involving the eyes.

Antimetabolite or chemotherapeutic drugs are compounds that typically inhibit some aspect of the synthesis of DNA. They are stronger than steroids in managing severe inflammation.

Drops also are used to treat glaucoma. Most glaucoma can be successfully treated with drops that reduce eye pressure and maintain the pressure at a safe level. Beta-adrenergic blocking agents in topical form commonly are used. Some examples of this type of eye drop include Timolol, Betagan, and OptiPranolol. Epinephrine drops or pilocarpine drops are sometimes used in combination with other medications.

Oral medications used to treat eye problems include antibiotics, anti-inflammatories, and those used to treat glaucoma. Your doctor may decide to prescribe oral medications instead of eye drops for a variety of reasons, such as the severity of an infection, or where the infection is located within the eye.

Oral medication also may be used for an eye disease that is secondary to a systemic inflammatory disease or infection. In some cases, depending on the severity of the problem, medications may be given intravenously or injected directly into or around the eye. Injections of antibiotics or anti-inflammatories in or around the eye are the most extreme use of medication to treat eye problems.

If a patient has developed endophthalmitis, a rapidly developing, severe intraocular infection in the back of the eye, for instance, a doctor may choose to use injections to treat it. This type of treatment normally is only done in very serious situations or for conditions that don't respond to other therapy.

LASER TREATMENTS

Possibly no other medical treatments have received more attention in recent years than procedures performed with lasers. Lasers have revolutionized treatment for blinding diseases such as diabetic retinopathy and are helpful in managing glaucoma and macular degeneration. Doctors and researchers are hopeful that treatments for these conditions will continue to progress. While lasers allow doctors to perform many procedures with greater precision, lasers do not perform miracles of themselves. Lasers are simply tools that help doctors do their jobs better.

Various types of lasers are used for different procedures in eye care. A fairly new type of laser, called the excimer laser, is used in photorefractive keratectomy (PRK) to permanently reshape the cornea by removing tiny amounts of tissue. It also is used in LASIK surgery to correct moderate to extreme nearsightedness, farsightedness, and astigmatism, and in phototherapeutic keratectomy (PTK). PTK is another surgical procedure that is used to remove cloudy scar tissue from the cornea. The excimer laser is referred to as a "cold laser" because it has the ability to remove tiny layers of tissues with very little or no heat damage to the surrounding tissue. It is important because of its precision, and is being considered for new uses and applications.

Another use of lasers in ophthalmology is to repair retinal holes, which, if left untreated, can cause retinal detachment. A laser can be used to seal a hole in the retina before detachment occurs. If the retina does detach, a retinal reattachment operation would be performed, and a laser may be used to secure the retina.

A new laser treatment called photodynamic therapy is being used for some patients with the wet form of age-related macular degeneration. This therapy, which was approved by the Food and Drug Administration in April 2000, involves a special dye that is injected into the patient and absorbed by the abnormal blood vessels in the eye. Once the dye has been absorbed, a low-level laser is used to activate it, causing the dye to block the abnormal blood vessels. This can be done without damaging other areas of the eye, which makes it a significant breakthrough in the treatment of ARMD.

Lasers also are used in some glaucoma surgery—to help manage tumors within the eye and for cosmetic surgery involving the eye or area surrounding the eye.

The laser, which stands for *l*ight *a*mplification by *s*timulated *e*mission of *r*adiation, was invented by Arthur L. Schawlow and Charles Townes, both scientists at Bell Labs, in 1958. Schawlow and Townes received a patent for the laser in 1960, and the first laser was manufactured the same year. They began to be used in eye surgery just a few years later.

Simply, a laser is a device that creates and amplifies a narrow, intense beam of coherent light. It allows surgeons to work with extreme precision and easily reach areas of the eye that otherwise would be very difficult to access. Surgery performed with lasers generally requires less healing time than traditional surgery.

SURGICAL TREATMENTS

While laser surgery in the area of eye care is making headlines, traditional surgery remains extremely important as well.

Some important areas of eye surgery include:

- Periocular and retrobulbar intraocular injections
- Cataract surgery

- Glaucoma surgery
- Cornea surgery
- Retina surgery
- Oculo-plastic surgery
- Pediatric ophthalmologic surgery

Periocular and Retrobulbar Intraocular Injections

Periocular and retrobulbar intraocular injections are specific injections into different parts of the eye. They are performed for very specific purposes, such as to administer anesthesia before surgery or before laser treatments. They may deliver antibiotics or anti-inflammatory medication as well.

Cataract Surgery

Cataract surgery is one of the most common surgeries performed in America today, and, in nine cases out of 10, it results in improved vision for the patient. A cataract is a clouding of the lens of the eye that can interfere with daily tasks such as reading, driving, or watching television. When clouding of the lens occurs, surgery can be performed to remove the cataract and clear the vision.

There are two main ways to remove a cataract. The first is called phacoemulsification, a procedure that uses ultrasound to emulsify, or liquify, the lens of the eye. In phacoemulsification, the doctor makes a small incision on the side of the cornea, then inserts a tiny probe into the eye. The probe emits ultrasound, which breaks up the lens. The lens is then removed by suction, and an artificial lens known as an intraocular lens is inserted. This method has been less commonly used in the last decade.

The other primary method of cataract removal is extracapsular surgery. This involves making a slightly larger incision in the eye, after which the doctor removes the hard center of the lens. Suction is used to removed the rest of the lens, and an intraocular lens is inserted.

> More than half of people 65 years or older have cataracts. They are considered a natural result of aging.

Glaucoma Surgery

While most glaucoma can be successfully managed with medication, some cases require surgery. Glaucoma is a condition in which pressure builds up inside the eye and damages the optic nerve. This can cause sight problems such as blind spots. If left untreated, the disease can completely destroy the optic nerve, at which point all sight would be lost.

The purpose of glaucoma surgery is to make a new opening, through which fluid can drain from the eye. This reduces the pressure inside the eye and helps to maintain it at a healthy level.

During surgery for glaucoma, a small piece of tissue is removed from the white part of the eye, the sclera. This makes a new channel through which fluid can drain.

Anyone can get glaucoma, but those who are 60 years or older, African American and 40 years or older, or who have a family history of glaucoma are at greater risk.

Cornea Surgery

The cornea, which is the transparent tissue that covers the front of the eye and is essential to good vision, is subject to various problems. If the cornea is damaged by a deep scratch, bacteria or fungi can pass into it and cause serious infection. Infection also can result from ocular herpes or herpes zoster.

Other conditions, such as keratoconus, Fuch's dystrophy, and Lattice dystrophy also cause corneal problems. If the cornea becomes too damaged, a doctor may decide to perform a cornea transplant. Ophthalmologists perform more than 40,000 cornea transplants in the United States each year.

Corneas are obtained from donors and stored in eye banks. During a cornea transplant, the diseased or damaged cornea is removed from the patient's eye, and the donor cornea is stitched into place. The stitches are removed after the eye heals, usually after several months.

A new type of cornea surgery is the insertion of small semicircular lenses into the cornea, outside the optical zone. These inserts, called Intacts, or Intrastromal Corneal Ring Segments, are designed to correct myopia (near-sightedness).

Retina Surgery

Surgery is sometimes necessary to repair the retina, the inner layer of the eye where images are focused. Focused inverted images are processed and sent as electrical signals to the brain via the optic nerve. Surgery may be needed to repair macular holes, retinal detachments, abnormal membranes, intraocular hemorrhage, or to treat endophthalmitis.

One method of repairing a retinal detachment, which most commonly occurs when the vitreous pulls away from the retina and causes the retina to tear, is a scleral buckle operation. During this procedure, the doctor places a piece of material implanted with silicone around all or part of the eye. This causes the wall of the eye to indent and counteract the force that resulted in the tear or detachment.

Another procedure is a vitrectomy, during which the vitreous is removed from the center of the eye and replaced with saline, silicone oil, or a gas bubble. The bubble or silicone oil pushes against the break in the retina and begins to seal it. Eventually, a gas bubble is absorbed by the body and replaced by the natural fluids of the eye. Silicone oil requires another operation for removal.

Oculo-Plastic Surgery

Oculo-plastic surgery combines ophthalmology and plastic surgery and is used to treat conditions and diseases affecting the eyelids, eyebrows, the tear system, and the bones around the eye.

The uses for this type of surgery range from children with congenital eyelid abnormalities to adults with droopy eyelids. Some common conditions that require oculo-plastic surgery include

- Eyelid skin cancer
- Thyroid eye disease that results in bulging eyes
- Ptosis (drooping of the eyelids)
- Tear drainage system disorders
- Orbital disease

Procedures used to correct these and other conditions include blepheroplasty, dacrocystorhinostomy, and ptosis repair.

Pediatric Ophthalmologic Surgery

Surgery sometimes is necessary to treat unique ocular problems of children, such as strabismus, which is commonly called crossed eyes, and amblyopia, which is known as lazy eye. In addition, children sometimes are born with cataracts that require surgery or develop cataracts due to trauma to the eye. Surgery also may be done for cosmetic purposes.

EXPERIMENTAL, NEW, AND FUTURE TREATMENTS

While there have been many significant advances in eye care during the past decade, research continues to find even better treatments and cures for various eye diseases and disorders.

There is great effort under way to find a way to stop, or at least slow down, the effects of macular degeneration. Researchers and doctors are looking at procedures such as macular translocation surgery, which would allow the healthy retina to be moved to a healthier part of the eye and keep its function; photo-dynamic therapy, which destroys abnormal damaging blood vessels; new medications for conditions such as diabetes; and the possibility of retinal pigment-epithelial transplantation for macular degeneration.

Retinal transplants and implantable retinal chips are important areas of research. Stem cell transplantation for retinal regeneration may radically alter the course of debilitating retinal disease, as will retinal transplantation. Genetic research is occurring in every area of ophthalmology and may alter the diagnosis and course of many genetic diseases.

New technologies may alter the course of cataract and refractive eye disease treatments, such as wave front technology, and new types of intraocular implants.

CHAPTER 5

LIVING WITH VISION PROBLEMS

If you are visually impaired, you already know that you face many daily challenges and frustrations. Hopefully, you also know that there are many sources of help and assistance to make those challenges less daunting.

There are many associations of and for the blind or visually impaired and many organizations that supply all kinds of tools and aids to make everyday life a little easier.

You will read more in the next chapter about how vision loss can affect a person emotionally, and the impact that it can have on not only him/her, but his/her friends and family as well.

In this chapter, however, we deal with means of coping with vision problems so that you can continue in as many tasks and activities as possible, as well as get the support that you need.

SOME INFORMATION YOU NEED TO KNOW

There are services and various types of assistance available to people who are blind or visually impaired. Some of them that you might want to know about are listed below.

- *Social Security disability benefits.* You may be eligible for social security benefits, even if you are not yet 65. If you are eligible for disability benefits, they will automatically convert to retirement benefits when you turn 65. Contact your local Social Security office to see if you qualify.
- *Medical assistance.* A blind person under age 65 who receives Social Security disability benefits is eligible for Medicare benefits after a two-year waiting period. A waiting period is not required for people who are 65 or older.
- *Library services.* Books and magazines, both in Braille or recorded on tape, are available through the National Library Service for the Blind and Physically Handicapped of the Library of Congress. There is no cost for this service, and the organization will loan you special machines on which to play the tapes. More information about this service is available by calling the National Library Service's toll-free number at 800-424-9100.
- *Large-print books and magazines.* Many libraries and bookstores carry large-print books and magazines. For a free catalog of books available in large print, contact The Large Print Book Club, G. K. Hall & Com-

pany, 70 Lincoln Street, Boston, MA 02111. Or, you can get a list of many different types of materials, all available in large print, by contacting the National Library Service for the Blind and Physically Handicapped of the Library of Congress. The address is 1291 Taylor Street, NW, Washington, DC 20542, and the toll-free number is 800-424-9100. Request the circular entitled *Reading Materials in Large Print.*

- If your community or county has an Association for the Blind, call to see what services may be available. Some groups will help you to organize your home, install special knobs on your stove, and so forth. Check your local phone directory to find out what might be available in your area.
- Each state has a Department of Rehabilitation that offers special services to the visually impaired. In some states, services such as mobility training and orientation are free. Check with your state department to see what's available.
- The National Federation of the Blind has a state-by-state list of resources that allows you to find out what is available for you. You can call the federation at 410-659-9314 or log onto its website at www.nfb.org and click on "Services and Resources."

There are many other resources and services available in addition to these. Be sure to contact a local or state agency or the National Federation of the Blind to find out what else might be available.

EQUIPMENT TO HELP MAKE LIVING WITH LOW VISION EASIER

If you have some vision but it is not good enough to allow you to get away with wearing your regular old glasses anymore, there are plenty of tools, equipment, and special items that you may find useful. From talking thermometers and scales to beeping wallets, electronic magnifiers, Braille playing cards, and low-vision sewing kits, there are hundreds of products available to help you. A few are listed below, and information on where to go to find about the rest is given.

- *A cane.* If your vision is severely impaired, you may want to consider using a cane. Called a white cane, or a long cane, this tool can help you greatly when traveling alone. Many visually impaired people feel a cane is crucial to their independence, although some resist using a cane. The technique for using a white cane isn't difficult, and can be learned in a very short time. You should, however, have instruction to make sure you're using the cane to its fullest advantage.
- *A dog guide.* Many blind or visually impaired people use dogs to guide them. Dogs were first trained as guides in the 1930s, and there now

are more than a dozen guide dog training schools across the country. If you choose to have a dog guide, you will be matched with a dog that has already been trained. You and the dog then will have to undergo training together to learn how to work as a team. Many visually impaired people say that using a dog guide gives them a great sense of confidence.

A lot of progress has been made, and continues to be made, in technology designed for visually impaired people. Listed below are brief descriptions of some reading-enhancement devices and computer equipment. If you're considering getting a reading-enhancement device, first check with your eye care specialist for advice about what is best for you.

- *Hand-held magnifiers.* These vary a lot, from low-power models that you can buy at your local drugstore to high-power ones that you order or get from a vision center. To magnify the print, you hold them over whatever you are reading.
- *High-powered reading glasses.* These are much different from the reading glasses to which you are probably accustomed. They are a lot stronger, which means you have to hold whatever it is you are reading very close to your face, or the print will look distorted. This is bothersome to some people, but the glasses are an effective aid.
- *Stand magnifiers.* These are magnifiers that lie directly on top of whatever you are reading. The advantage is that you do not have to hold the material up close to your face, and you do not have to hold the magnifier. It does, however, limit the area that you can read from without having to move the magnifier.
- *Telescopes.* Telescopes are great for seeing faraway objects. Various models are available, some of which can be clipped or fastened onto eyeglasses. In many states, it is even legal to use telescopes to drive, under certain conditions. Many people have found telescopes to be very useful in situations such as watching a baseball game or working on a computer.
- *CCTV.* A closed-circuit television system that uses a hand-held or stand-mounted video camera to scan reading material and project it in an enlarged version onto a television screen. There are controls for magnification, brightness, focus, and contrast.
- *Computer equipment.* There is lots of specialized equipment to make computers usable for blind or visually impaired people. There are technologies that enable you to magnify text and graphics programs on your computer screen, and those that convert the material on the screen to sound (this often can be added to a computer you may already own). There also are computer programs that translate Braille, and printers that print in Braille.

An ever-increasing number of high-tech products are available for people who are blind or visually impaired, and more will come as technology continues to advance.

There also are many items designed to help with daily household tasks and activities. These include large-print cookbooks, black plastic measuring cups that provide high contrast, large-display digital clocks, bingo cards with raised letters and numbers, audio-equipped balls, hand-held talking compasses, talking scales and thermometers, phones and remote controls with large push buttons, magnifying tweezers, prescription bottle magnifiers, and large-symbol playing cards.

These are just a few examples of the hundreds of items available to help people with low vision. Some sources for these and other items are listed below.

SOURCES FOR PRODUCTS

- Accessibility Products, Inc.
  Call 800-428-9234 for a catalogue, or visit online at www.accesstoday.com.
- Lighthouse International
  Call 800-829-0500 for a catalog, or visit online at www.lighthouse.org/prodpub_products.htm.
- Independent Living Products
  Call 800-377-8033 for a catalog, or visit online at www.ilp-online.com/index.html.
- Maxi-Aids
  Call 516-752-0521 for a catalog, or visit online at www.maxiaids.com.
- LS&S Group, Inc.
  Call 800-468-4789 for a catalog, or visit online at www.1ssgroup.com.
- Sight Connection
  Call 800-458-4888 for a catalog, or visit online at www.sightconnection.com.

For a comprehensive listing of resources and special products, go online to the Disability Mall at www.disabilitymall.com.

STRATEGIES FOR COPING WITH VISION LOSS

People coping with vision loss, or impending loss, often wonder how they will manage to accomplish daily tasks and activities. They wonder if they will be able to cook for themselves, or handle their money, or measure a window for curtains, for example.

With rehabilitative training, visually impaired people can learn to do all of these things and many more. Some tips and strategies for daily living are outlined below.

What About Money?

Money is important, there's no question about it. So, how does a visually impaired person know how much to pay for that hamburger she orders? Coins are identified by touch. Bills of different denominations can be folded differently and kept in a designated pocket or wallet. She may need to ask for help to check the bills she gets back as change.

Visually impaired people who handle large amounts of money regularly sometimes use a talking paper-money identifier to keep track of bills. Generally, though, this is not necessary.

What About Measuring?

There are Braille rulers and special tape measures for typical measuring jobs. There also is a tool called a Rotomatic that assures accurate measuring. For measuring while cooking, use different colored measures to quickly differentiate what they are, or dark-colored ones that provide contrast to milk, flour, sugar, and other light-colored substances.

You also can get a product that squeezes out of a tube, then hardens into raised dots on the item onto which it has been squeezed. You can use such a product (one is called Hi-Marks) to identify various measuring cups and spoons.

What About Cooking?

Organize the kitchen so that you can easily find what you're looking for. Put all the canned soups on one shelf, for instance, and fruit on another shelf. Always return items to the same place when you have finished using them. If you share the kitchen, make sure the other person does the same.

When you put a small item, or several small items, in the oven, place them on a baking sheet first. This allows you to pull out the entire sheet instead of feeling around in a hot oven. Use a black marker to write the purchase date on perishable items. Use Hi-Marks or another substance to identify markings on the stove and oven dials.

What About Personal Hygiene?

Buy products like shampoos and conditioners in different sizes or differently shaped containers so that you can tell them apart. Find soap that is attached to a rope that you can anchor onto the tub or shower. If you cannot get your toothpaste squeezed out onto your brush, buy a tube just for yourself and squeeze it directly into your mouth or try the newer stand-up dispensers that allow you to put your toothbrush directly against them.

Use a magnifying mirror with a bright light to apply makeup or do your hair, and use light-colored makeup for easier blending. If you have trouble seeing colors, buy neutral-colored clothing and use brightly colored accessories.

What About Health and Medicines?

Be sure to label all medications so you know what you are taking. Use color codes, tactile markings, braille, or large print—whatever works best for you. Wrap rubber bands around a medication bottle to indicate the number of daily doses required or buy a pill organizer with an alarm that reminds you when it is time to take a medication.

Ask the pharmacist to put similarly shaped pills into different sized containers. If you are diabetic or have other health problems, consider getting an alarm system that allows you to press a button if you require medical assistance. Keep track of all medications you are taking and pertinent information relating to them. Be sure to take a record of medicines you are taking with you when you visit your doctor to help avoid the possibility of drug interactions.

What About Household Chores?

Separate items you need for different jobs and store them in buckets of different colors. That way you will have everything you need to clean the kitchen (or whatever) all together before you start the job. Get an automatic watering system for houseplants.

Use a criss-cross method for chores such as vacuuming, mowing grass, dusting, and washing dishes. Work down, and then across. This is most efficient. Run a soft mop around baseboards and in corners where you suspect dust and webs might collect.

What About Recreational Activities?

Paint large objects on large canvases. Buy or borrow large-print books and magazines, or listen to books on tape. Buy large-type crossword puzzles. Find out about keyboards with oversized keys. Learn to play a musical instrument, such as a guitar, for which sight isn't necessary. Look for special computer games.

Travel with a friend until you are comfortable traveling alone. Continue participating in activities that you enjoy. Look into getting a good pair of sports glasses that magnify up to two and a half times. Use them at sporting events or the theater.

These are just a few suggestions for coping with the challenges of low vision. You'll come up with many, many more on your own, or you can benefit from support groups and rehabilitative services. To learn more about what is available in your area, call Lighthouse International, a well known and valued resource on vision impairment and rehabilitation, at 800-829-0500.

Look for support groups that may be available in your area. These sometimes are offered through a local Association for the Blind. Websites that can connect you with support groups are listed in an appendix at the back of this book.

As devastating as vision impairment is, know that you are not alone. Low vision affects about 14 million Americans—that is one out of every 20 people—and the number is expected to increase as the population ages. There are an estimated 135 million people with low vision throughout the world. Do what you can to locate the support and resources that are available to you. Talk to a friend, family member, counselor, or minister or rabbi if you feel that you are having problems coping. Visual impairment can be incredibly frustrating and can impact greatly on your confidence and your life, but remember that there is help available, and many people who understand what you are experiencing.

CHAPTER 6

HELPING A LOVED ONE TO COPE WITH VISION PROBLEMS

People with significant vision problems face many challenges that those with normal vision do not. If your sight is normal, take a minute and try to imagine what it would be like to be visually impaired. Imagine going to a restaurant and not being able to read the menu or see your plate when your meal arrives. Imagine not being able to read the thermostat in your living room to see at what temperature your heat is set or see anything smaller than the large headlines in your daily newspaper. Imagine listening to television without being able to see the images.

Try to understand what it would be like to know that someone has entered the room where you are but not be able to see who it is, or hear someone walking behind you on the street but be unable to look back and see who it is. Or have a neighbor wave to you from across the street and not be able to recognize which neighbor it is. Think about looking at the latest photos of your children or grandchildren and seeing only dim shadows instead of the details of their faces. One woman who was losing her sight said she became distraught and sad when the time came that she could no longer prune her roses—something she had done every year and always enjoyed.

Those of us with normal vision probably can't really imagine what it is like to be visually impaired. We can, however, be supportive toward those who are, and help family and friends with significant vision impairment to get on with their lives and be as independent and self-sufficient as possible.

ATTITUDES TOWARD BLINDNESS AND VISUAL IMPAIRMENT

History has not been kind to people who are blind or visually impaired. Many misconceptions about blindness and vision impairment have caused those affected to be discriminated against and thought of as somehow less than those with sight. There's an old proverb that originated in the Middle East concerning blindness: "When you see a blind man, kick him. Why should you be any kinder to him than God has been?"

Most people today understand that blindness and vision loss are the results of disease, accidents, or genetic conditions, and not curses from

God. For some, however, the misconceptions linger on, and negative attitudes concerning blindness and vision loss continue.

Blindness has been badly understood throughout history. A blind person was considered to be helpless and dull-witted. Literature and film have portrayed blind people as being evil, helpless, grouchy, or stupid. Gloucester, a character in Shakespeare's *King Lear* is foolish and gullible. In Robert Louis Stevenson's *Treasure Island* the character Blind Pew is evil. A 1934 movie called *The Gift* included a stereotypical blind character who was clumsy, helpless, and irritable.

Tragically, similar stereotypes and misconceptions are passed along to children via cartoons such as *Mr. Magoo*. Mr. Magoo, a near-blind cartoon character, frequently bumps into things and speaks to objects that he thinks are people. While children laughed at Magoo's antics, the negative stereotypes concerning blind people were reinforced.

It is nice to think that these stereotypes are lessening, but as recently as 1991 ABC aired a show called *Good & Evil* that featured a blind character. The character, a psychologist, was inordinately clumsy, and his blindness caused him great embarrassment. He broke things all the time, he caressed a man who he thought was a woman; he hugged a coat rack. The show was taken off the air following protests from organizations affiliated with blind and visually impaired people.

Negative attitudes and stereotyping toward any group pave the way for discrimination, and blind and visually impaired people have been no exception. In some states, blind people may not serve as jurors. Blind students have been prevented from running for class officer. Astonishingly, between 70 and 79 percent of blind people are estimated to be unemployed.

Advocates of the blind and visually impaired explain the extremely high rate of unemployment as follows. Sighted people cannot imagine how they would do their jobs if they could not see. They are certain they would never be able to navigate an office or perform job-related tasks—and they are probably right. But because someone who is blind has learned different ways to work and complete tasks, an average blind person who is trained for a job is equally as competent to do it as the average sighted person.

This lack of understanding and stigma has taken its toll on the blind and visually impaired. Parents would (and probably some still do) tell their visually impaired children to not let anyone know they could not see well. Many blind people have refused to carry canes, use dog guides, or learn to read Braille, seeing these activities as shameful. Nearly all blind or visually impaired people have in some way felt the effects of these negative attitudes. Attitudes may be changing and improving, but there is still a long way to go.

Many blind and visually impaired people say there are certain thoughts and feelings they would like to pass along to sighted people in order to foster better understanding. Some of those thoughts include the following:

- Don't feel that you must avoid words like *look* and *see* in conversation. Blind people use those words too.
- Announce who you are when you come into a room, and let the person know when you are leaving.
- Say your name when you start a conversation, even if you have met the visually impaired person you are addressing before. Voices are often difficult to recognize.
- If a visually impaired person is a guest in your home, show him or her where things are located.
- Never interfere with a dog guide being employed by a blind or visually impaired person.
- If you're going to help a blind person to get from one place to another, do not grab her arm or pull her along. Allow her to take your arm and to follow a bit behind you.
- Look at the visually impaired person's face when you talk to him, and do not speak louder than normal. He be able to tell from your voice if you're looking somewhere else while talking to him. And, his trouble is with his eyesight, not his hearing.

UNDERSTANDING HOW A
VISUALLY IMPAIRED PERSON MIGHT FEEL

If somebody you care about—a parent or other family member, friend, coworker, or whoever—is losing or has lost their eyesight, don't assume that you understand how he or she feels.

Different people react differently to all kinds of situations, including the loss of their eyesight. Some people will be angry, while others will experience terrible self-pity. Nearly everyone will be very much afraid. Gallup polls indicate that blindness is the most feared condition, next to cancer.

Many people also will feel a great sense of loss, a response that is fully understandable. Someone who is told that she is going to be blind knows she is not only losing her sight but her life as she knew it. That is not to say that life for a blind person cannot be, or will not be good. But it is certainly going to be different than it was for that person when she could see.

Loss of vision often brings with it a loss of confidence—at least temporarily. Many visually impaired people say they're afraid to go out or try to participate in the activities that they enjoyed when they had their sight.

A woman who nine years ago lost her sight completely due to a genetic retinal disease shared her feelings about the experience. She wrote:

I became legally blind, left work, and began collecting Social Security disability income. For a year I struggled with clinical depression, the encroaching fog in my vision poured over into my spirit. My whole world was slowly closing, and no matter how much I wanted to, I couldn't change what was happening to me. I could not work. I was afraid to go out. I could not participate in the activities I loved because of my visual loss. I stopped doing the things that I loved, like drawing, reading, and writing. My insecurities increased and my self-esteem suffered. My loss was shocking and unexpected and I grieved over it like a lost child. I felt as if I could no longer believe in myself.

Depression among people who are becoming blind or have become blind is common. Some are so devastated that they consider suicide. Others withdraw from the people they love. Some people feel that they are being punished with the loss of their eyesight for sins or wrongdoings. Others rage against whatever god they know.

It is important to understand that a person who loses his or her vision is, indeed, suffering a significant loss. Dean W. Tuttle, Ph.D., wrote a book entitled *Self-Esteem and Adjusting with Blindness: The Process of Responding to Life's Demands* (Charles C. Thomas: Springfield, Ill., 1996). In it, he discusses an adjustment process that is necessary when vision loss occurs. Just as a person who is dying experiences stages, a person who is losing, or has lost, his or her eyesight will pass through different levels of emotions and feelings. Some of the stages that Tuttle identifies are shock, denial, a "what hit me?" feeling, depression, mourning, and withdrawal.

As a family member or friend of a person who is losing or has lost sight, it is extremely important to try to understand the sense of loss the person is experiencing and to allow him to share his feelings. Don't minimize the experience by saying something like, "well, it could be worse," or, "at least you are still alive." It could be that the visually impaired person doesn't feel very lucky to be alive at that moment.

Often, a person losing her eyesight will withdraw from friends and family, preferring to stay home and be alone. Family and friends might use this time to hook up with a support group or association for family and friends of the blind and visually impaired, or to find a social worker or counselor who might be able to offer assistance. If your loved one is open to it, you might suggest that she find some help as well.

THE PRACTICAL ASPECTS OF VISION LOSS

In addition to the emotional and psychological aspects of vision loss, your family member or friend is going to have to deal with all kinds of practical matters.

How will he take care of himself when he can't read the label on the soup can or read how much laundry detergent must be added to the washer? What if he has a headache and wants to take some pain medication but cannot be sure that the bottle in his hand is the right one? How will he be able to tell if the hamburger he is cooking is done? There are hundreds of practical matters that will need to be addressed and dealt with. Even though most of the kinds of situations mentioned above can be resolved rather easily if the person is willing to be innovative and resourceful, the thought of getting along without sight is very frightening.

Family and friends can be encouraging and helpful. Offer to help, but don't assume that the person losing his sight can do nothing for himself. Allow him to be as independent as he can be. If he's not aware of the many organizations and assistive devices available, do steer him in that direction. Be positive about his future, and willing to discuss situations that apply to him.

BE AN ADVOCATE

People who have lost their vision often report feeling isolated and alone. If somebody you know is facing this experience, let her know that you are there to help her. If you can, help the person get in touch with others in the same position. Experts say that this restores confidence and makes the person feel that she is not alone.

You also can help her to get necessary information about issues such as Social Security benefits or rehabilitation opportunities. Contact the National Federation of the Blind or another agency for information concerning these and other such topics, such as employment, scholarships, civil rights, products and aids, free reading matter, publications, education of blind children, and library services.

Help your family member or friend to figure out how she will organize things within her home, and how she will accomplish tasks such as shopping, cooking, and laundry when she no longer has much vision. Be there for her. Do not, however, be overly protective. While it is good to offer help and support, you don't want to make a person who is losing his sight feel helpless or incapable of getting around on his own.

Of course there will be times and places when and where a sightless person will need your assistance. However, helping someone too often can cause him to become dependent and fearful when you are not there. If you are not sure if he wants your help, go ahead and ask. But do not insist that he needs it, or force him to accept your help if he doesn't want it.

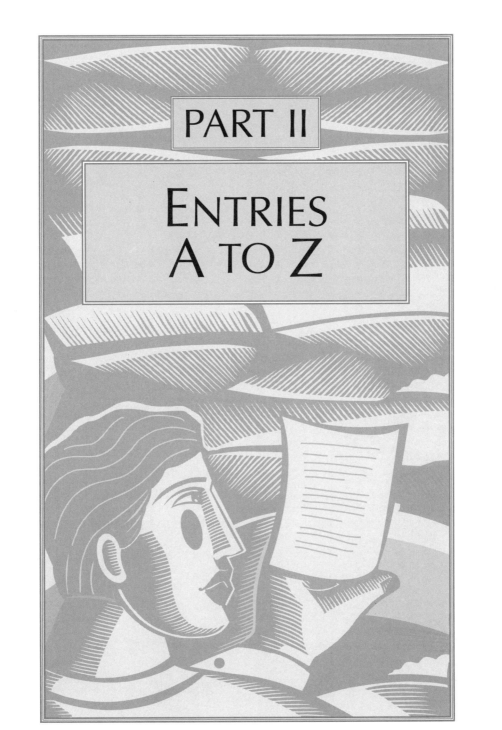

PART II

ENTRIES
A TO Z

A

abacus   The abacus is used to teach mathematics skills to blind and visually impaired students. The Cranmer abacus is an adaptive device that has a backing behind the beads to prevent accidental movement or sliding.

It is used to add, subtract, multiply, and divide whole numbers and decimals. Calculations can be done faster on a talking computer or a calculator, but the Cranmer abacus is considered to be faster and easier to use than a BRAILLE WRITER, TAYLOR SLATE, or pegboard. Schools for blind students offer courses in the use of the Cranmer abacus.

accessibility   The ability to enter and navigate through a building or environment and to use all its facilities or services. To ensure integration of disabled persons into all aspects of society, Congress has issued laws and regulations that prohibit those who accept federal funds from discriminating against disabled persons by limiting accessibility.

Federal accessibility standards are outlined by the American National Standards Institute (ANSI) in the document "The American National Standard Specifications for Making Buildings and Facilities Accessible to, and Usable by, the Physically Handicapped." Compliance with the standards is monitored by the Architectural and Transportation Barriers Compliance Board, an organization within the Department of Health, Education and Welfare.

Although ANSI works with architects, public officials, organizations that serve the disabled, and disabled individuals, the federal requirements may not be the complete solution to accessibility. The standards represent only minimum levels of accessibility and do not encourage efforts to exceed these levels. Federal regulations do not solve problems that result from the conflicting needs of two or more types of disabilities; for example, street crossing curb cuts that serve wheelchair users may be hazardous for visually impaired persons.

Accessibility requirements for visually impaired persons may be inadequate as well. The standards are generally misunderstood and underdeveloped because blind people and those working professionally in services for the visually impaired have been unable to reach a consensus on accessibility needs. Excellent methods of orientation and mobility have been developed to enable visually impaired persons to successfully compensate for their sight loss. As a result, the visually impaired segment of the disabled community may lack the urgency felt by other members who cannot compensate for physical barriers.

Groups representing blind and visually impaired persons are in place and working to improve accessibility. The World Wide Web Consortium is in the process of finalizing accessibility guidelines to assure that all people have equal access to the Internet. These efforts are a collaboration of industry, disability, and research organizations, as well as various governments from around the world.

For more information about federal accessibility standards and ANSI, contact:

American National Standards Institute
1819 L Street, NW, Suite 600
Washington, DC 20036
212-642-4900
www.ansi.org

Act to Promote the Education of the Blind   Passed by Congress in 1879, this act mandates that the American Printing House for the Blind, a nonprofit agency, produce and distribute specially designed and adapted educational materials to blind students in public schools in America.

Such materials are necessary so that blind students have equal access to public education, and include textbooks in Braille and large type, tangible teaching devices, educational tests, and special instructional aids, tools, and materials adapted for students who are legally blind. The American Printing House for the Blind received federal funding to produce and distribute materials.

acyclovir   Acyclovir, also known as ACV or Zovirax, is an ANTIVIRAL DRUG used to treat ocular herpes. The drug suppresses the enzyme thymidine kinase, which is vital to the virus. Acyclovir is distinctive in that, unlike other antiviral medications, it attacks the viral cells only and disregards normal cells.

adaptive aids   Adaptive aids (or daily-living aids, independent-living aids) are devices and tools that have been adapted or invented to enable visually impaired persons to perform sight-related tasks independently. Often, an unadapted tool or utensil is marked with raised dots, braille, or large print to become an adaptive aid. Other aids are equipped with voice simulators.

Adaptive aids may require prescription by an ophthalmologist or low-vision specialist and may require special training for use. Adaptive aids are available through adaptive-aids catalogs or are constructed or adapted by the users themselves.

Health aids are instruments that can be used by visually impaired persons to monitor their health or administer medicine. Devices for monitoring temperature, blood pressure, pulse, and glucose are marked in braille or announce the measurement in a synthesized voice. Pill splitters divide pills into even halves, and guides are available for measuring liquid medications. Diabetes-related devices measure insulin to preset levels and serve as needle guides. Many syringes are marked in large print.

Household aids include cooking devices, such as a liquid level indicator (which hooks over the lip of a cup and beeps or vibrates as the liquid nears the top of the cup), one-cup beverage makers (which heat liquids for soup, coffee, etc.), electromagnetic stoves (which heat food without flames or heating elements), elbow-length oven mitts, and knife slicing guides.

Other aids for the home include self-threading needles, sewing-machine magnifiers, magnetic padlocks (which require no combination and open with a magnetic sensor), raised large-print telephone dials, one-button automatic telephone-dialing systems, and brailled clothing tags.

Magnification aids, or magnifiers, include hand-held devices such as a bar magnifier, which enlarges one line of print, and hand-held aspheric magnifiers, which magnifies three to 10 times the normal size. Magnifiers may lie on the page as a sheet magnifier, may be held by stands at a precise distance from the page or object, or may be attached to spectacles and swung down into place when needed. Magnifiers may be telescopic and enable the user to see street signs or other distant objects.

Electronic magnifiers or visual aids include closed-circuit television (CCTV), which employs a camera and a zoom lens to magnify a page of print 60 times normal size. Portable models are available and constantly improving.

Nonoptical or *environmental aids* improve vision but do not use lens magnification. These factors improve the environment rather than the device or object of regard. They include illumination, light transmission, reflection control, and contrast.

Illumination is improved through use of brighter or dimmer room lighting, as needed according to the cause of disability. Light transmission is improved through lenses, filters, and absorptive lenses, which reduce glare and highlight contrast.

Reflection is controlled by visors, sideshields, specially treated lenses, and typoscopes. Contrast is enhanced by using highly contrasting colors near one another, such as black ink on white paper or fluorescent strips on stair risers.

Talking aids, or *auditory aids,* allow the user to access information by the sense of hearing. They are devices that play or read the text, message, measurement, or degree according to a preset interval of time or on activation of the voice.

Tape recorders are used to play and/or record communications and recorded materials such as talking books. Some models are available with stop/start foot pedals to allow for typing while listening. Many tape recorders and players contain variable speed adjustments to reduce the time spent listening.

Speech compressors are machines that control the speed of the audio of a tape by deleting portions of the pauses between words or by shortening vowel sounds. The material is rerecorded in the shorter version, and the sound of the speech is not affected.

Accelerated speech is text that is recorded at normal speed but reproduced and played at an accelerated speed. Highly accelerated speech may produce a distortion in the sound of the voice, although some models contain pitch-controlling options.

Talking books and other recorded texts are available through talking-book programs or the Library of Congress. Books on cassette tape are also available through commercial publishers.

Synthetic speech is the computerized production of sounds into words and is used in the voice output of reading machines and computers. The Kurzweil Reading Machine is a talking device that uses a computer-controlled camera to scan lines of print. A voice synthesizer "reads" the print to the user.

Talking adaptive aids are tools that supply a voice reading of the information normally gained by sight. Such aids include the talking scale, clock, watch, timer, blood-pressure monitor, thermometer, blood-glucose monitoring kit, talking wallet (which identifies bills of $1–$10 denominations), label makers, calculators, and computer-speech output.

Tools and instruments include rulers, yardsticks, and tape measures with raised tactual readings or braille markings, saw guides with raised markings at specific degree points, drill guides and squares, calipers, and micrometers with raised-dot markings. Light probes and metal or voltage detectors locate light or flame, metal objects, or live electrical current and sound an audible signal to alert the user.

Travel aids allow the user to move in an environment safely and independently. These include canes, folding or rigid, and electronic travel aids that are prescribed by an optometrist or ophthalmologist and include the laser cane, the Pathsounder, the Sonic Guide, and the Mowat Sensor, all of which require specialized training to use.

Electronic travel aids send out light beams or ultrasound waves that come into contact with objects in the path. When the beam or waves hit an object, the device responds by vibrating or emitting a sound. They are used by approximately 1 percent of all visually impaired persons.

Orientation aids familiarize a visually impaired traveler to the layout of a particular building or site. Orientation aids include tactile maps, three-dimensional maps that include raised lines and are read with the fingertips, models, three-dimensional scale representations of the site, and verbal recordings of site descriptions or travel routes.

Watches, clocks, and timers are available in a variety of forms. Watch covers are designed to open so the user can feel the hands in relation to the raised dots at each hour. Time pieces may be tactually marked with dots at each hour or at set intervals on the dial. Many feature large print or bold, high-contrast numbers. Some designs announce the time audibly at the touch of a button, and others automatically announce the time at set intervals.

Writing and communication aids enable users to perform writing and reading tasks independently. Braille books, magazines, musical materials, and maps are available to those who read braille. Large-print materials employ larger lettering for use by those with partial vision. Written materials are recorded on tape or gramophone and are available to visually impaired persons.

A script-writing guide is a template with an opening that corresponds to one line of space on a lined page. The device can be lowered one line at a time as the writer progresses down the page. Many designs allow adaptations for drawing vertical lines and for use on nonstandard-size paper.

Bold-line paper is lined writing paper with heavy, dark lines in place of standard light blue lines. The bold lines (often used with a thick-tipped felt pen) may be all that is necessary to allow persons with low vision to write independently.

Templates or stencils are available in myriad forms for tasks that range from envelope addressing to check writing. They are made from plastic or metal and have openings or windows that correspond to the type of document. Many templates can be made to order to suit the user's needs or documents. A signature guide is a template that has one opening to place on the signature line.

A raised-line drawing kit involves a penlike stylus for forming letters or drawings on special plastic paper or mylar covering a drawing board. Drawn lines are visible and can be tactually traced. A similar device, a dot inverter, involves embossed dots that can be used to make simple maps or figures.

Thermoform is a system that uses an oven to heat plastic sheets. The heated sheets can be embossed into dots or shapes including braille letters or maps. The thermoform sheets can be used to duplicate braille pages from a master sheet.

Label makers include designs that make adhesive-backed or magnetic labels in large print, braille, raised-line letters, or "talking" labels.

Three-D markers allow writing three-dimensional letters or figures that can be felt with the fingertips. The ink may be brightly colored and may be used on cloth, plastic, and metal.

Braille writers or braillers are used to type braille. A slate and a stylus are portable writing devices for printing braille.

The Optacon is a reading device used by those who read braille. The user sweeps a line of print with a small camera held in one hand. The other hand rests on a console that receives the print and converts it to a series of vibrating pins that simulate print letters.

Standard typewriters or word processors can be used for those with touch typing skills. Computers that print braille or standard print are available with speech output.

Many advances in computer access for visually impaired persons have been made in recent years. Special tools are available that convert documents into text, which can be read by a screen-reading program that synthesizes text as audible speech.

In some cases, regular computers can be converted and made accessible to blind or visually impaired users.

advocacy   An advocate is one who pleads the case of another. Advocacy among persons with disabilities often centers on working to change legislation, to fill unmet needs or to take advantage of denied opportunities or rights ensured by law. Advocacy measures may involve issues of legislation, medical rights, housing rights, fair compensation, nondiscrimination, employment rights, educational rights, use of public transportation or facilities, and rights of privacy.

The Rehabilitation Act of 1973 established the discretionary creation of advocates or client assistants at the state level. These assistants work as ombudsmen with disabled individuals and service providers to ensure that individuals receive the services they seek. Many states have established specific state protection and advocacy agencies to serve as advocates. Local governmental social service offices may provide additional help in gaining appropriate services and aid.

Professional, consumer, and advocacy organizations and agencies for the blind and visually impaired on the national, state, and local level serve as self-advocates by informing and educating lawmakers, providing services and information to the public, and offering referral services.

Parents of disabled children frequently merge to form advocacy groups. Whether working individually for their own children, or in groups to represent the needs of similarly disabled children, parents are an effective force. For example, during the epidemic of cases of retrolental fibroplasia in the 1940s and 1950s and later in the 1960s following an epidemic of rubella, parents formed advocacy groups that forced schools to provide special education for their visually impaired and multihandicapped children and to include these children into public schools and mainstream classes.

A parents advocacy group active today is the National Organization of Parents of Blind Children, affiliated with the National Federation of the Blind. It can be accessed on the Internet at www.nfb.org/nopbc.

Successful advocacy usually includes phases of preparation, action, and evaluation. During the preparation phase, the advocate identifies the specific need, researches the existing organizations that provide services and aid and identifies which agency or individual is best prepared to fill the need.

In the action phase, the advocate contacts the agency or individual, convinces the individual of the needs of the disabled person and the ability, appropriateness or responsibility of the agency to provide for those needs, works with the individual to target specific methods to meet needs and develops a timetable or plan for fulfilling the needs.

During the evaluation phase, the advocate determines whether the needs have been met according to the agreement and remains in contact with the agency until the needs are met.

aging   More than 50 percent of all individuals with severe vision impairments are over 65. In addition, a study by Lighthouse International showed that one in six people age 45 or older report some type of visual impairment. More than half of these people describe the impairment as severe. Changes with age occur both in the external and internal portions of the eye. Externally, the globe itself may seem to have sunken into the skull. This is the result of a breakdown or natural degeneration of the retrobulbar fat that supports the globe in the bony socket. Fortunately, the bony socket, called the orbit, is not susceptible to osteoporosis, as are other bones in the body. The orbit does not weaken or become thin and brittle with aging.

The eyelids may lose elasticity and tone causing PTOSIS (drooping eyelid). This may cause a reduction in the area of visual field.

ENTROPION (a turning inward of the eyelid) and ECTROPION (a turning outward of the eyelid) are common complaints associated with aging. Both conditions can be successfully treated with surgery if they produce discomfort or a threat to vision.

The CONJUNCTIVA, or white portion of the eye, becomes slack and more susceptible to chronic inflammations with age. As it slackens, a section may become caught between the lids during blinking. Harmless degenerative plaques may appear on the white of the eye.

ARCUS SENILIS may appear on the margin of the cornea. This harmless white circle bordering the cornea is a common occurrence in the elderly. Composed of cholesterol and its derivatives, the presence of arcus senilis does not necessarily indicate an overall raised cholesterol level.

Most aging eyes become presbyopic, a condition in which the hardened lens is unable to bend and focus effectively on objects at close range. Presbyopia usually surfaces near age 45 and affects both nearsighted and farsighted eyes. The condition is treated with reading glasses or bifocals.

The lens often becomes opacified with age. Degrees of OPACIFICATION vary and are not termed cataract until a significant opacification develops. The lens may yellow and cause color vision changes and nearsightedness.

The pupil loses its ability to accommodate quickly with changing light. The pupil becomes smaller and reduces the light entering the eye to approximately 30 percent of normal levels.

The vitreous of the aging eye may contain opacities that become visible to the individual as floaters, or spots that bounce or float in the field of vision. The vitreous may collapse or detach from the retina. This may cause a more serious condition, retinal detachment, and vision loss.

The arteries and veins of the retina become narrower with age, reducing the flow of blood. The aging retina is duller and exhibits a less responsive light reflex. The optic disc may be paler also.

VISUAL ACUITY, or the ability to see small objects under normal lighting and contrast conditions, may suffer with age. The reduction may occur as a result of the smaller pupil and/or the aging, opacified lens. Decreased visual acuity may affect the ability to perform tasks such as reading or driving.

The aging eye requires more light than a younger eye. It is estimated that for every 13 years of life, twice the amount of light is needed to function effectively. This may be due to the smaller pupil and less transparent lens.

CONTRAST sensitivity and spatial perception reductions may occur with age. The ability to detect and recognize contrast is controlled by the neural circuitry of the retina and brain. As neuronal changes occur, contrast sensitivity decreases. Spatial perception depends on contrast detection, so any reduction in contrast perception affects this ability as well.

Adaptation, the ability to be sensitive to changing light levels and adjust to them, is diminished by age. An elderly eye may require more time to recover from glare or a bright light such as a flashbulb or car headlights. This is a result of the smaller, less adaptive pupil and the opacified lens.

Color vision may fade or change with age. The yellowing lens tends to absorb and scatter blue light, rendering blues darker and less intense. The unimpeded red and yellow light is allowed to pass through and cast a warm, reddish glow onto objects.

In addition to visual changes, vision loss occurs as a result of diseases that are associated with aging. The four leading causes of vision loss among elderly individuals are age-related maculopathy, cataracts, glaucoma, and diabetic retinopathy.

Age-Related Maculopathy (ARM) is a progressive disease in which the macula, or area of sharpest central sight, deteriorates. Central vision and contrast enhancement is lost but peripheral vision often remains intact. Some types of macular disease may be treated with laser therapy, and other advances in the treatment of ARM are occurring rapidly. Doctors and scientists are optimistic about new treatments for ARM, and are working hard to find a cure for this disease.

Cataracts are opacifications or cloudy spots on the lens of the eye. Senile cataracts, those associated with aging, are usually progressive and may exist for several years before requiring surgical removal. Removal of cataracts is highly successful, and entails removal of the lens. The lens is replaced by an artificial intraocular lens or by a contact lens or glasses. The results of cataract removal, although generally successful, vary from person to person.

Glaucoma is an increase in the intraocular pressure. This occurs when the eye produces an overabundance of AQUEOUS FLUID or when the eye fails to drain the fluid adequately. The increase in pressure may damage organs of the eye and result in vision loss. Glaucoma can be treated and controlled with medication or surgery.

Diabetic retinopathy is an eye disease that results from diabetes. The small blood vessels that support and nourish the retina become damaged and weak. These may hemorrhage and cause an accumulation of fluid in the retina that limits or alters vision. New, weaker vessels may proliferate, hemorrhage and form vision-limiting scar tissue. The scar tissue may trigger a retinal detachment, and permanent vision loss may result.

Aging eyes may benefit by changes in the environment and lifestyle of the individual. Increased lighting and color contrast coupled with reduced glare may aid residual vision, increase effectiveness in the performance of tasks, and enhance safety. ADAPTIVE AIDS may improve or enhance remaining vision, aid in the performance of skills and tasks, and increase independence. Biannual eye examinations for those over 40 may uncover an eye disorder at its earliest and most treatable stage.

American Foundation for the Blind. *Aging and Vision.* New York: AFB, 1987.
Carroll, Thomas J. "A Look at Aging," *The New Outlook* (April 1972): pp. 97–103.
Denby, Dorothy. "Aging and Blindness," *Aging and the Human Condition,* New York: Human Services Press, Inc. 1982.
Galloway, N. R. *Common Eye Diseases and their Management.* Berlin: Springer-Verlag, 1985.
American Society on Aging. Visual Disorders and Aging. www.asaging.org/ameritech/V002_visual_disorders.html, 2000.

AIDS   Acquired immunodeficiency syndrome, or AIDS, is a disease of the immune system characterized by a deficiency of thymus-derived lymphocytes. These lymphocytes, identified by the phenotypic marker T4, function as helpers to the immune system. The lack of T4 lymphocytes leads to a breakdown in the immune response and allows the body to become host to opportunistic infections and neoplasm (tumor) development. AIDS is caused by a virus called HIV (human immunodeficiency virus). Having HIV is not the same as having AIDS. AIDS is the late stage of HIV infection.

Visual disorders or disturbances affect over 50 percent of AIDS patients. One-third of these patients have cytomegalovirus retinitis, an infection of the retina caused by the cytomegalovirus (CMV). Cytomegalovirus is a member of the herpes virus family and may cause primary, latent, and persistent infections.

Cytomegalovirus retinitis progressively destroys tissue that leads to scar formation, and possible retinal detachments. Symptoms of the condition include blind spots, blurred vision, and loss of peripheral vision, although the infection may be present without any apparent symptoms. The infection progresses rapidly and may cause blindness if left untreated.

Current treatment for cytomegalovirus retinitis involves the use of two ANTIVIRAL DRUGS: ganciclovir and foscarnet. Ganciclovir stops the progression of the disease and may save the residual vision. The drug is contraindicated for use with AZT. The drug is given by daily intravenous infusion, but an oral form has recently been developed and is in testing.

Foscarnet also stops the progression of the infection. It is given intravenously but can be taken in conjunction with AZT. Foscarnet may be less effective in preventing relapses of CMV retinitis after the initial high-dose induction phase of treatment. Foscarnet may have the additional advantage of being effective in combatting HIV activity.

air bags   Protective devices that are installed in many cars. Air bags, also known as inflatable restraint systems, are designed to inflate immediately upon impact, in the course of an automobile accident. They are designed to prevent the driver and front-seat passenger from being thrown against the steering wheel, dashboard, or window or from being thrown from the car.

Although they are credited with saving lives and preventing many injuries, there are risks, including eye injuries, associated with air bags. This is particularly true with regard to children.

An article in the August 2000 issue of *Ophthalmology,* the journal published by the American Academy of Ophthalmology, concluded that air bags can cause serious eye injuries to children and that to avoid such injuries, children should not be permitted to ride in the front seat of an automobile.

Some possible eye injuries that could result from air bag deployment include cataracts, glaucoma, blood in the front chamber of the eye, alkali burn, temporary loss of consciousness and visual acuity, laceration of the eyelid, inflammation of the iris, corneal lesions and abrasions, black eye, and swelling and hemorrhage of blood vessels under the outer surface of the eyeball.

albinism   A hereditary condition in which all or part of the body lacks pigment. Albinism may affect the skin, eyes, and hair of the individual. It is thought to be caused by an enzyme deficiency involving the metabolism of melanin during prenatal development.

There are two major types of albinism: oculocutaneous albinism and ocular albinism. Oculocutaneous albinism involves a lack of pigmentation in the eyes, skin, and hair. The condition is subdivided into two groups, tyrosinase-positive or tyrosinase-negative, according to the presence or absence of the enzyme tyrosinase in the hair bulbs. Tyrosinase inhibits the formation of pigment in the body. Tyrosinase-negative individuals have white hair, pink skin, and pale blue eyes, and tyrosinase-positive individuals produce some melanin and vary as to physical condition and coloring.

Ocular albinism involves the lack of, or reduced amount of, pigmentation of the eye. Individuals with ocular albinism may exhibit no lack of pigmentation of the skin and hair.

Those with ocular albinism and tyrosinase-negative oculocutaneous albinism usually experience severe visual disorders. These may include a visual acuity of 20/200 or less, NYSTAGMUS (an involuntary movement or jerking of the eyes), amblyopia (a condition in which the brain does not receive information from one or both eyes as a result of a failure of the vision development as an infant or child), iris transillumination (the ability of light to pass through the normally pigmented iris), lack of fundus pigmentation, and PHOTOPHOBIA (a sensitivity to light).

Albinism cannot be cured. Symptoms such as loss of visual acuity, nystagmus, amblyopia, and photophobia may be treated with therapy, surgery, corrective lenses, or light-reducing lenses.

alcohol amblyopia   A visual condition unique to alcoholics or those who have a history of chronic, severe drinking problems. The disorder involves lost vision, including SCOTOMAS (blind spots) and decreased visual acuity within the central portion of the visual field. The painless, bilateral sight loss gradually worsens. The disorder is caused by the toxic effects of alcohol on the optic nerve. The toxicity causes optic neuropathy, a condition in which the optic nerve swells.

Alcohol amblyopia may be linked with a thiamine (vitamin B_1) deficiency, a condition that can lead to optic-nerve damage. Alcohol consumption may interfere with the absorption or activation of nutrients and vitamins within the body, including thiamine and zinc.

Alcohol amblyopia may be treated with proper diet and vitamin supplements. The condition is usually reversible but may lead to permanent vision loss if untreated.

Burde, Ronald M., Peter J. Savino and Jonathan D. Trobe, *Clinical Decisions in Neuro-Ophthalmology.* St. Louis: C.V. Mosby Company, 1985.
Havener, William H. *Ocular Pharmacology.* St. Louis: C.V. Mosby Company, 1970.
O'Brien, Robert, and Morris Chafetz. *The Encyclopedia of Alcoholism.* New York: Facts On File Publications, 1982.

amaurosis   The loss of sight due to disease.

ametropia   A vision problem caused by the eye's inability to focus properly. Ametropia occurs when the cornea and the lens of the eye cannot effectively focus light, and the resulting image, onto the retina. This focusing impairment is also called REFRACTIVE ERROR.

Refractive errors such as hyperopia (farsightedness), MYOPIA (nearsightedness), astigmatism (distorted image) or presbyopia (aging eyes) result in blurred vision. Ametropia can be diagnosed in a routine ophthalmologic examination and is usually corrected with eyeglasses or contact lenses.

Amsler grid   A specialized testing device, invented by Professor Marc Amsler and used to detect disorders and SCOTOMA (blind spots) in the central field of vision. It is routinely used to screen patients for age-related maculopathy during the ophthalmologic exam.

The Amsler grid is a black-on-white grid of 400 squares. It is composed of 20 horizontal squares by 20 vertical squares. A black dot is in the center of the grid where the two central horizontal and vertical lines intersect.

With one eye covered, the patient is asked to look at the center dot. The patient is asked whether the center dot is visible, all the sides are visible, the entire grid is visible, any lines are wavy or bent, there are any blurs, color differentiations or distortions within the grid. If any lines appear wavy, if some of the lines disappear, or if all four corners are not visible, scotomas or age-related maculopathy may be present.

aneurysm   A diseased or weakened section of a blood vessel that fills with blood and dilates. Aneurysms may occur within blood vessels throughout the body.

Aneurysms within the blood vessels of the brain may be the result of ARTERIOSCLEROSIS. They may rupture and bleed into the cerebral fluid, a condition called a subarachnoid hemorrhage. A subarachnoid hemorrhage may cause increased pressure within the brain and decreased blood supply, resulting in a STROKE. Paralysis of the limbs, sudden changes in the field of vision, speech and memory disorders and thinking or reasoning problems may follow.

Aneurysms of the eye's retina may occur as a result of another disease or disorder such as diabetic retinopathy. In this disease, the retinal vessels are weakened by diabetes. They tend to bulge and leak, hemorrhaging into the retina and causing vision loss. As the disease progresses, neovascularization occurs producing weakened blood vessels that rupture, hemorrhage and may cause retinal detachment and scar tissue resulting in permanent vision loss.

aniridia   Aniridia (or irideremia) is the absence of the IRIS within the eye. It is a congenital or acquired condition. Congenital aniridia is a genetically determined condition. In many cases, a vestigial portion of the iris root or margin is present. The congenital condition is usually bilateral and often seen in conjunction with congenital cataract. Glaucoma tends to develop in early adolescence in approximately 25 percent of congenital aniridia cases, due to the abnormal angle of the anterior chamber and blockage by the iris root.

Individuals with congenital aniridia are photophobic and may experience amblyopia (loss of vision in one eye due to disuse) and NYSTAGMUS (involuntary jerking of the eyes). Associated retinal abnormalities or malformations may exist. The condition, which develops at about the 12th week of pregnancy, is very rare, affecting 1 in 500,000 to 1 in a million children.

Acquired aniridia occurs as a result of trauma or injury. The iris is dislodged or torn from the CILIARY BODY. It contracts into a small pellet and moves to the outlet of the anterior chamber, where it may form a blockage and cause secondary glaucoma.

The glaucoma of both types of aniridia is treated with medications or with surgical procedures such as goniotomy or trabeculotomy if the medication proves ineffective. The prognosis for the vision of those with aniridia is generally poor.

anisocoria   A condition in which the pupils differ in size. Average-size pupils range from three to four millimeters.

All pupils are small at birth. Differences in size become more apparent as the individual grows and achieves maximum pupil size by adolescence. The pupil may become smaller with advancing age.

Approximately 17 percent of the population have minor amounts of anisocoria, but only 4 percent have pronounced cases. The difference in size may vary from minute measurements to noticeable degrees. The size difference may be variable during the course of a day.

On the average, women tend to have larger pupils than men have, and blue or less pigmented irises are larger than brown, more pigmented irises. Myopic (nearsighted) individuals usually have larger pupils than those with hyperopia (farsightedness).

Anisocoria may be congenital or acquired, as from ingestion of oral contraceptives. The condition may be a first indication of pupillary defects but may also exist in the absence of ocular disorder. One or both anisocoric pupils that fail to properly react to light may indicate neurological problems.

anisometropia   A common condition in which the eyes have unequal refractive power or unequal ability to focus and see. The degree of anisometropia can be determined during an ophthalmologic examination. Anisometropia is corrected by prescribing a stronger prescriptive lens for one eye than the other to equalize the eyes' refractive powers. Contact lenses often can greatly reduce the effects of anisometropia.

Without correction, anisometropia can cause amblyopia in children. The weaker anisometropic eye sends less reliable information to the brain than does the stronger eye. The visual cells of the brain ignore the information of this eye, become dysfunctional and cause the eye, however healthy, to become amblyopic.

anterior chamber   A section of the eye between the cornea and the lens. The chamber is filled with a clear liquid called AQUEOUS FLUID.

The cornea and the lens of the eye lack blood vessels, which deliver nutrients and carry away waste. The aqueous fluid, produced by the CILIARY BODY, provides these services as it circulates within the anterior chamber. The aqueous fluid leaves the chamber through the Schlemm's canal, a channel where the IRIS and the cornea meet. If the channel becomes blocked, fluid may build up in the eye and cause a rise in intraocular pressure, a condition known as glaucoma.

antibiotics DRUGS that fight infections caused by bacterial microorganisms. They are commonly prescribed for those who have a bacterial eye infection or who undergo eye surgery. Antibiotics are often taken prior to surgery to avoid the possibility of infection.

Antibiotics may be topical (applied outside the body) or systemic (taken internally). Antibiotics prescribed to treat eye disorders may be in ointment, eye-drop, or pill form.

Antibiotics are classified as one of two types, bacteriocidal or bacteriostatic. Bacteriocidal antibiotics, such as penicillin, ampicillin, and amoxicillin, disrupt the natural cell formation of microorganisms to eliminate them. Bacteriostatic antibiotics, such as tetracycline, doxycycline, and erythromycin, hinder reproductive chemical processes to eradicate the unwanted microorganisms.

When an infection is suspected in the eye, a culture may be taken from the conjunctival sac. A wide-spectrum antibiotic may be prescribed until the cause of the infection is isolated. Once the cause is determined, both systemic and topical antibiotics may be required.

antiviral drugs DRUGS that fight viruses that infect the body. Viruses that affect the eye usually result in inflammation or infection. These infections may lead to serious, vision-limiting conditions such as KERATITIS (corneal inflammation) or IRITIS (inflammation of the IRIS).

Since HERPES SIMPLEX is a major cause of viral infection in the eye, several antiviral drugs have been developed for the purpose of treating this condition. Drugs most often prescribed include IDOXURIDINE, TRIFLURIDINE, ACYCLOVIR, and ARA-A.

A new group of drugs, including acyclovir and ARA-A, has since been developed that attack only the viral cells and leave the body's healthy cells intact. These drugs, also known by the names ACV, Zovirax, vidarabine, Vira-A, and adenine arabinoside, are less toxic and can be prescribed in drop, ointment, injection, or pill form.

None of these drugs is a cure for the herpes simplex virus. They can treat the virus only when it is active in the body. The drugs discourage the virus from generating new cells, and the virus then retreats into the ganglion of the body where it remains latent. The drugs are ineffective against the virus during periods of latency. The drugs cannot stop the virus from becoming active, which could occur at any time.

Antibiotics may also be used to treat viruses. TRACHOMA, a leading cause of blindness in the world, is often successfully treated with tetracycline hydrochloride ointment.

aphakia   Aphakia refers to an eye without a lens. After cataract surgery, during which the lens of the eye is removed, the eye is aphakic. A monocular aphake is a person without the lens from one eye. A bilateral aphake is a person missing both lenses.

Without the lens, the eye is unable to accommodate or adjust to focus on an object. Commonly, elderly cataract surgery patients experience limited accommodation before surgery and therefore surgery-induced aphakia minimally affects their vision. People with aphakia are at a greater risk for some types of retinal detachment than those who are not aphakic.

Aphakia also distorts the size of objects, makes images appear larger, and may bend or curve straight lines. Distance judgment problems may result. Changes in color-perception may also occur. Colors may appear brighter, pinker, or bluer.

Aphakia can be corrected with glasses, contact lenses, or intraocular lenses, also called IOLs.

appetite suppressants   Systematic use of appetite suppressants, including amphetamines, dextroamphetamines, methamphetamines, and phenmetrazine compounds, can affect the eyes, causing such side effects as pupil dilation and impaired vision. These drugs also can cause difficulty with accommodation and convergence, which can make reading difficult. Persistent use of these drugs also can lead to closed-angle glaucoma in some people.

aqueous fluid   The aqueous fluid (or aqueous humor) is the clear liquid that fills the ANTERIOR CHAMBER of the eye, located between the cornea and the lens. The cornea and lens must be transparent to function and, therefore contain no blood vessels. The aqueous fluid functions as blood vessels by delivering the nutrients and antibodies and carrying away the waste normally.

The clear, thin fluid is produced by the ciliary body at a rate of approximately two cubic millimeters (about one drop) per minute. The nutrients and antibodies are pumped from blood vessels within the ciliary body and mix with the aqueous.

The aqueous flows from the CILIARY BODY, behind the iris, across the lens, through the pupil into the anterior chamber, and along the back surface of the cornea. It circulates in the anterior chamber, bringing nutrients and carrying away waste from the avascular cornea and lens.

The aqueous fluid drains from the eye at the base of the cornea, an outflow channel called the Schlemm's canal. The aqueous fluid is strained of waste and collected in the canal. It then flows to small veins in the sclera and joins the body's blood stream.

When the draining channels become blocked or if the eye overproduces aqueous, the fluid may build up. Intraocular pressure builds within the eye, damaging the nerve endings of the retina. This condition is known as glaucoma.

ARA-A   An ANTIVIRAL DRUG prescribed in the treatment of ocular herpes. Available in ointment and pill form, it is also known by the names vidarabine, Vira-A and adenine arabinoside. Unlike IDU or TFT, drugs that attack healthy as well as infected cells, ARA-A is less toxic and attacks only viral cells.

architectural barriers   See ACCESSIBILITY.

arcus senilis   Arcus senilis is a grey or white ring or arc that appears on the edge of the iris, or colored part of the eye, where it borders the SCLERA, or white part of the eye. The ring is actually located on the margin of the cornea, the clear, protective covering of the eye.

The condition is caused by aging and is most often noticed in dark-eyed people. Arcus senilis is a harmless condition that does not affect vision and is not a sign of another eye disorder. Arcus senilis also is known as a cornea ring.

argon laser   The argon is a laser often used to treat diabetic retinopathy, a leading cause of blindness in the United States. A complication of diabetes, diabetic retinopathy occurs as a result of damage to retinal blood vessels that leak or hemorrhage. The retinal tissue loses oxygen normally brought by the vessels and develops new vessels (neovascularization) that tend to be weak and bleed. Continuous leaking and the formation of retinal scars may lead to blindness.

If neovascularization has occurred, unhealthy, oxygen-deprived tissue is treated with the laser. The directed energy of the laser causes scarring and prohibits the tissue from forming new, weak vessels.

The argon laser, which was invented in 1964 by William Bridges, a scientist at Hughes Aircraft, may be used to treat subretinal neovascularization, a disorder caused by age-related maculopathy (ARM), a major cause of blindness associated with aging. ARM produces scarring of the macula, the region of the retina that allows for sharpest vision. Subretinal neovascularization is caused by a break in the pigment epithelium, a layer below the retina. A collection of blood vessels below the retina bleeds into the retina through the break and causes scarring.

During argon laser treatment, burns are placed around the neovascularization areas to cauterize the bleeding. However, the bluegreen light of the argon laser is absorbed by the pigment of the inner retina, above the deeper affected layers. This may cause damage to the inner retina.

The red krypton laser is often substituted for the argon on this procedure since it is absorbed only in the melanin pigment of the deepest layers of the retina where the neovascularization occurs. Treatment with the krypton laser is preferred since it allows the inner, unaffected retinal layers to remain untouched while treating only the deep, affected layers.

Laser therapy called laser trabeculoplasty may be an alternative to surgery in the treatment of glaucoma, a disease in which the intraocular fluid fails to properly drain from the eye, accumulates and causes elevated intraocular pressure. If untreated, glaucoma causes a loss of peripheral vision and eventual blindness.

When medication fails to lower the intraocular pressure, laser trabeculoplasty with the argon may be used to open the drainage area located where the cornea meets the iris. A series of burns are placed in the drainage area, which causes scarring and openings within the meshwork of drainage channels. The fluid drains more easily from the eye, and intraocular pressure is reduced.

Berland, Theodore, and Richard A. Perritt. *Living With Your Eye Operation.* New York: St. Martin's Press, 1974.

Eden, John. *The Eye Book.* New York: Penguin Books, 1978.

Krames Communications. *The Retina Book.* Daly City, Calif.: KC, 1987.

Reynolds, James D., "Lasers in Ophthalmology." *HealthNet Library.* Columbus: CompuServe, 1989.

Shulman, Jules. *Cataracts.* New York: Simon and Schuster, 1984.

arterial occlusion   A blockage of the arteries of the retina. When this occurs, blood is prevented from reaching the retina, and vision is threatened. Arterial occlusions may be caused by carotid artery stenosis, retinal artery emboli, retinal artery occlusion and temporal (also called giant cell) arteritis.

Arterial occlusion occurs most frequently in people between the ages of 50 and 80.

Carotid artery stenosis occurs when one of the carotid arteries, which lie on each side of the neck and supply blood to the brain, becomes narrowed with arteriosclerotic plaque. The blood flow to the brain and the eye is decreased, and a TIA, transient ischemic attack, or ministroke may occur.

TIAs are warning signals of more serious impending strokes and include the symptoms of tingling in the face or limbs, difficulty speaking, headache, dizziness, vision disturbances, inability to swallow, mental confusion, and loss of memory.

During a carotid artery stenosis or TIA, vision may be suddenly lost in one eye. The loss is usually painless and generally lasts for a short period of time. Temporary loss of vision of this type may be accepted as a symptom or warning sign of a TIA.

Individuals with any symptom or combination of symptoms of a TIA should be examined by a physician immediately. Treatment for carotid stenosis may include anticoagulants or a surgical procedure called carotid endarterectomy, which removes arteriosclerotic plaque from the carotid artery.

Retinal artery emboli are small particles of blood clots that enter the blood's circulation and become wedged in a retinal artery. These emboli may cause obstructions that result in vision loss.

The loss of vision is usually swift and painless. If treatment is not begun within minutes, vision may be permanently lost. Results from current treatments to restore vision are often disappointing. Therapy should include treatment of the underlying cause such as arteriosclerosis, hypertension, and heart disease.

Retinal artery occlusion is a blockage of the retinal artery that does not involve emboli. This is most common in hypertension patients as a result of ARTERIOSCLEROSIS. The sight loss is usually sudden, painless and permanent. Treatment is directed to the underlying hypertension and arteriosclerosis.

Temporal or giant-cell arteritis is a chronic condition that involves inflammation of all the body's arteries. The inflammation causes the artery walls to thicken, which may block the flow of blood to vital organs, including the eyes. Symptoms include dizziness, headache, weight loss, scalp tenderness, jaw pain, depression, low-grade fever, and vision loss. Vision loss may be sudden and permanent.

The disease may be diagnosed with a blood test that reveals the presence of giant cells and a biopsy. The disease is treated with corticosteroids. Vision in one eye may be lost before the diagnosis is made but careful monitoring and treatment of the unaffected eye may prevent further loss of vision.

Temporal arteritis may last from two to three months and is rarely seen in patients under 50 years of age. Approximately 25 percent of cases result in permanent blindness.

(See STROKE and VENOUS OCCLUSION.)

American Heart Association. *1989 Stroke Facts.* Dallas: AHA, 1988.

Galloway, N. R. *Common Eye Diseases and Their Management.* Berlin: Springer-Verlag, 1985.

Gurwood, Andrew S., Alan G. Kabat, and Joseph W. Sowka. "Handbook of Ocular Disease Management." *Review of Optometry Online,* Jobson Publishing, 2002.

Reynolds, James D. "Ocular Artery and Vein Occlusion." *HealthNet Library,* Columbus: CompuServe, 1989.

arteriosclerosis   A condition in which the arteries become narrow and blocked, also known as hardening of the arteries. The condition is a leading cause of stroke and is associated with heart disease and other disorders. Arteriosclerosis produces fatty material, called plaque, that accumulates and lines the artery walls. The arteries become smaller in diameter, then clogged. This results in decreased blood circulation or cessation of the blood flow. As the body's organs receive less blood and oxygen, they may fail to function properly. When the blood flow is blocked, blood fails to reach the brain, and a STROKE results.

Arteriosclerosis is a factor in the formation of blood clots. Platelets, blood-clotting cells in the blood, tend to adhere to the arteriosclerotic plaque and further block the arteries. When the clot of platelets is jarred loose from the artery, it is termed an embolism. The embolism can travel through the blood stream, become wedged into a smaller blood vessel and cause a stroke.

Arteriosclerosis may also cause heart attacks, heart failure, heart disease, angina, kidney damage, poor circulation, and vision loss. It is associated with aging and high blood pressure, or hypertension, and is linked to obesity, improper diet, smoking, stress, and lack of exercise.

Arteriosclerosis may affect the eyes as the blood vessels of the retina become constricted. A normal retina, the light-sensitive layer in the back of the eye, gathers light information about an object and encodes it into electrical impulses. The impulses travel along the optic nerve to the brain where they are translated into an image. A retina impaired by arteriosclerosis cannot function adequately, and vision may be blurred or lost.

Retinal arteriosclerosis, when coupled with hypertension, is a condition called hypertensive retinopathy. Although the condition alone is rarely vision-threatening, it may lead to other eye diseases such as age-related maculopathy.

Age-related maculopathy (ARM) is a condition in which the macula, the center of the retina and point of clearest vision, deteriorates. As the macula degenerates, central vision is lost. ARM may be caused by heredity, chronic sun exposure, or arteriosclerosis. It is a progressive disease without a cure but that can sometimes be treated with photocoagulation or laser treatments.

Arteriosclerosis is often present without symptoms. The condition may be detected during a medical or ophthalmologic examination. It is treated with medication for high blood pressure or anticoagulants that increase blood circulation and discourage the accumulation of plaque. Patients are often urged to make changes in diet and exercise and to reduce smoking and stress.

arteritis   See ARTERIAL OCCLUSION.

artificial tears   Artificial tears are used to treat dry eye, a condition brought about by allergy, keratoconjunctivitis (corneal and conjunctival inflammation), extreme vitamin-A deficiency, TRACHOMA, chemical burns, and disorders and diseases, such as BELL'S PALSY. Many artificial tears are available without prescription.

These drugs are known by the generic names hydroxyethylcellulose, hydroxyproplycellulose, hydroxypropl methylcellulose, methylcellulose, polyvinyl alcohol, and other polymeric solutions. Numerous trade names include Clerz, Lacrisert, Isopto Alkaline, Muro Tears, Methopto, Methulose,

Aqua Tears, Liquifilm Tears, aqua-FLOW, Refresh, Adapettes, Comfort Drops, Moisture Eyes, and Hypo Tears.

Henkind, Paul, Martin Mayers and Arthur Berger, eds. *Physicians' Desk Reference for Ophthalmology 1987.* Oradell, N.J.: Medical Economics Company Inc., 1987.

artificial vision system   A system that uses technology to produce images that can be detected and recognized by blind people. Developed by Dr. William H. Dobelle, the device is battery operated and weighs about 10 pounds. It works through a miniature digital video camera and an ultrasonic distance sensor, which are built into a pair of sunglasses. The sensor connects through a cable to a small computer, which the blind person wears around his or her waist.

The computer processes the video and distance signals, then uses computer-imaging technology to transmit the image to the person wearing the device. Once the image has been transmitted, the computer triggers a second computer, which sends pulses to 68 platinum electrodes that have been surgically implanted onto the part of the brain that controls vision. The second computer is screwed into the wearer's skull bone, with its shaft protruding through the skin.

When the electrodes are stimulated, they generate a display of phosphenes, which are bursts of light caused by pressure on the eyeball. Phosphenes appear as black-and-white images, and the wearer of the device possibly can learn to recognize patterns and distinguish images. Reportedly, one blind man who received the artificial vision system made such progress that he was able to recognize different character sets commonly used in visual acuity tests. The system also has an electronic interface that is a radio frequency. It can replace the camera and allows patients to watch television and use a computer.

The artificial vision system, also called a visual prosthesis, is still in the testing stages, but is expected to be available on a limited commercial basis sometime in 2002. Dobelle, who heads the Dobelle Institute at Columbia Presbyterian Medical Center in New York City, and the Institute Dobelle AG in Zurich, Switzerland, has been working on the vision system for 30 years.

Reuters Health. "Artificial Vision System Gives 'Sight' to the Blind." *Rx.com Magazine,* January 18, 2000.

A-scan   An A-scan is a test that uses ultrasonic waves to determine the length of the eye. An A-scan is performed prior to cataract surgery to predetermine the power of an intraocular lens implant or to ascertain whether an implant is necessary.

The average eye is approximately 24 millimeters from the cornea to the retina. A shorter eye is usually farsighted, or hyperopic. A longer eye is usually nearsighted, or myopic. A shorter eye needs a stronger lens to focus properly. A longer eye needs a weaker lens to focus. An extremely long eye may not require an implant.

The information from this painless test is analyzed by a computer along with the results of KERATOMETRY. The computer evaluates the information and determines the power of the needed implant.

B

Bell's palsy   A disorder involving unilateral facial weakness or paralysis. The condition usually has its onset over a two- to five-day period. During that time, the patient may experience a loss of facial sensation, a numbness, drooling, delay in blinking, inability to close the eye, excessive tearing, paralysis of one side of the face, or noticeable drooping of the mouth or face. Half of those with Bell's palsy experience pain behind the ear, but the condition does not cause hearing impairments.

The symptoms of Bell's palsy, named for Sir Charles Bell, the 19th-century physician who first described the disease, may be confused with those of a stroke. Bell's-palsy symptoms, however, usually affect the entire side of the face from forehead to chin, whereas stroke symptoms are usually located below the eye. Bell's-palsy symptoms do not include classic stroke indications, such as weakness in limbs, slurred speech or double vision.

Bell's palsy is caused by a swelling of the facial nerve due to immune disorders or a viral disease. The nerve is constricted, the blood supply is limited and the nerve becomes ischemic, or anemic, due to lack of blood flow. Nerve degeneration may follow.

Individuals who contract Bell's palsy are typically in good health, but a history of DIABETES, SARCOIDOSIS, or LYME DISEASE has been linked to the disorder. It has been associated with influenza, colds, and headaches and may be triggered by such illnesses. Bell's palsy may occur to either sex at any age but is most prevalent after the age of 40.

Bell's palsy poses the greatest threat to the eye's cornea, the clear, protective cover of the eye. When the eyelid, which normally protects the cornea, functions incorrectly, the cornea becomes dry and is vulnerable to the elements. Constant exposure may result in KERATITIS (corneal infection), ulceration or injury, causing a loss of vision.

The eye may be treated with occasional applications of ARTIFICIAL TEARS such as methylcellulose solution during the day and a lubricating cream or ointment such as Lacri-Lube S.O.P. at night. The eye may be taped shut or protected with an eyeshield.

Dryness or irritation, increased sensitivity to light or symptoms of infection may develop and require further treatment. A partial TARSORRHAPHY, a surgical procedure in which the upper and lower eyelids are stitched together at the corner, may be performed. The tarsorrhaphy is reversible and may be temporarily effective but may cause corneal breakdown, irritation to the cornea from eyelashes or scars along the lashline.

The treatment of Bell's palsy may include physical therapy, a combination of heat application and facial massage or facial exercises. In severe cases, corticosteroids may be prescribed for 10–14 days.

In 85 percent of cases, recovery begins to occur within 10 days to 3 weeks. The remaining 15 percent of cases may require up to 12 months to recover. The condition tends to recur in 10 percent of cases and usually affects the opposite side of the face. Pregnancy has been linked to recurrences, as has multiple sclerosis.

Dyke, Peter J., Gunter Haase and Mark May. "Diagnosis and Care of Bell's Palsy." *Patient Care* (October 1988): 107–118.
The Bell's Palsy Network Frequently Asked Questions. www.bellspalsy.net, 1997.

bifocals   Bifocals or bifocal lenses contain two prescription lenses put together in one lens. Each contact or eyeglass lens has two focusing abilities, one for seeing near objects and one for seeing distant objects.

Bifocals are usually needed after age 40. They are a common aid in the treatment of presbyopia, aging eyes. As the eye ages, its lens loses the ability to focus on close objects.

Prescription of reading glasses alone would solve the problem, but the wearer would have to remove the glasses to see distant objects. The wearer requiring a distance vision correction would have to constantly switch between reading glasses and distance glasses. Bifocals eliminate the necessity of swapping glasses when changing tasks.

Although modern bifocals are essentially the same two pairs of glasses combined into one frame that Benjamin Franklin invented, today's lenses are custom-designed for the wearer. The reading and distance segments of each lens may be small or large and placed high or low in the frame. The lens size and placement are determined by the needs of the wearer. Using an updated method of polishing, bifocals today can be made without a noticeable line. These are called "blended bifocals," and are preferred by many people.

The clerk whose job requires copious amounts of reading and occasional distance viewing will need a large reading segment and a smaller section for distance at the top of the lens. The factory supervisor who manages a long assembly line will need a smaller reading section located low in the lens to avoid obstructing a distance view.

Bifocal wearers must adopt new head movements to use bifocals correctly and safely. The wearer may have to raise his chin when reading something at a level higher than normal or learn to lower his head, rather than just his eyes, when navigating a cluttered path.

biomicroscope   The biomicroscope (or slit lamp) is an instrument used to examine the eye. It magnifies the ANTERIOR CHAMBER of the eye, including the cornea, iris, and lens.

A biomicroscope examination is one step in a routine eye exam. It is painless. The patient places his chin on a chin rest centered at the bottom of an open square-shaped frame. A bright light in front of the frame shines a vertical beam of light through the cornea. The light that is reflected back gives an illuminated, magnified cross-section of the front part of the eye.

The biomicroscope examination is used to check for abrasions, erosion or scarring, inflammation, presence of blood vessels, or change of shape in the cornea; inflammation or thinning of the SCLERA, inflammation or irregularities of the iris; and subluxated or shifted lens and cataracts.

The biomicroscope may also be used to examine the eye during tests such as those to determine intraocular pressure (TONOGRAPHY) or the junction of the cornea and the iris (GONIOSCOPY). It also is used as a tool in some laser treatment procedures.

bioptics   Optical aids that consist of small telescopes fused onto the upper portion of spectacles, on one or both lenses. The bottom portion of the spectacles contains the individual's corrective prescription.

The bioptics involving both eyes enable the low-vision user to view distances when walking or driving or to view closer objects or material if magnification is needed. The bioptics that involve one eye only are used for near and intermediate distance viewing for reading material.

Bioptics are prescribed by an ophthalmologist or low-vision expert and must be properly centered to the eyes of the wearer. Magnification may extend to six times normal size when used for distance viewing. Wide-angle lenses may be incorporated into the device. Thirty states permit driving with the aid of bioptics. Regulations vary from state to state.

blepharitis   Blepharitis is a common condition of the eyelids. The margin of the eyelid becomes swollen and red with inflammation, and a crusty discharge may gather at the base of the lashes. Some lash loss may occur, but in milder cases the lashes grow back. In severe cases, the lash follicles are destroyed and permanent lash loss results.

Causes of blepharitis, sometimes called eyelash dandruff, are unknown. It is often associated with allergies, a disorder in the lipid layer of the tear film or seborrhoea of the scalp. Although blepharitis is a difficult condition to treat, it rarely results in loss of vision.

It is important to keep the eyelid area very clean in order to cut the buildup of secretions. Ophthalmologists may treat the symptoms of blepharitis with ANTIBIOTICS, but since there is no cure, the disorder may become chronic. Chronic blepharitis may involve CONJUNCTIVITIS and inflammation of the cornea.

blindisms   Stereotypical mannerisms or behaviors of blind children or infants are commonly called "blindisms." The term is misleading, since the same mannerisms are also stereotypical of children with other disabilities, such as autism.

These stereotypical behaviors include rocking, shaking or turning the head, shaking the hands, mouthing the hands or objects, and eye poking or pressing. The repetitive and unconsciously performed mannerisms are most often found in those who are congenitally blind but may be acquired by those with adventitious blindness.

Some studies indicate that children create these mannerisms of self-stimulation to compensate for the lack of sensory stimulation and activity in their lives. Others cite the lack of opportunity and ability of blind children to imitate the acceptable behaviors of others and to develop a sense of unacceptable behaviors.

Behaviors related to the vision loss may appear to be blindisms. A child may hold the head unnaturally to one side in order to make the best use of residual vision or a reduced visual field or may grimace in an effort to see an image.

Blindisms may lead to social segregation if the mannerisms are considered distracting or unsightly. They may falsely indicate to others the presence of mental retardation, autism, or emotional disorders. Blindisms may become injurious to the individual, since eye rubbing and poking can cause bruising and callous formation.

Blindisms may be prevented by the use of stimulating, physical activity (including the use of motion furniture such as rocking chairs and swings), development of an interest in the environment and frequent opportunities for new experiences.

Established blindisms may be corrected if the child is given a substitute activity for the physical movement. The effort of flapping the hands may be redirected to playing an instrument or fondling a stuffed toy.

Bonfanti, Barbara H. "Effects of Training on Nonverbal and Verbal Behaviors of Congenitally Blind Adults," *Journal of Visual Impairment and Blindness* (January 1979): 1–9.

The Canadian National Institute for the Blind. *The Impact of Vision Loss on the Development of Children from Birth to 12 Years.* www.cnib.ca/pamphlets_publications/vision, 2000.

Eichel, Valerie J. "A Taxonomy for Mannerisms of Blind Children." *Journal of Visual Impairment and Blindness* (May 1979): 167–177.

Fraiberg, S. *Insights from the Blind.* New York: Basic Books, 1977.

Harper, Florine Watson. "Gestures of the Blind." *Education of the Visually Handicapped* (Spring 1978): 14–20.

Hoshmand, Lisa T. "Blindisms: Some Observations and Propositions." *Education of the Visually Handicapped* (May 1975): 56–59.

Miller, Barbara S., and William H. Miller. "Extinguishing 'Blindisms': A Paradigm for Intervention." *Education of the Visually Handicapped* (Spring 1976): 7–14.

Scholl, Geraldine, ed. *Foundations of Education for Blind and Visually Handicapped Children and Youth.* New York: American Foundation for the Blind Inc., 1986.

Warren, D. H. *Blindness and Early Childhood Development.* New York: American Foundation for the Blind Inc., 1984.

blind spot   The blind spot is a point of blindness or blocked vision found in normal peripheral vision. This spot is caused by the OPTIC DISC. The optic disc is the spot on the retina where the optic nerve meets the eye.

The retina is the light-sensitive layer of the back of the eye. It contains cells called rods and cones, which receive light and provide information about the viewed object. The retina encodes this information into electrical impulses. The impulses are sent to the brain via the optic nerve, a cord of nerve fibers that connects the brain to the eye and supplies blood to the retina. The brain translates the impulses into an image. The optic nerve is joined to the retina at the optic disc. The optic disc is devoid of photosensitive rods or cones and is unable to collect information about an object. As a result, the disc is "blind."

Since the blind spot is small and located within the peripheral (side) field of vision, it does not interfere with normal vision. The optic disc may be observed during an ophthalmologic exam or by moving an object into the field of the blind spot.

This is easily accomplished by marking a piece of white paper with an *X*. Approximately two inches to the right of the *X*, mark a dark circle. Close the left eye and look directly and steadily at the *X*. Move the paper forward or back until the circle disappears. This circle lies in the sphere of the optic disc.

The blind spot does not affect normal vision. Constant eye movements deflect attention from the blind area and the brain compensates for its lack by completing any incomplete lines and filling in any gaps.

braille   A tactile language made up of a system of raised dots. The reader of braille feels the dots to recognize the letter. Braille makes reading, writing, note taking, and communicating possible for visually impaired, blind, and deaf-blind users.

Braille was invented in 1824 by LOUIS BRAILLE, a blind French student. He based his system on a method of raised dots and dashes called night writing or Sonography. Sonography was developed by Charles Barbier de la Serre to enable soldiers to read messages passed during night maneuvers. Braille and Barbier met to discuss possible alterations to the system. When Barbier insisted that the method remain unaltered, Braille developed a new system that involved raised dots in a fresh configuration.

Although the braille system was met with enthusiasm by blind users, the system was not first accepted officially by educators until 30 years later, in 1854. This may have been caused by resistance to change from the proven methods of instruction, a lack of willingness on the part of sighted instructors to learn a new method, or the simultaneous development and promotion of other new language systems for the blind.

The braille system is based on a cell, a configuration of dots forming two columns of three dots each. Each letter of the alphabet and each punctuation mark is made up of one or more of the possible six dots that make up a cell. Sixty-three combinations or patterns are possible.

In addition to the alphabet, there are 189 contractions and short forms or abbreviations for words that are formed in the cells. These same braille cells are also assigned different meanings to write music, foreign languages, numbers, and science terms.

Different forms or grades of braille are available. Grade 1 braille is the form developed by Louis Braille and utilizes one character per each letter of the alphabet. It contains no contractions. Grade 2 braille was developed in England and contains over 200 contractions and short forms for common words. In 1932, Grade 2 or Standard English Braille was officially adopted as the braille of choice for English-speaking nations. Grade 3 braille is an expansion of Grade 2. It extends the list of contractions and deletes vowels. Grade 3 is used most often for ease in writing rapidly or for taking notes.

Braille is embossed onto thick paper or plastic sheets by a braille press, braille writer or brailler, braille computer printer, or manual slate and stylus. Because braille requires a large amount of space, the braille edition of a book or magazine is several times longer than the print edition.

Braille is read with the finger tips of the index finger and/or middle finger or ring finger of one or both hands. An average reading speed of a reader using one hand is approximately 104 words per minute. Ambidextrous readers may increase the rate to 200 or more words per minute.

Braille is not used by all visually impaired or blind people. Some visually impaired persons have sufficient remaining vision to read with the use of an optical aid such as a magnifier. Others with less useful residual vision may opt to forgo learning braille due to physical problems such as diabetic neuropathy (decreased sensitivity in the fingers due to diabetes) or because of advanced age.

The wide availability of recorded books, other reading materials and synthetic speech output for computers may have had an effect on the willingness of visually impaired persons to learn braille. However, braille reading is accepted as a necessary skill for learning the basic literacy skills of reading, grammar, and diction.

Braille, Louis   Louis Braille is the inventor of braille, a language of raised dots read by the fingers and used by visually impaired persons.

Braille was born in 1809 in Coupvray, France, the son of a harness maker. At the age of three, he injured his eye while playing with his father's leather-working tools. The initial injury became infected, spread to both eyes and left him completely blind.

He was sent to the Royal Institution for Blind Youth in Paris when he was 10. The students in the school were taught orally through lessons repeated to them by their instructors or through books printed in embossed letters in a system developed by the founder of the school, Valentin Haüy. Later, the school adopted Sonography, an adaptation of a system of night writing developed by an army captain, Charles Barbier de la Serre. The night-writing system was used to write messages and maneuver instructions that could be read in the dark by the fingertips.

Sonography employed a complicated system of raised dots and dashes that spelled words phonetically. It was based on a 12-dot cell for each letter that used considerable space on a page. Braille began to experiment with the writing system, making changes and improvements. Braille met with Barbier, who rejected the changes and insisted that the system remain as introduced.

Over the next three years, Braille worked continuously to develop his own language of dots. In 1824, at the age of 15, his work was complete. He had developed a reading and writing system of dot patterns or characters based on a six-dot cell. Each character represented one letter of the alphabet or one numeral. He went on to adapt systems that could be used for musical notation and a method for drawing letters using a slate and stylus, called Raphigraphy.

Although the Braille method was immediately adopted by pupils at the school, it was officially rejected. This may have been for reasons of fear on the part of sighted teachers, hesitancy to revamp current teaching methods, and reluctance to make obsolete teaching tools that had been difficult and expensive to purchase.

It was not until 1843, at the inauguration of the new building of the Institution for Blind Youth, where an exhibition of the system was given, that braille gained official recognition. In 1854, at the insistence of the students and blind teachers, braille was adopted as a teaching method by the school. Acceptance for the system spread throughout Europe. It was first taught in America in about 1859 or 1860 at the St. Louis School for the Blind. Today, braille is universally used as a language of reading and writing for the blind and visually impaired.

Louis Braille did not live to see the acceptance of his writing system. He died in 1852 of tuberculosis. A century later, in 1952, his remains were moved from his native Coupvray for reburial in the Pantheon, the highest honor that can be bestowed on a French citizen. (See BRAILLE.)

American Foundation for the Blind. *A Different Way of Seeing.* New York: AFB, 1984.
American Foundation for the Blind. *Louis Braille.* New York: AFB, 1987.
American Foundation for the Blind. *Understanding Braille.* New York: AFB, 1970.
Davidson, Margaret. *Louis Braille,* New York: Hastings House Publishers, 1971.
Kugelmass, J. Alvin. *Louis Braille.* New York: Julian Messner, 1951.

braille music   Music printed in braille traditionally was produced manually by a limited number of people who specialized in the service. Musicians often were frustrated by having to wait weeks, sometimes months, to have their music transcribed.

In 1997, a company called Dancing Dots Braille Music Technology introduced a braille music translator program that allows music to be produced locally by sighted copyists. The service is based on a software program called GOODFEEL. With this program, braille music can be produced by people with no special training. Braille scores are produced from the same computer music files that are used to print staff notation.

The technology was spearheaded by Bill McCann, president and founder of Dancing Dots, who is also a blind musician and programmer. The company also offers other music-related products for visually impaired people.

Contact:

Dancing Dots Braille Music Technology
1754 Quarry Lane
P.O. Box 927
Valley Forge, PA 19482-0927
610-783-6692 (ph)
610-783-6732 (fax)
info@dancingdots.com
www.dancingdots.com

braille writer   A braille writer, or brailler, is a machine used to write braille. Similar to the function of a typewriter, braillewriters come in manual or electric forms. They are more practical for large writing tasks than a slate and a stylus, which is the equivalent of paper and a pen for a sighted person. The first brailler, the Hall Braillewriter, was introduced in 1892 by Frank H. Hall, superintendent of the Illinois School for the Blind.

Braille writers have six keys and a space bar. Each key corresponds to a dot of the six dot braille cell. To form a braille letter, the user simultaneously pushes the keys corresponding to the needed dot combination. The dots are pressed onto lightweight manila tag paper. Users can attain writing speeds of up to 60 words per minute.

Braille writers vary in size by maker but generally are approximately 15″ × 9″ × 5″ and weigh 10 pounds. Current braille writers include the Perkins Brailler, the Lavender Braillewriter, and the Hall Braillewriter.

Brailon   The trade name for the paper used in a thermoform duplicator. Each plastic sheet is placed atop a page of brailled paper or tactual paper and inserted into the thermoform machine. The machine heats the Brailon plastic sheet and creates a duplicate of the tactual sheet.

Brailon is used to make duplicates of braille books and other tactual materials such as tactile maps. The Brailon exchange is the agreement of many educational agencies or organizations for the blind to provide a braille copy of a book in exchange for an equal number of Brailon sheets.

B-scan   A test performed prior to cataract surgery to view the retina. The retina is usually examined with a binocular indirect ophthalmoscope, but in some cases, the cataract is dense enough to obstruct the view of the retina. In these instances, a painless, ultrasonic B-scan affords a picture of the hidden retina.

The health of the retina must be determined before cataract surgery to rule out the possibility of a detached retina. Without this knowledge, the surgery could successfully remove the cataract, only to reveal a non-functioning eye.

Business Enterprise Program   (BEP)   A federally supported program administered by each individual State Department of Rehabilitation. The program was established by the Randolph-Sheppard Act in 1936 and amended in 1974. The program provides employment opportunities to qualified blind persons, licenses blind vendors, and establishes vending facilities in federal, state, county, and some private buildings.

Vending facilities may sell newspapers, periodicals, confections, tobacco products, foods, beverages. and other articles or services. The articles or services may be dispensed automatically or manually and are prepared on the premises. The facility may also be a cafeteria, snack bar, or a dry/wet facility.

To qualify for the BEP training program, an applicant must be a citizen of the United States, legally blind, emotionally and physically qualified to operate a vending facility as verified by medical and vocational evaluation, have independent living skills, and have a reasonable expectation to succeed in the program.

An applicant entering the BEP program must complete a training program. Those who have had prior management experience in food service may be eligible to demonstrate their skills by completing two months on-the-job training with another vendor and passing the final exam covering all the training program material with a grade of 85 percent or better.

The standard training program is seven months long and consists of pretraining evaluation, basic training, and on-the-job practical experience. All trainees must pass a comprehensive final exam.

Those who complete the program are certified as eligible for licensing as a BEP vendor. As locations become available, students are notified and can apply for a specific location. Applicants are interviewed by a selection panel of business people who decides which vendor is to be assigned. Selection is based on prior work experience, education, training, experience, and performance on the oral interview. Vendors are considered trainees until the first year of vending has been completed.

The income from vending machines that compete with BEP vendors may be accrued to a maximum and paid to the vendor. The income may be used to establish a fund for sick leave, vacation, or retirement benefits.

C

cancer Cancer of the eyes is relatively rare. According to the American Cancer Society, ocular cancer is responsible for approximately 2,500 new cases of cancer each year and for approximately 400 deaths from cancer each year as compared with lung and breast cancers, which are responsible, respectively, for 144,000 and 115,000 new cases of cancer each year.

Cancer of the eyes usually develops into tumors. The tumors may be found in the eyeball, the orbit, or the eyelids. Because ocular tumors are often hidden deep in the eye and therefore resist biopsy, it is often difficult to differentiate a malignant tumor from a nonmalignant or benign tumor.

Cancerous or malignant tumors differ from benign tumors in several ways. The cancerous cells are different from their surrounding tissue, often grow quickly and uncontrollably, rarely stop growing, and tend to spread or metastasize to other parts of the body. Malignant tumors threaten life as well as vision.

The three most common types of malignant tumors are malignant melanoma, retinoblastoma, and metastatic tumors. Each is a serious disorder that benefits from early and appropriate treatment.

MALIGNANT MELANOMA is the most common of all tumors that originate in the eye. This type of tumor grows from melanin-laden cells in the eye's CHOROID, iris, or CILIARY BODY. It generally affects one eye only and may develop spontaneously or from a mole within the eye. It is usually slow to grow and metastasize. The onset may be at any age and is more common among whites than blacks. They occur more often in people who have skin melanoma.

Symptoms of malignant melanoma include redness, inflammation, loss of vision, and glaucoma. Pupil distortion may be present in melanoma of the iris. Little is known about the cause and progression of these tumors.

Malignant melanomas are generally treated by enucleation, or removal of the entire eye. An uncertain diagnosis may lead to a period of observation augmented by chemotherapy or radiation treatments. Melanomas of the iris are extremely slow-growing and are often treated during observation. Approximately 60 percent of those diagnosed and treated for malignant melanomas are alive five years after treatment.

RETINOBLASTOMA is the most common type of malignant intraocular (inner eye) tumor in children. It occurs in one out of every 12–20,000 children. This tumor develops in the eye's retina. Retinoblastomas may be hereditary or may develop sporadically. The less common hereditary type is usually present at birth and has its onset near one year of age. In both types, the condition is almost always expressed by age five. It is often bilateral (affects both eyes).

Although hereditary retinoblastomas are present in family histories, any occurrence of bilateral retinoblastoma should be considered hereditary and capable of being passed to further generations. Infants of hereditary families should be screened regularly for tumors.

Sporadic tumors are not hereditary. They are generally unilateral (affecting one eye only) and appear at approximately two years of age.

The first symptoms of retinoblastoma include redness, pain, and inflammation. As the tumor grows, the eyes may cross and the pupil may change from black to white or gray, a condition called leukokoria. The light color is the hue of the tumor visible through the hole of the pupil.

Retinoblastoma is treated by enucleation, radiation, or cryotherapy (freezing treatments). In bilateral cases, the more affected eye may be removed and the other eye may receive chemotherapy or radiation treatments. If left unchecked, the tumor could grow and spread up the optic nerve to the brain.

The cause of retinoblastoma is due to the absence of both retinoblastoma genes on the 13th chromosome. Although it has the one of the highest rates of spontaneous regression among all tumors, little is known about the cause of regression. The cure rate for retinoblastoma ranges from 85 percent to 90 percent.

Metastatic tumors are malignant tumors that originate in other parts of the body and spread to the eyes. Among those that can metastasize to the eyes are tumors of the lung, breast, kidney, and prostate. These secondary tumors are bilateral approximately 25 percent of the time.

Symptoms of metastatic tumors may include redness, pain, vision loss, or glaucoma. Often, symptoms of the ocular tumor may present themselves before those of the primary tumor. Because metastatic tumors look much like primary ocular tumors, diagnosis can be problematic.

Once a metastatic tumor has been diagnosed, the primary tumor can be appropriately treated. Depending on the size and growth rate of the ocular tumor, treatment may include surgery, chemotherapy, or radiation treatments.

Malignant tumors of the eyelids include the basal-cell carcinoma and the squamous-cell carcinoma. The more common basal-cell carcinoma, the result of sun damage to the skin, first appears as a slight bump on the eyelid. It develops into a saucerlike shape with a raised edge.

Since the tumor is on the eyelid, it is easy to remove and submit to biopsy. If left untreated, the tumor may spread to the underlying bone. Advanced basal-cell carcinomas are treated with radiation therapy.

Squamous-cell carcinomas appear in observation much like basal-cell carcinomas but can be identified through biopsy. This type of tumor tends to spread to the lymph nodes of the upper or lower eyelid and may metastasize to other parts of the body.

Rhabdomyosarcoma is a highly malignant tumor of the orbit. It is a rare tumor that develops in children. The tumor spreads rapidly but can be detected by a biopsy taken through the eyelid. Treatment may include radiation or chemotherapy. Cure rates for rhabdomyosarcoma range from 30 percent to 40 percent.

central vision   Central vision is the "straight-ahead" vision in the visual field. Central vision is controlled by the macula, a tiny section of the retina. Although the macula occupies only 1 percent of the retina, it is responsible for distinguishing all detail in vision.

The retina is the light-sensitive layer between the choroid and the vitreous gel. It contains rods and cones that receive light information about an object in view. The rods react to faint light, movement, and shape, and are responsible for peripheral or side vision. The cones distinguish color and detail but require high levels of light to function. They are responsible for central vision.

The retina encodes the information from the rods and cones into electrical impulses. The impulses are sent via the optic nerve to the brain, where they are translated into an image.

The cones of the retina are concentrated into a central section called the macula. Within the macula is an indentation called the FOVEA. The fovea contains the greatest concentration of cones and is the site of sharpest vision. Light is focused by the cornea and the lens onto the macula, and specifically onto the fovea. When the macula or fovea are damaged, central vision is affected.

Macular disease is a common problem affecting central vision. It may be caused by an injury, heredity, other diseases such as arteriosclerosis, or aging.

Age-related maculopathy (ARM) is the most common form of this disease. It is a progressive disease in which the macula deteriorates, and central vision is lost. ARM may in some cases be treated with laser therapy, but there is no cure for the disease. It is seldom responsible for total blindness, since some peripheral vision usually remains intact.

ARTERIOSCLEROSIS, or hardening of the arteries, may cause macular degeneration. In this condition, the arteries become clogged and smaller in diameter. Blood circulation slows, and the body's organs are denied oxygen. In some cases, the retinal blood vessels become clogged and the macula degenerates.

Amblyopia of disuse, or lazy eye, is a condition that affects central vision. It is a condition of childhood in which one eye is misaligned to the other. The eyes are unable to focus together and double vision occurs. The vision of the misaligned eye is suppressed by the brain, which accepts only information from the aligned eye. In effect, the unused eye ceases to develop and becomes "blind" or amblyopic. In the treatment of amblyopia, the aligned eye is usually patched to encourage the amblyopic eye to function. The central vision of the amblyopic eye is affected, but it usually retains some peripheral vision.

TOBACCO AMBLYOPIA is a condition in which the excessive use of tobacco impairs central vision. The condition usually rights itself when tobacco use is discontinued or drastically reduced.

The cones responsible for central vision need light to function and to survive. Eyes denied light for long periods may lose central vision. A complete lack of vitamin A in the diet may also result in cone or retinal dysfunction and cause blindness.

cerebral palsy (CP) Cerebral palsy (CP) is not a disease, but rather a group of conditions caused by damage to the motor area of the brain before, during or directly following birth. The condition affects about 500,000 persons in the United States and is the most prevalent lifelong disability in the country.

Over one-third of those with CP are teenagers or young adults. Each year, approximately 5,000 babies are born with CP and an additional 1,500 acquire CP before the age of five.

The condition usually involves nerve and muscle dysfunction and may exhibit such characteristics as difficulty in walking; loss of muscle coordination or manual dexterity; spasms; seizures; tremors; hearing, speech, or vision impairments; learning disabilities; mental retardation; and psychological or behavioral problems.

There are five types of cerebral palsy: spastic, athetoid, rigid, ataxia, and tremor. Spastic CP, the most common type, involves the trait of tense, contracted muscles. Athetoid CP entails uncontrollable, constant movement of the head, limbs, and body. Rigid CP is characterized by contracted muscles that resist movement.

Ataxia encompasses coordination and balance problems. Tremor CP is the most rare and is similar to the athetoid type since it involves uncontrollable tremors or trembling of the limbs that hinders balance and coordination. Most individuals with CP are affected by more than one type of CP, a condition termed "mixed type."

Brain damage that results in CP can be caused by acute or chronic anoxia or oxygen deprivation, a result of premature separation of the placenta from the uterine wall, improper birth position, prolonged or abrupt labor, complications during labor, or obstruction by the umbilical cord.

Other congenital causes may include maternal viral infections such as rubella (German measles), Rh and A-B-O blood-type incompatibilities, poor health, excessive smoking or alcohol consumption by the mother, premature birth and untreated jaundice of the newborn causing kernicterus, a disease that involves damage to the nervous system and is also caused by Rh-factor incompatibility.

Acquired CP is a more rare occurrence and results from an injury to the head due to trauma or infection. Cerebral palsy is not hereditary. It is not a progressive condition and is not communicable. Each case of CP is unique. The amount of damage to the brain, the site of damage and the degree to which the nervous system is involved produce varying symptoms.

Vision may be affected if the damage affects the portion of the brain that controls the eyes or the parts of the eyes that process or transmit information such as the retina or optic nerve. Corrective lenses or surgery may be necessary to improve or correct vision.

Early detection and treatment of CP are essential in achieving the best possible management of the condition. Symptoms of CP in infants may include irritability, difficulties in feeding or sucking, and abnormally delayed development of muscle control or coordination. Less noticeable symptoms may be detectable by a pediatrician during a medical examination.

Cerebral palsy currently cannot be cured, but management or treatment may reduce the limitations it imposes. Treatment may include physical, occupational, speech, language, hearing, or behavioral therapy. Neurological or orthopedic surgery may increase control over muscles. Braces may strengthen and support the body and correct deformities. Medications may reduce rigidity and ease nerve-damage problems.

Congenital cerebral palsy can often be prevented. Pregnant women can maintain good nutrition, avoid alcohol, smoking, and unnecessary X rays or medications, and control diabetes and anemia. Routine tests for Rh incompatibility in the mother and immunization with Rhogam within 72 hours after delivery can eliminate problems in future pregnancies.

Infants with blood incompatibility may receive a blood transfusion. Premature infants and those at high risk can be monitored closely in neonatal intensive care units. Infants and young children can of course be protected from trauma.

There is much help available for those suffering from cerebral palsy and for their families. The United Cerebral Palsy Association, founded in 1949 as a voluntary organization, has more than 150 state and regional affiliates. The agency, through its affiliates, serves more than 30,000 children and adults with cerebral palsy and other disabilities every day. It offers assistive technology training, community living, referrals, employment assistance, advocacy, early intervention programs, therapy, and so forth.

To find out more about the organization that serves your area. Contact:

United Cerebral Palsy Association
1660 L Street, NW, Suite 700
Washington, DC 20036-5602
800-872-5827 (ph)
202-973-7197 (TTY)
202-776-0414 (fax)
www.ucpa.org
Listings of local affiliates are available from the website.

Mann, Richard C. *Diagnosis: Cerebral Palsy.* Oklahoma City: United Cerebral Palsy of Oklahoma, 1986.
United Cerebral Palsy Association. *What Is Cerebral Palsy?* New York: UCPA, 1978.
UCP Net. Cerebral Palsy-Facts and Figures, www.ucp.org, 2001.

chalazion   An inflammation of the eyelid gland. It is caused by a blockage of the meibomian gland duct.

A chalazion appears as a bump or swelling on either the top or bottom eyelid. It is painless and may develop slowly over many weeks. Treatment of chalazion may include warm compresses and sulfonamide eye drops.

Once the chalazion has grown large enough to press on the eyeball, it may cause damage to vision by producing an astigmatism. In such cases, surgery to remove the chalazion may be required. The eye is patched after surgery, and antibiotic eye drops are often prescribed.

Chalazions may become chronic. Prevention may be achieved through strict hygiene and the application of warm compresses at the first sign of inflammation. If they do reoccur, it could be an indication of a more serious condition and should be checked.

children   See DEVELOPMENT OF BLIND CHILDREN.

chlamydia   A type of sexually transmitted disease that can cause conjunctivitis, both in adults and babies, who are affected at birth. Caused by a bacterium, chlamydia is the leading sexually transmitted disease in the United States. About 4 million new cases occur each year.

Early symptoms include abnormal genital discharge or pain when urinating, but symptoms can be very mild and may not even be noticed. As the disease progresses, it can cause eye infection and proctitis and urethral infection in men.

Newborns affected while in the birth canal may develop conjunctivitis or pneumonia. Typically, symptoms of eye problems will occur within the first 10 days of life. The eye infection can be treated with antibiotics in both newborns and adults. Many doctors advise that all pregnant women be tested for chlamydial infection because of the risk it presents to newborns.

chorioretinitis   A secondary condition caused by CHOROIDITIS, a swelling of the CHOROID (also called posterior UVEITIS). Chorioretinitis occurs when the inflammation of the choroid spreads to the underlying retina.

The choroid is the pigmented tissue layer between the retina and the SCLERA (white part of the eye). It is the posterior section of the uveal tract, a vascularized tissue layer that supplies blood to the eye and that includes the iris and CILIARY BODY in the anterior section.

The retina is the light sensitive layer at the back of the eye. The retina receives light information from the rods and cones located there. It converts the information into electrical impulses that it sends to the brain. The brain transforms the impulses into an image.

Symptoms of choroiditis include redness of the eye, light sensitivity, and lost or blurred vision. The symptoms of choroiditis may not be noticeable to the patient if they are located in the areas of peripheral vision.

Choroiditis may occur spontaneously. It may also be linked to viruses, injuries, TOXOPLASMOSIS, arthritis, tuberculosis, venereal disease, parasites, and SARCOIDOSIS.

Because of the close proximity of the choroid and the retina, the inflammation of choroiditis often spreads to the overlying retina, resulting in chorioretinitis. When this occurs the vision becomes acutely blurred. If the inflammation involves the macular region of the retina, permanent central-vision loss could occur.

Chorioretinitis may be treated with systemic (given orally) or local corticosteroids.

choroid   The choroid is the dark, middle tissue layer between the retina and the SCLERA, or white part of the eye. It is the back portion of the uveal tract, a vascularized tissue layer that supplies blood to the eye. Blood circulates through the choroid layer to nourish and support the eye.

The UVEA or uveal tract contains the pigmented portions of the eye. These consist of the iris, the CILIARY BODY, and the choroid. When uveitis, or inflammation of the uvea occurs, the choroid may be involved.

Inflammation of the choroid is called CHOROIDITIS or posterior UVEITIS. Symptoms of choroiditis may include pain, redness of the eye, and light sensitivity. However, choroiditis is often present without symptoms, and since it may be present only in the peripheral field, it may persist unnoticed. The inflammation may spread to the retina and the vitreous, in which case, the vision becomes blurred.

Choroiditis may be caused by parasites (as it is in TOXOPLASMOSIS), viruses, or other diseases such as tuberculosis or syphilis. Choroiditis and posterior uveitis are usually treated with steroid pills, drops, or ointments.

choroiditis   Choroiditis is an inflammation of the CHOROID, the vascular layer between the retina and the SCLERA. It is a type of UVEITIS, an inflammation of the uveal tract, and is sometimes referred to as arthritis of the eye.

The uveal tract is composed of the iris, the CILIARY BODY, and the choroid. The iris is the colored part of the eye that controls the pupil and enables it to open and shut to control the amount of light entering the eye. The ciliary body produces aqueous fluid and moves the lens to focus properly by changing its shape. The choroid, which supplies blood to the eye, is a vascular layer between the retina and the sclera.

Uveitis is categorized as either anterior or posterior. When the iris and ciliary body are involved, the condition is termed anterior uveitis. When the choroid is involved, it is termed posterior uveitis, or choroiditis.

Choroiditis is usually less painful than anterior uveitis. It may be accompanied by redness of the eye, light sensitivity, and lost or blurred vision. The symptoms of choroiditis that occur in the areas of peripheral vision may not be noticeable to the patient.

Choroiditis may occur spontaneously. It may also be linked to viruses, injuries, TOXOPLASMOSIS, arthritis, tuberculosis, venereal disease, parasites, and SARCOIDOSIS. If choroiditis is not treated, it may spread to the retina, a condition called CHORIORETINITIS, and to the vitreous. Once in the retina, it may affect the macula, and result in a loss of central vision.

Choroiditis is treated with steroid pills or drops. Immunosuppressive medications may be prescribed in severe cases. It tends to reoccur.

ciliary body   The ciliary body is the group of ciliary muscles that are attached to the ZONULE, a group of fibers that hold the lens in place. The ciliary muscles change the shape of the lens when focusing, and they open and shut the pupil.

The ciliary muscles contract to bulge the lens forward and focus on a near object. The muscles expand to flatten the lens and focus on a distant object.

The ciliary body also produces the aqueous fluid of the eye. The aqueous fluid flows through the anterior chamber of the eye where it nourishes the lens and cornea and carries away waste. Changes in the ciliary body may affect the production and flow of the aqueous fluid, which can result in an increase in intraocular pressure and glaucoma.

Iritis, an inflammation of the iris, can cause inflammation of the ciliary body, known as CYCLITIS. This results in pain, redness, light sensitivity, and constricted pupil. Iritis and cyclitis are usually treated with steroid pills, eyedrops, or ointments.

Civil Service Reform Act   The Civil Service Reform Act of 1978 authorized widespread changes in federal employment practices. Among other reforms, the Act allowed agency directors to hire assistants for visually impaired or hearing-impaired employees to enable them to do their jobs effectively. These assistants included reading aides for visually impaired employees and interpreters for hearing-impaired employees.

U.S. Department of Education. *Summary of Existing Legislation Affecting Persons with Disabilities.* Washington, D.C.: USDE, 1988.

coloboma   A cleft or notch in the iris, retina, and/or CHOROID due to incomplete formation or closure of the optic cup during gestation. The cleft produces a section of missing iris, retina, and/or choroid that may extend from the optic disc to the periphery of the FUNDUS.

Coloboma most often appears as a keyhole-shaped pupil. The condition may be bilateral, but usually one eye is more acutely affected than the other. If the iris is minimally affected, vision interference may be insignificant. However, if the retina (particularly the macular area) and choroid are involved, vision loss could be serious.

Coloboma is a birth defect that is inherited in a dominant pattern. It sometimes is accompanied by other developmental flaws. There is currently no treatment to correct coloboma.

color blindness   Difficulty in recognizing or distinguishing one color from another. It may be one of two types, hereditary or acquired. The hereditary variety is the most common. It is present at birth in 1 out of 12 men and 1 out of 200 women. It is a genetic defect that affects both eyes and does not change in severity over a lifetime.

The retina contains photoreceptor cells called rods and cones. They change light energy into information about the object in view. The retina changes the information into electrical energy that is sent to the brain and translated into an image.

Each cone contains visual pigments that are sensitive to one of the three primary-color light wavelengths. One group of cones recognizes green, one red and one blue. By blending these three colors, the eye is able to distinguish all the colors of the spectrum. This is known as normal trichromatic color vision.

Color blindness occurs when one group of cones does not recognize its color properly. This may be caused by a lack of visual pigment, called an anopia, or by faulty visual pigment, known as an anomaly. Individuals lacking visual pigment are termed dichromats; those with faulty pigment are termed anomalous trichromats.

Most people with color blindness see some color. Many see all three primary colors but in the wrong proportions and may require brighter shades to recognize a particular hue. Other individuals may be red or green blind. A person with red blindness sees reds and oranges as shades of gray or black. A person with green blindness sees reds, oranges, and greens as much the same shade and cannot distinguish between them. Blue blindness is extremely rare, as is complete color blindness, a condition usually attributable to other visual problems.

Color blindness may be detected during the routine ophthalmologic examination. A common screening device called the Ishihara Test uses circles of different sizes and hues to form a mosaic picture. The picture shows a two-digit number in a background field of circles. Those with normal color vision are able to see the number formed with colored circles. Those with color blindness cannot detect a number from the background field.

There is no cure or treatment for hereditary color blindness although some experimentation is being done with tinted contact lenses, such as the X-CHROM LENS, and filters. The individual may not be able to see color with the lenses but may be able to distinguish between colors better as a result of wearing them.

Acquired color blindness can occur as a result of aging or disorders such as retinal optical-nerve conditions, TOXIC AMBLYOPIA, macular disease, cataract, glaucoma, and diabetic retinopathy. The diseased eye is generally the only eye affected, and effective treatment of the illness may result in an improvement in color vision.

Drugs can temporarily alter an individual's color vision. Barbiturates given as sedatives and large doses of vitamin A may affect the yellow or yellow-green vision, and caffeine has been shown to affect and alter all colors. The popular drug Viagra also has been found to cause temporary changes in blue/green colors and increased sensitivity to light in some cases.

conjunctiva   The conjunctiva is the transparent mucous membrane that covers the inside of the eyelid and the SCLERA, the protective white part of the eye. Conditions that are commonly associated with the conjunctiva include CONJUNCTIVITIS, hemorrhage, pinguecula, and pterygium.

Conjunctivitis, or "pink eye," is an inflammation of the conjunctiva. It may be caused by allergies, viral infections, bacterial infections, or overexposure to light. Symptoms of conjunctivitis may include redness of the eye, itching, burning, or discharge.

A hemorrhage in the conjunctiva, called a subconjunctival hemorrhage, may occur due to an injury, excessive rubbing, or coughing and sneezing. A hemorrhage shows itself as a bright red mark on the sclera (white of the eye). The hemorrhage looks frightening but rarely has any long-term effect and generally goes away without treatment.

Pinguecula is a small, yellowish, raised mark on the sclera. It is usually associated with age and is a harmless condition.

Pterygium is a patch of raised vascular tissue on the sclera. If the pterygium grows into the cornea, it may block vision.

conjunctivitis   Conjunctivitis is a common infection of the CONJUNCTIVA. Conjunctivitis can be caused by large doses of ultraviolet light, as in snow-blindness, by allergies to pollen, medications, food or smoke, or by bacteria or viruses. While all forms of conjunctivitis are commonly referred to as "pink eye," only the viral form is pink eye in the true ophthalmic sense.

Conjunctivitis caused by overexposure to light can cause redness of the SCLERA and a burning sensation. Treatment involves shielding the eye from excessive light and allowing it to heal with time.

Viral conjunctivitis—which is truly pink eye because it does, indeed, cause the eye to become pink, as opposed to bright red or yellowish from discharge—is caused by one of the viruses responsible for the common cold. It is extremely contagious. This form of conjunctivitis usually occurs seven to 10 days after contact with an infected person, and causes the eye to become itchy and watery. Like a cold, this form of conjunctivitis can linger for weeks. It can be treated with antihistamine eye drops and cold compresses on the eye to relieve swelling but, generally, it simply has to run its course. Avoiding viral conjunctivitis is difficult because it is so contagious. It can be spread by a pillowcase, towel, washcloth, article of clothing, tissue, and so forth.

Bacterial conjunctivitis normally is characterized by eyes that are noticeably inflamed, bright red, and discharge a thick yellow mucous. It is easy to contract because bacteria are so easily introduced into the eyes. While the conjunctiva, just like the mouth, normally contains bacteria, those bacteria that cause conjunctivitis are not normally present there. Antibiotic eye drops generally are prescribed to treat bacterial conjunctivitis. In some cases, oral antibiotics may be necessary.

Allergic conjunctivitis, which can be caused by a host of irritants ranging from pollen to rabbit fur, results in the eyes becoming red, itchy, swollen, and teary. Some eye-care products, such as the preservatives used in eye drops, also can cause allergic conjunctivitis. Pollutants and chemicals also can cause allergic conjunctivitis. This condition normally is treated with antihistamines and cold compresses. Over-the-counter pain relievers may be used to relieve discomfort.

Conjunctivitis can produce serious damage and should be treated by a physician.

contact lenses   An alternative to eyeglasses, contact lenses are small, thin discs of plastic that rest in place on the cornea. Held in position by the natural moisture of the cornea, contacts have several advantages over glasses. Many people find contacts to be more comfortable and convenient than glasses, and they provide better peripheral vision than glasses do. Because the lens rests directly on the eye, size differences that sometimes occur with glasses are minimized, giving a more natural appearance to what you see.

Contacts have become increasingly popular since 1972, when soft lenses were first introduced, but the idea for them has been around for centuries. In fact, Leonardo da Vinci is credited with having come up with the idea for contact lenses in about 1550. It was a scientist in Switzerland, however, who actually made the first contact lens out of glass in the late 1800s. These glass lenses were not successful because they were very uncomfortable to wear. Plastic lenses, which we still use, were introduced in the 1940s, although many innovations and improvements have been made since then. Contact lenses are made today to correct almost any vision problem, and there are many varieties. Basically, however, they are divided into two major categories: hard and soft.

Hard contacts, the kind that were first introduced in the 1940s, can correct nearsightedness, farsightedness, and astigmatism. Hard lenses were much improved upon during the 1970s, when a gas-permeable model was developed. Gas permeable lenses are hard but allow air to flow through them to the eye. They are more flexible than the earlier hard lenses, and they generally fit better. They are made with computer-controlled lathes and can be ground to correct various vision problems. They also can be made into bifocal lenses. Gas-permeable lenses also can be used to correct corneal problems that cause vision to be distorted.

Soft contacts are available to correct nearsightedness, farsightedness, astigmatism, and presbyopia (the inability to focus at near distances). They are flexible, and they absorb and hold water. Soft contacts are sometimes called hydrogels. Many more people can wear soft lenses today than in the past, due to advances in the way they are made. Soft contacts also can be made into bifocal lenses.

Daily-wear contact lenses are those designed to be placed in the eye in the morning and taken out at the end of the day. Extended-wear contacts are those that can be worn for more than 24 hours. Extended-wear lenses are designed to allow the eye to receive sufficient oxygen, so they can be worn even while the wearer is sleeping. Flexible-wear lenses can occasionally be worn overnight, but they are not designed to be worn constantly. Disposable extended-wear lenses have been available since the late 1980s and are just what they are called—disposable. They are designed to be placed in the eye, worn for about a week, and then thrown away. Lenses that are disposed of after one day of use were introduced in the mid-1990s.

All contact lenses should be kept very clean in order to avoid the risk of infecting the eyes. There are three basic methods of disinfecting contact lenses: with heat, chemicals, or a peroxide oxidative disinfectants. Heat systems destroy bacteria on the lenses with high temperatures. Lenses are first cleaned and rinsed, then they are placed into a heat unit, during which time bacteria are destroyed. Using heat to kill bacteria is a fairly quick process, and there is no need to use solutions that contain preservatives and chemicals, to which some people are allergic. A downside to heat cleaning is that it can cause coatings to build up on the lenses. Also, heat cleaning is not safe for all types of lenses.

Chemical disinfectants kill bacteria over a period of several hours. They are effective at cleaning and disinfecting lenses, but, as mentioned above, can cause allergic reactions in people with sensitivity.

Peroxide oxidative disinfectants were developed in the early 1980s and are considered to have some advantages over heating or chemical systems. Although the disinfectants are based on a hydrogen peroxide solution, they have built-in neutralizers that break down the peroxide so that it does not remain on the contact lenses. Because of the neutralization, there are no chemical residues. Nor is it necessary to heat the lenses.

Bifocal contact lenses are available in both hard and soft lenses and contain two prescriptions to correct refractive errors. Crescent bifocal lenses are similar to traditional bifocal spectacles in that the prescription for distance is at the top part of the lens and the prescription for close vision is in a crescent segment at the bottom. The lenses are either weighted or truncated (flattened) at the bottom to keep them from rotating out of position.

Concentric bifocal lenses differ in that the close vision prescription is in a ring around the inner circle of distance vision prescription. This design circumvents the problem of rotation.

Toric contact lenses are soft lenses that correct astigmatism. In the past, astigmatism had to be corrected with hard lenses because the soft lenses tended to mold themselves to the irregularities of the cornea. The toric lens provides the correction of the hard lens and the comfort of the soft. Like bifocal lenses, toric lenses require a predictable, nonrotating position in the eye. They are often weighted or truncated to discourage rotation. Toric lenses are typically more expensive than other lenses.

The *X-Chrom lens* is a contact lens for those with red-green color blindness. It is a deep red lens worn in the nondominant eye and intensifies the color of red and green objects. This allows the nondominant eye to feed information to the brain about colors it could previously not determine. The dominant eye continues to relate information about colors that it normally sees. The lens is not a cure for color blindness, but rather an aid in the improvement of color perception.

As compared with glasses, contact lenses have the advantage of providing more natural, distortion-free vision, unaffected by weather (raindrops and snowflakes), steam or glasses' frame obstruction. In the presence of high myopia (extreme near-sightedness), APHAKIA (loss of natural lens due to cataract surgery) or corneal diseases, contacts correct vision better than glasses.

Because the contact lens is a foreign substance in the eye, complications such as tearing, redness, itching, corneal abrasions, or infections can arise.

contrast   Contrast enhancement is a non-optical, or environmental, aid that maximizes residual vision. Contrast is enhanced by using dissimilar colors or brightness levels to make an object more visible. Highly contrasting colors near one another enhance contrast. Complementary colors that can be used together to create improved contrast include reds with greens, blues with oranges, and yellows with violet hues.

Light objects on a dark background or the re-verse improve contrast. Light plates on a dark tablecloth improve visibility. Black letters on a white or yellow page are more readable than blue letters. Dark stairs are more easily seen when next to a light wall or when lined with a fluorescent strip.

Other aids can be used to improve contrast. A sheet of yellow or amber acetate can be placed over pale or bluish print to increase visibility. A typoscope, or slit reader, isolates one line of print to reduce the page glare and add contrast.

convergence   The coordinated movement of the eyes to focus together on a near object. Convergence is tested in an eye examination by slowly bringing a light or object close to the bridge of the nose. The patient is instructed to keep the object in focus as long as possible.

As the object moves closer to the nose, the eyes turn inward to a cross-eyed position. Divergence occurs when the object can no longer be seen as one image and the eyes move from the convergent position.

The near point of convergence is the last point at which the object could be seen as one image. This point is measured in millimeters as the distance from the bridge of the nose to the object. A normal near point of convergence is approximately 50 millimeters.

corneal degeneration   The term for the breakdown of the cornea. Corneal degenerations are fairly rare disorders that may be caused by genetic or environmental conditions. Most disorders that cause corneal degeneration are inherited. Among these hereditary diseases are the two most common, *keratoconus* and FUCH'S ENDOTHELIAL DYSTROPHY.

Keratoconus is a disorder that may be inherited from a recessive trait. The disorder affects both eyes and is usually seen in children or adolescents. In this condition, the central part of the cornea thins and eventually protrudes forward into a cone shape. Distortion and loss of vision result. It is estimated to affect one of every 2,000 persons in the general population.

Keratoconus is a chronic, progressive disease that develops slowly. It can be corrected in mild forms with spectacles and, more advanced forms, with contact lenses.

Advanced conditions of keratoconus may be corrected with corneal transplants, called KERATOPLASTY. Keratoplasty to correct keratoconus is a highly successful procedure since the cornea remains relatively free of blood vessels.

Fuch's dystrophy is an uncommon hereditary disorder. It is more common in women than in men, and normally appears only after a person is 50. In this disease, the endothelium layer degenerates and impairs vision. Fuch's dystrophy may cause further complications such as corneal edema, a rise in intraocular pressure. Corneal transplantation may improve or restore vision.

Little is known about the causes and development of corneal degenerations. It is thought that some degenerations may result from irregularities within corneal fibroblasts, the cells that develop into fibrous tissue. The fibroblasts are central to the processes of healing a corneal injury.

In addition, some corneal degenerations may be caused by environmental influences. They may result from corneal infections or inflammations (KERATITIS) or from accidental injuries such as alkali burns.

corneal edema   A condition in which the cornea becomes overly hydrated. In order to remain transparent, the cornea is normally kept relatively dry through oxygen supplied in tears and the drain of water by the corneal endothelium. Any changes to the dehydration process or an influx of fluid can impede the process and allow fluid to accumulate.

Symptoms of corneal edema included blurred vision or the appearance of halos around lights. Later symptoms include severe pain as corneal nerves are damaged. Since the early symptoms are similar to those of cataract, an ocular examination is necessary for proper diagnosis.

Corneal edema may be caused by infection, corneal endothelial dysfunction (FUCH'S ENDOTHELIAL DYSTROPHY), a viral corneal inflammation (KERATITIS), a rise in intraocular pressure (as in glaucoma), postoperative changes, trauma, overwear of contact lenses, and ill-fitting contact lenses.

The condition is treated according to its cause. Edema caused by an infection or a corneal endothelial disorder may be treated with STEROIDS or other medications. Viral KERATITIS may be treated with ANTIVIRAL DRUGS. A rise in intraocular pressure may be controlled by glaucoma medication or surgery. Postoperative conditions and trauma may be treated with medications and properly fitted and worn contact lenses may alleviate the symptoms related to their use.

Corneal edema may become a chronic condition. As the condition progresses and worsens, the corneal nerves become ruptured and exposed, causing extreme pain. Treatment of acute edema may include a TARSORRHAPHY, in which a portion of the lids are stitched together, or a corneal graft.

corneal transplant   A corneal transplant, or keratoplasty, is the most common form of human transplant surgery performed today. There are more than 40,000 corneal transplants done each year in the United States. Keratoplasty uses a donor cornea to replace a diseased cornea. Although cornea transplants are generally successful in restoring vision, about 10 percent of transplanted corneas are rejected. Most rejections, however, can be prevented if treated early. Signs of rejection include sensitivity to light, redness, persistent discomfort, and changes in vision. Immunosuppressive drugs are available to reduce the possibility of cornea rejection, including an oral vaccine developed especially for that purpose.

Donor transplants come from people who have decided that when they die they want their corneas to be donated to others. The donor transplants are often kept in eye banks that help match appropriate corneas to needed hosts.

Donor transplants are selected according to age, cause of death, condition of the eye, and time between death and transplant surgery. Blood and tissue typing are not required as with kidney or heart transplants but time is a critical factor since the cornea should be transplanted within four days of donation.

Donor corneas are most desirable from individuals between the ages of 25 to 35 and who died from injury or disease. The donor corneas are screened for eye disease and the presence of venereal disease.

An individual becomes a candidate for a corneal transplant when all vision in that eye is lost due to injury, corneal dystrophy diseases such as KERATOCONUS, chemical burn, or infection. A transplant also may be performed to repair injuries or tears in the cornea, to relieve chronic pain, or to correct a cosmetically unattractive eye.

A normal cornea is avascular, or lacks blood vessels. In order to perform a successful keratoplasty, the transplant must be placed into the eye in a manner that discourages vascularization, or the growth of blood vessels, into the cornea. Vascularization of the transplant may destroy it.

Certain disorders or diseases such as keratoconus, or a bulging cornea, lend themselves best to corneal transplants because of the lack of corneal blood vessels involved with this disorder. Other conditions, such as corneal scars, are less effectively corrected with transplants because of heavy vascularization present in the cornea.

The surgery may replace part or all of the host cornea. A section of donor cornea is measured to the precise needs of the host with an instrument called a trephine. This section is removed from the donor cornea with scissors. A corresponding section of host cornea is measured with the trephine and removed with scissors. The donor cornea is placed into the remaining cavity and sewn into position with small sutures.

The procedure is performed with either local or general anesthesia and may take from an hour to an hour and a half. It is often done on an outpatient basis, but many patients require a day or two of hospitalization.

For several weeks after surgery, the patient is discouraged from bending, lifting, or straining. The patient wears a protective eye patch or shield and is treated with eye drops for several months. The stitches are removed after a period of six months to two years. Ophthalmologists recently began using artificial corneas is certain transplant cases. (See EYE BANK.)

corneal ulcer   Corneal ulcers occur when the cornea is worn down or damaged by injury or exposure and bacterial, viral, or fungal infections. Ulceration may lead to scarring and loss of sight. It is a common cause of blindness around the world.

Injuries or overwear of contact lenses usually result in minor corneal abrasions or scratches. The symptoms are extreme pain with a feeling of a foreign body within the eye. Anaesthetic drops may be administered to examine the eye that is then generally bandaged shut. The eye may be allowed to heal itself or an antibiotic ointment may be prescribed to avoid infection.

Ulcers due to exposure occur in cases of injury, facial palsy (Bell's palsy) or unconsciousness in which the lid does not adequately protect the cornea, allowing bacteria to enter and infection to result. Exposure-related ulcers may be treated with eyepads and/or anesthetic ointments.

Ulcers caused by bacteria are often associated with the staphylococcus or streptococcus bacterias. Other bacterias may infect the eye when the cornea is weakened by disease or additional infections. Bacterial ulcers are usually treated with ANTIBIOTICS or antibiotic-steroids.

Ulcers due to viruses are most often caused by the HERPES SIMPLEX virus. In infants, the virus is passed from the mother to the child as it travels through the birth canal. A rash may appear around the eyelids of the newborn, and the child may develop a fever.

The condition is serious and may result in death, blindness, or damage to other organs of the body. The virus is treated with ANTIVIRAL DRUGS and antibiotics.

The herpes virus may appear in adults after development of another illness. The virus, which had remained latent in the body, is reactivated and settles in the eye. This gives rise to KERATITIS, or inflammation, and the formation of star-shaped, or dendritic, ulcers. As the ulcers heal, they may leave scars that could impair vision.

An antiviral drug such as IDOXURIDINE, TRIFLURIDINE, or ACYCLOVIR along with an antibiotic may be prescribed as treatment. These drugs cannot cure the herpes simplex virus, but they effectively stop the reproduction of viral cells and prevent infection. STEROIDS are not recommended since they impair the body's rejection of the herpes simplex virus.

Fungal-related ulcers are most often caused by yeasts. The condition may require hospitalization and treatment with antibiotics. Healing of these ulcers often results in scarring of the cornea.

Damage to the corneal nerve, a vitamin-A deficiency, or the onset of other diseases or disorders may also trigger corneal ulcers. Any situation in which the cornea is inflamed (corneal keratitis) should be monitored for ulcers.

cortical blindness   Cortical blindness is a rare condition that occurs as a result of lesions on the occipital lobes where the visual cortex is located. The lobes control the visual field of each eye.

A lesion on one occipital lobe may result in HEMIANOPSIA, loss of half the field of vision, but does not affect the central vision acuity. Lesions on both lobes cause bilateral loss of vision with normally reactive pupils. This is known as cortical blindness.

Cortical blindness can be a congenital problem, but is most commonly seen in aging eyes affected by vascular disease. There may be a history of cerebrovascular incidents and loss of cerebral function. Cortical blindness may be a temporary condition that follows a cerebrovascular embolism or circulatory occlusion caused by a stroke, myocardial infarction, or heart surgery.

cortisone   A steroid hormone used in drugs to treat eye disorders. Cortisone may be an ingredient in prescribed eye drops, ointments, or pills. It is often used to combat inflammation and prevent scarring, as in corneal disease.

Cortisone must be used with caution since it increases the eye's susceptibility to infection. Antiviral or antibacterial drugs are often taken at the same time to augment the eye's natural defenses.

Cortisone should be used in the eyes for the prescribed period of time only. Long-term use of cortisone may cause glaucoma or cataract.

cortisporin ophthalmic antibiotic   A drug used to treat bacterial eye infections. It may be prescribed in drop or ointment form. Equivalent products include Triple-Gen and triple antibiotic. Side effects from use of this drug may include burning or stinging of the eyes, redness, blurred or reduced vision, and headache. Eye pain, changes in vision, and headache indicate a serious problem that should be checked by a physician.

The drug should not be prescribed for fungal or viral eye infections or those that involve the back sections of the eye. Those with an allergy to hydrocortisone or any other ingredient, as well as those with tuberculosis, should not use this drug. Those with inner-ear problems, myasthenia gravis, or kidney disease should use the drug with caution.

The eye infection should be monitored during the time the drug is taken, even if the drug is used for a short period of time. If the drug is used long-term, the eye should be examined regularly for the development of cataract or a secondary infection.

cryosurgery   Cryosurgery is a procedure that uses very low temperatures to induce adhering scars in tissue. Cryosurgery employs a cryoprobe, a pencil-like probe with a tip that is cooled to a tempera-ture between 30 and 70 degrees below freezing. Cryosurgery is used to repair retinal detachments.

A retinal detachment occurs whenever the retina is disconnected to the back layers of the eye. The retina normally adheres closely to the pigment epithelium and is supported by the vitreous gel. When the retina detaches or separates from the epithelium layer, vision is threatened and surgery is needed to reattach it.

In order to reattach the retina, the CHOROID, which lies just below the epithelium and the retina, must be irritated to form adhering scar tissue. The surgeon may use surgical diathermy, a procedure in which a needle transmitting high-frequency electrical current is touched to the SCLERA.

The heat of the electricity is transmitted to the choroid, which is stimulated to form scar tissue.

An alternative method uses cryosurgery. The cryoprobe is touched to points on the sclera, which is unaffected by the procedure. A hypodermic needle is then inserted to drain any fluid that has accumulated under the retina.

The surgeon may then make an indentation in the back of the eye and place a silicone buckle or band around the eye to indent it slightly inward. This pushes the epithelium into contact with the retina. Adhering scar tissue forms in the frozen area and ensures that the retina will remain in position. The band remains permanently in the eye but is neither seen nor felt.

Berland, Theodore, and Richard A. Perritt. *Living With Your Eye Operation.* New York: St. Martin's Press, 1974.

Eden, John. *The Eye Book.* New York: Penguin Books, 1978.

Krames Communications. *The Retina Book.* Daly City, California: KC, 1987.

Reynolds, James D. "Lasers in Ophthalmology," *HealthNet Library.* Columbus: CompuServe, 1989.

crystalline lens   The crystalline or natural lens is the transparent, elastic lens of the eye located behind the posterior chamber. The lens changes shape to focus light that enters the eye through the pupil. The lens is held in place by fibers called ZONULES. The zonules are attached to ciliary muscles, which contract or expand to change the shape of the lens. The lens bulges forward to focus on a near object and flattens to focus on a distant object.

The crystalline lens is subject to common eye disorders. It may become subluxated or develop cataracts. A subluxated lens is one that has shifted out of place due to a birth defect or an injury. The placement of the lens, usually downward from its normal position, determines the degree of affected vision.

Cataracts are a clouding or opaque spot on the surface of the lens that may develop over long periods of time. Most cataracts, termed senile cataracts, are those associated with aging. Cataracts may also be caused by birth defects, injuries, over-exposure to light, medications, diabetes, Down's syndrome, Marfan's syndrome, and other diseases.

Cataracts may be removed surgically. In some procedures, a portion of the crystalline lens is removed, and an artificial, plastic lens is placed in the eye. This intraocular lens, or IOL, replaces and serves as a permanent substitute for the removed section of natural lens.

See also IOL SURGERY.

cyclitis   An inflammation of the CILIARY BODY of the eye. The ciliary body lies behind the iris and is attached to ZONULES, which hold the LENS in place. The ciliary body produces AQUEOUS FLUID, which flows into the anterior chamber to nourish the cornea and lens and carry away waste matter. It also moves the lens, allowing it to focus properly.

Cyclitis is associated with UVEITIS, an inflammation of the uveal tract that sometimes is referred to as arthritis of the eye. The ciliary body, the iris and the CHOROID make up the uveal tract. When the choroid becomes inflamed, as in CHOROIDITIS, it is termed posterior uveitis. When the iris or ciliary body becomes involved, it is termed anterior uveitis. Since the ciliary body is linked so closely to the iris, the inflammation soon spreads from one to the other. Because of this, cyclitis is often seen in cases of IRITIS, or inflammation of the iris.

The symptoms of cyclitis include extreme pain, contracted pupil, blurred vision, light sensitivity, and redness of the eye. It may develop quickly within a 24-hour period.

Cyclitis may develop spontaneously. It has been linked to other conditions such as arthritis, tuberculosis, venereal disease, SARCOIDOSIS, sinus disorders, viruses, and injuries. An ophthalmologic examination plus X rays of the sinuses, skull, and chest, as well as blood tests may be involved to determine the cause of the condition.

Treatment of this condition usually involves steroid eye drops and cycloplegic eye drops to dilate the pupil. Untreated cyclitis may spread to the choroid, retina, and vitreous, or may result in secondary glaucoma.

cycloplegic drops   Cycloplegic, or mydriatic, drops are eye drops that dilate the pupils. Cycloplegics are most often used during the ophthalmologic examination to observe the back of the eye. Most drops reach a maximum effect after 15 minutes and last approximately three hours. Stronger cycloplegics may last for 24 hours and are frequently used in young children or for lengthy examinations.

In diseases in which the lens and the iris have developed adhesions, such as IRITIS, cycloplegics may be used to suspend accommodation, or movement, of the pupil. Atropine, a drug commonly administered in such cases, may last up to seven days.

Occasionally, the instillation of cycloplegic drops induces glaucoma. This occurs when the dilated pupil further constricts the space in an unusually narrow anterior chamber. This impedes the flow of AQUEOUS FLUID from the eye, and intraocular pressure rises. Pilocarpine or other meiotics, drugs that constrict the pupil, can reverse the problem.

In rare instances, the patient may have an allergy to an ingredient in the cycloplegic eye drops. This may result in irritation, redness of the eye or dermatitis that should dissipate as the effectiveness of the drug wears off.

cytomegalovirus retinitis   See AIDS.

dacryocystitis An inflammation of the tear drainage sac caused by an infection. It usually affects one eye only and may become a chronic disorder. It is most commonly found in adult females.

Dacryocystitis may be caused congenitally, from a blockage or obstruction of the tear duct or from a trauma or injury. The resulting infection is caused most often by bacteria such as *Staphylococcus aureus* and beta-hemolytic *Streptococcus* and by fungi such as *Candida albicans*.

Symptoms may include constant tearing, swelling, discharge and tenderness of the eye. A culture of the discharge may identify the infecting agent. The condition can be difficult to treat because the sac is located deep within the tissues surrounding the eye. Also, the condition can be hard to pinpoint and sometimes remains undetected for long periods, leading to scarring and tearing problems.

Dacryocystitis is usually treated with warm compresses and topical or systemic ANTIBIOTICS. Blocked nasolacrimal ducts of infants may be massaged to encourage dilation. If the duct fails to open, it may require surgical dilation. If the condition produces an abscess, it may be drained.

deaf-blind Deaf-blind persons are those who have a severe hearing impairment in addition to a vision impairment. The combination of severities varies according to the individual and often results in some residual hearing or vision. Deaf-blind individuals may retain enough residual hearing or sight to benefit from hearing aids or prescriptive lenses.

Deaf-blindness may be caused genetically and be present at birth, may develop over time as a result of RUBELLA or USHER'S SYNDROME or may be the result of aging. Usher's syndrome is a leading cause of deaf-blindness and responsible for approximately 10,000 of the deaf-blind individuals in the United States.

Deaf-blind infants may exhibit autisticlike tendencies and are often misdiagnosed as retarded or emotionally ill. Parents of deaf-blind infants and children are urged to hold their children as much as possible to provide the information that someone is close by. They are encouraged to talk, sing, and hum to their children and to hold the children near their chests to allow them to feel the vibration of the sounds.

If a child has some residual hearing, he can be encouraged to make sounds. Parents can expose the child to as many vibrations as possible, from the vacuum cleaner to the stereo speaker. Parents can place their hands on the child's face and bend to the child's face level while talking to the child.

Children can be stimulated with toys or movement to avoid unwanted mannerisms (see BLINDISMS). Playing with drums, whistles, or other vibration instruments may be helpful. If the child has some residual hearing, the association of sounds and actions or sounds and people helps to define the world.

Deaf-blind children can be gently urged to sit up, crawl, stand, and walk with encouragement from parents. The child should always have support until he can stand by himself. Self-care activities such as eating, toilet training, and dressing can begin early and should be consistent and reasonable in practice. Specific movements or signals may be used to cue activities such as meal or bath time.

Once the child learns that motor movements can be used to communicate, language development begins. The individual's residual vision and hearing and fine motor skills will determine which method of communication is used.

Some individuals who retain enough hearing or become deaf after learning to speak can use speech. Those without residual hearing may use fingerspelling, American Sign Language (ASL) or Signed English, three sign languages that can be used by deaf and totally blind persons.

In order to communicate with sighted and hearing individuals, the deaf-blind person may use the alphabet glove, the Braille Alphabet Card, or the Tellatouch device. The alphabet glove is a thin, cotton glove printed with the letters of the alphabet at specific spots that are memorized by the wearer. The user or sighted person spells out words by touching the letters on the glove.

The Braille Alphabet Card is a pocket-size card that has both braille and printed letters on it. The deaf-blind individual must read braille to use the card. The user or the sighted person spells out the words by touching the letters on the card.

The Tellatouch is a small, typewriterlike device that raises braille letters under the deaf-blind readers fingertip as the other communicator types on the keyboard. The device also includes braillewriter keys for use by blind persons.

Education for deaf-blind children can begin through early intervention programs or preschools for deaf-blind persons. Those children with greater hearing and less sight may be placed in programs for visually impaired students. Those with greater residual vision and little or no hearing may be placed in programs for the hearing impaired.

Deaf-blind children entering kindergarten are protected by the Education for All Handicapped Children Act, which ensures them a free, appropriate, public education in the least restrictive setting, which includes special education according to each child's needs. A leading advocacy group for deaf-blind people is the American Association of the Deaf-Blind.
Contact:

American Association of the Deaf-Blind
814 Thayer Avenue
Silver Spring, MD 20910

800-735-2258 (ph)
301-588-8705 (fax)
301-588-6545 (TTY)

American Foundation for the Blind. *The Preschool Deaf-Blind Child: Suggestions for Parents.* New York: AFB, 1974.
American Foundation for the Blind. *What to Do When You Meet a Deaf-Blind Person,* New York: AFB, 1985.
Esche, Jeanne, and Carol Griffin. *A Handbook for Parents of Deaf-Blind Children.* Lansing, Michigan: Michigan School for the Blind, 1980.
McInnes, J. M., and J. A. Treffry. *Deaf-Blind Infants and Children.* Toronto: University of Toronto Press, 1982.
Scholl, Geraldine T. *Foundations of Education for Blind and Visually Handicapped Children and Youth.* New York: American Foundation for the Blind, 1986.
Walsh, Sara R., and Robert Holzberg, eds. *Understanding and Educating the Deaf-Blind/Severely and Profoundly Handicapped.* Springfield, Illinois: Charles C. Thomas Publisher, 1981.

development of blind children   Visually impaired and blind children develop according to the same patterns and stages that govern the development of sighted children. The effect the loss of vision has on each child depends on the severity, the type of loss, the age at which the loss occurred and the child's overall functioning level.

Each visually impaired child is an individual; therefore, there is no typical visually impaired child. Each develops according to his own timetable and abilities. However, many visually impaired children have certain traits and needs in common.

Blind or visually impaired children may depend more on their parents initially. They rely on their parents to bring the world to them. Parents need to fill the gaps presented by the lack of sight with experiences involving all the senses, including making the best use of any residual vision.

Severe impairments may require the children to be hospitalized and separated at birth from their parents for extended periods. At the end of such time, the children may resist cuddling and not like to be held. The parents and children may respond negatively to the lack of eye contact.

Parents of visually impaired babies and children may need to hold, stroke, and talk to their children more than normal in order to reassure the children that someone is near. Although some visually impaired children react negatively to being held or picked up from the crib, this is not a rejection of affection, but may rather be a reaction to the sudden interruption. Babies who lie quietly in the crib may be concentrating on sounds in the environment and become frightened or confused at a sudden jostling. Parents may substitute voice contact for eye contact by speaking and crooning to the children and imitating sounds the children make.

The lack of vision may also affect the ability of children to distinguish between self and nonself. Sighted children develop the concept by use of vision. They are able to see themselves as separate from their environment and from others by watching others come forward or move away. Parents may encourage their visually impaired children to develop this concept through auditory means by talking to their children as they enter and leave a room.

Up to age four months, visually impaired children and sighted children vary little in their development. At about four months of age, the sighted child may become fascinated with watching his hand, an activity that the visually impaired child may miss. This hand-watching encourages the child to direct his attention to the outside world.

Because of the impairment or lack of sight, visually impaired children may not reach out to explore their world and depend on their parents to bring objects to them. Blind or visually impaired babies may mouth objects for a longer period of time during development (extending into childhood) than their sighted peers. An abundance of tactile sensors in the lips makes this a logical way to gain information in the presence of a sight loss.

Vision provides useful stimulation for motor development, motivating babies to hold their heads up, reach for objects, sit, participate in imitative activity, crawl, and walk. Parents of babies with a sight loss may have to develop creative ways to motivate their children into movement to teach them these actions. Babies without this stimulation may become passive.

As the children grow, they may be encouraged to participate in the same activities and sports as their sighted peers, including group games, jump rope, skating, running and riding a tricycle. Visually impaired or blind children who are physically active tend to show little difference in gross motor skills as compared with their sighted peers and have a better awareness of body image and spatial orientation than blind or visually impaired children who are not physically active.

If visually impaired children lack sufficient opportunities for movement, they may develop stereotypical behaviors, sometimes called "blind-isms." These movements include rocking, head swaying, and poking or rubbing the eyes. Often described as a reaction to a need for stimulation and activity, these behaviors may be curtailed by providing a stimulating environment and ample opportunities for movement, including such activities as climbing and riding a rocking horse.

Fine motor skills such as using a crayon, tying shoes, and playing with blocks or pegs should also be stressed. These skills help children explore the world and prepare them for learning to read and write.

Abstract concepts are more difficult for children with a sight loss, since they are often linked to visual concepts. Concepts such as dirty and clean, in and out, open and shut, up and down, and forward and behind are crucial to the full development of any child. Parents of visually impaired children may have to try methods based on other sensory experiences, in repeated exposures, to teach these concepts to their visually impaired children.

Language and speech development tend to be comparable in sighted and visually impaired children. If children have had a limited amount of gross motor experiences, however, language development may be delayed.

Visually impaired and blind children may repeat or echo what other people say for a longer period of time than their sighted peers. This repeating, called *echolalia*, may be an attempt to practice linking words to the concepts they stand for.

Nonverbal communication develops in sighted children when they smile in response to smiles by others. Later, they imitate and experiment with facial expressions to determine the kinds of reaction they can elicit. Visually impaired children may not participate in this kind of imitative activity, which may limit their development of nonverbal communication. As children grow, they can be instructed verbally as to the kinds of facial expressions and postures that are socially acceptable in order to avoid embarrassment and misunderstandings in social interaction.

During preadolescent and adolescent years, the emphasis of development is placed on educational and social needs. Visually impaired and blind children are entitled by law to a free and equal EDUCATION, including special education programs to fit each child's needs, in the least restrictive environment. Children may go to school in a variety of settings and may begin to use ADAPTIVE AIDS and devices to complete their studies.

Social needs center on feelings of belonging. Group participation in activities such as Girl or Boy Scouts, and school sports and clubs increases feelings of confidence and acceptance by peers. Self-acceptance should be stressed and children should actively participate in determining their own activities and future pursuits.

American Foundation for the Blind. *Is Your Child Blind?* New York: AFB, 1975.
American Foundation for the Blind. *Parenting Preschoolers.* New York: AFB, 1987.
American Foundation for the Blind. *Touch the Baby.* New York: AFB, 1987.
National Association for Visually Handicapped. *Family Guide: Growth and Development of the Partially Seeing Child.* New York: NAVH, 1985.
Warren, David H. *Blindness and Early Childhood Development.* New York: American Foundation for the Blind, 1977.

diabetes   Diabetes or diabetes mellitus (DM) is a name for a group of inherited medical conditions or diseases in which the body is unable adequately to process and store glucose. According to the American Diabetes Center, 15.7 million Americans are afflicted with this serious disease. It is the sixth major cause of death by disease.

Diabetes, specifically diabetic retinopathy, is one of the chief causes of blindness in the United States. Approximately 150,000 diabetics in the United States experience a significant degree of vision loss, and 3 percent have a severe vision loss as a result of this condition.

Diabetic retinopathy, a disease of the retina, is a complication of a general circulatory problem caused by diabetes. This disorder causes the blood vessels that nourish the retina, a light-sensitive inner lining in the back layer of the eye, to weaken, disintegrate, or become blocked. The vessels may leak fluid, bleed, grow unnaturally, bulge, or stop functioning completely.

According to the National Institute of Health, 12 percent of diabetics have experienced cataracts, or opacities of the lens, and an additional 11 percent have been diagnosed with glaucoma, a condition in which intraocular pressure builds within the eye and causes vision loss. These rates are over twice those for the general population.

Those most at risk of developing diabetes include members of families with a history of diabetes, women (by a two-to-one margin over men), obese or overweight people, people over 40, blacks, Hispanics, native Americans, and those from low-income groups.

The disease affects many organ groups and causes complications such as retinopathy (disease of the retina), nephropathy (disease of the kidney), neuropathy (disease of the nerves), arteriosclerosis (hardening of the arteries), and skin disorders.

Carbohydrates are broken down into glucose by the body's digestive juices. When glucose enters the blood stream, the beta cells of the pancreas produce and release insulin, which helps the body tissues absorb the energy-producing glucose.

Diabetes is present when the beta cells fail to react to the elevated glucose level in the blood. As a result, the blood glucose level rises above normal, the liver produces sugar from protein in the body, glucose appears in the urine, and the individual experiences frequent urination, constant thirst, and weight loss. If untreated, the disease can cause dangerous levels of acid in the blood and diabetic coma.

Three main types of diabetes exist. Type I, insulin-dependent diabetes mellitus (IDDM), is characterized by insulin dependency; the presence of HLA, DR3 and DR4 genetic markers; the appearance of circulation antibodies that attack the cells of the pancreas; and a predisposition to acquire ketoacidosis, high levels of ketones, fatty acids, and glucose in the blood.

Type I diabetes is also called juvenile-onset diabetes and occurs in children and adolescents. The onset of the disease often follows an infection or virus. Several viruses including rubella, mumps, coxsackie B, and Echo viruses are being explored as possible links to a cause.

Type II, noninsulin-dependent diabetes mellitus (NIDDM), occurs generally in middle-aged adults. NIDDM patients secrete insulin, lack HLA genetic markers, are insulin resistant, and are usually overweight.

Since six out of seven Type II patients who develop the disease after age 45 are overweight, studies are being conducted to determine whether inheritance may interact with obesity to trigger the disease.

Type III diabetes is a milder form of the disease. It is non-progressive and has no known cause beyond inheritance. It affects young and old alike.

Treatment for diabetes may include dietary measures, exercise, oral drug treatment, insulin injections, daily monitoring of blood glucose levels in the blood or urine, and regularly scheduled medical examinations. It is extremely important that anyone who has diabetes get regular, thorough eye exams. The severity of many diabetes-related eye problems can be reduced if the problem is detected early.

U.S. Department of Health and Human Services, NIH. *Facts About Insulin-Dependent Diabetes.* NIH Publication No. 80-2098. Washington, D.C.: Government Printing Office, 1980.
National Diabetes Data Group, NIH. *Diabetes in America.* NIH Publication No. 85-1468. Washington, D.C.: Government Printing Office, 1985.
American Diabetes Association, Diabetes Facts and Figures, ADA website, 2000.

diopter   A unit of measurement for the power of a lens. It measures the extent light rays will bend as they pass through the lens.

Diopters are written in prescriptions as O.D. or O.S. followed by a plus or minus sign and a number. The O.D. stands for the Latin *oculus dexter,* or right eye. The O.S. stands for *oculus sinister,* or left eye.

Plus signs indicate convex or farsighted lenses. Minus signs stand for concave or nearsighted lenses. A +3.00 prescription calls for a 3 diopter convex lens for a farsighted eye. A -1.5 prescription requires a 1-1/2 diopter concave lens for a near-sighted eye. The stronger the lens is, the higher the number.

Prescriptions to correct astigmatism employ cylindrical lenses that are often incorporated into a convex or concave lens to curve it more in one direction. Astigmatism prescriptions indicate the diopter degree of near- or farsightedness, plus the word "axis" and a number from 1 to 180. The axis number refers to the number of degrees on a protractor and determines to which degree the cylindrical lens must be oriented.

The prescription -3.25–2.00 axis 95, calls for 3-1/4 diopters of nearsightedness with 2 diopters of astigmatism. The axis 95 indicates the degree at which the cylindrical lens must be oriented (95 degrees in this case).

diplopia   The term for double vision. Diplopia is often confused with blurred vision when cited as a patient complaint. Blurred vision is a cloudy or hazy image, but diplopia is the sighting of two separate images at the same time.

Diplopia may be constant or intermittent and binocular or monocular. Monocular diplopia occurs if the double image persists when one eye is closed. This is a common form of diplopia and is often caused by cataract. Binocular diplopia occurs when the diplopia is corrected when one eye is closed.

Diplopia may go unnoticed in adults or children due to poor general vision or suppression of image. Children often accommodate to the double image by suppressing the image of one eye, a condition called amblyopia. This condition may lead to vision loss.

Diplopia is a serious symptom and requires examination of the eyes. The examination involves testing of the gross eye movements to check the degree of separation of images in various positions. The Hess chart, red-glass test, or the cover-uncover test may be used.

The Hess chart test involves placing a red filter in front of one eye and a green filter in front of the other. The patient looks at a screen of small white dots. The patient is asked to point to specific dots with a pointer. The amount of mislocation is measured.

The red-glass test involves placing a red glass in front of the right eye and a green glass in front of the left. The patient looks at a light 20 feet away and then at a separate light 14 inches away. The patient tells the examiner if separate red and green lights are seen while fixating on the near or far light.

During the cover-uncover test the patient looks at a letter or object at 20 feet. One eye is covered and the other is observed to see whether it moves to fixate on the object. If the eye moves, a disorder is present. The other eye is tested at 20 feet and then both are tested at 14 inches.

Diplopia may be caused by misalignment of the eyes, as in strabismus (or a latent strabismus from childhood), an ocular muscle imbalance; third, fourth or sixth cranial nerve palsy; orbital lesions; muscle lesions; cataracts; nerve lesions; multiple sclerosis; myasthenia gravis; injury to the orbit; thyrotoxicosis, in which extraocular muscles become inflamed; stroke; or intracranial tumor.

Diplopia may often be treated with corrective lenses, surgery or medication therapy of the underlying cause.

Burde, Ronald, Peter J. Savino and Jonathan D. Trobe. *Clinical Decisions in Neuro-Ophthalmology.* St. Louis: C.V. Mosby Company, 1985.

Eden, John. *The Eye Book.* New York: Penguin Books, 1978.

Galloway, N. R. *Common Eye Diseases and their Management.* Berlin: Springer-Verlag, 1985.

Phillips, Calbert I. *Basic Clinical Ophthalmology.* London: Pitman Publishers Limited, 1984.

disability   There is no complete consensus on terms concerning the topic of blindness and vision impairment. Rehabilitation experts, doctors, educators, and other leaders in the field determine and define terminology according to their own preferences and viewpoints. In recent years, those involved in the field of blindness and vision impairment have made efforts to standardize terms such as disability to eliminate confusion or misinterpretation.

A disability may be defined as the way an impairment (a diagnosed defect or malfunctioning of a body part or organ) affects an individual's ability to function. It is the limitation, restriction, or disadvantage due to the malfunction.

See TERMINOLOGY.

divergence   Divergence is the movement of the eyes from a convergent position. Convergence is the turning-in movement of the eyes to focus on a near object. When the object is too close to the nose to be seen as one image, the eyes diverge, or move from the convergent position.

dog guide laws   All of the 50 states, plus Puerto Rico, have enacted statutes that regulate dog guides. All states guarantee the legal right of a blind person to be accompanied by a trained dog guide on all public transportation and in all public accommodations.

Public transportation is described as all modes of public conveyance and includes airplanes, trains, boats, buses, taxis, and elevators. Public accommodations are anywhere the public is invited. They include city streets, stores, restaurants, hotels, lodging places, resorts, amusement parks, educational institutes, and public buildings. The blind person cannot be charged a fee for the dog guide but is liable for any damage to the premises that the dog might cause.

Violation of the law by a person or organization generally results in a fine or imprisonment. Some states allow dog-guide users who are denied their civil rights to take the offending parties to court.

Although the above minimum statutes apply in all 50 states and Puerto Rico, some dog-guide laws designate specific restrictions while others extend rights. Some states require the dog guide to be in harness or compel the owner to muzzle the dog guide upon request. Others specifically note that dog guides may not occupy a seat or that the blind person must carry and show, on request, the identification card issued by the school that trained the dog. Others allow dog guides to be exempt from licensing regulations or fees.

In Hawaii, dog guides, like all dogs entering the state, must undergo a 120-day quarantine. However, dog guide users may stay with their dogs in special cottages on quarantine grounds. Dog guides are not exempt from the regular quarantine fee.

Some state laws order drivers to use every safeguard to avoid injury or endangerment to a dog-guide user traveling the streets. Drivers must yield the right of way to a crossing user and bring the car to a stop if necessary.

Many states include in the dog-guide law assurances that dog-guide users have the right to equal accommodation in commercial housing. The definition for commercial housing varies greatly from state to state. It may be described as one or more of the following: a self-contained dwelling unit; property offered for rent, lease, or compensation; group homes; residential communities; or public-assisted housing. Many states make specific exceptions for single-family private homes that offer one rental room only. Some stipulate that a fee cannot be charged due to the presence of the dog guide; others allow the landlord to levy a limited security deposit against possible damage incurred by the dog guide.

Some states express the right of dog-guide users to have equal employment opportunity in state employment, public schools, or any employment supported by public funds, so long as the person is qualified to perform the job.

A number of Canadian provinces have enacted dog-guide laws that closely resemble the basic statutes of those in the United States. Dog-guide users must carry a current health record for the dog guide, including proof of rabies vaccination, when crossing the Canadian-American border. Users are advised to include an identification card from the dog-guide training school and a muzzle, because in many provinces muzzling is required.

dominant eye   In normal, healthy eyes, one eye is usually in some degree dominant over the other. Eye dominance follows the same principle as right- or left-handedness and often complies with hand dominance.

In normal vision, both eyes focus on an object. Each eye sends a slightly different view of the sighted object to the brain where the two views are processed into one three-dimensional image. The normally dominant eye is the sighting eye that finds and focuses on the object, whereas the nondominant eye focuses just off center, the dominant eye is usually used unconsciously to look through a telescope, into a microscope, or through the sight of a camera. To find the dominant eye, punch a hole in a piece of paper and then, without thinking, quickly look through the hole. The eye used to look through the hole is the dominant eye.

Overdominance of one eye may affect or limit vision. If one eye or its muscles are weakened or impaired by conditions such as MYASTHENIA GRAVIS, MULTIPLE SCLEROSIS, brain tumor, STROKE, or infection, the eyes may become uncoordinated and fail to focus on the same object. When this occurs, DIPLOPIA, or double vision, results.

When one eye turns in (esotropia) or out (exotropia), a condition called strabismus, or crossed-eyes, occurs. The aligned eye becomes the dominant eye over the misaligned eye. Diplopia occurs as a result of strabismus. Strabismus may occur at any age but generally is present in young children. Strabismus may affect over 1.6 million children in the United States.

As the brain receives two images from the misaligned eyes, it relies increasingly on the dominant eye for information about the object viewed. It may begin to suppress the information from the nondominant eye, causing the vision to deteriorate from lack of use of the eye. This condition is known as amblyopia. The suppressed or amblyopic eye may become less functional or lose vision due to lack of light stimulation. Amblyopia usually occurs in young children and affects over 2.5 percent of all children in the United States.

An overdominant eye can often be corrected with surgery to repair or reinforce weakened eye muscles, or with nonsurgical techniques such as glasses, exercise therapy, or patching of the dominant eye. Early diagnosis generally results in the most favorable results.

double vision   See DIPLOPIA.

Down's syndrome   Down's (or Down) syndrome, or mongolism, is a genetic condition produced by a chromosomal abnormality involving an additional 21st chromosome. Down's syndrome is marked by mental retardation, mongoloid facial characteristics, small stature, heart abnormalities, and obesity. Down's syndrome occurs most often in children born to women over 35.

Ocular conditions associated with Down's syndrome include high MYOPIA (nearsightedness), hyperplasia of the iris, strabismus, narrow palpebral (eyelid) fissures, epicanthus (vertical folds of the eyelids), and cataract. Cataracts may be slight or serious enough to warrant surgical removal.

dreams   Dreams of the blind have long been a subject of interest to psychologists. Research, however, has been sparse, and few investigations have been launched into the activities and objects in dreams of the visually impaired.

Two early studies, Heermann (1838) and Jastrow (1888), drew four major conclusions that are still widely held today. They discovered that no visual images exist in the dreams of the congenitally blind, nor for those blinded before age five, but that the dreams of those who become blind between five and seven may or may not contain visual imagery and that most optical imagery tends to fade markedly with time.

McCartney (1913) discovered that dreams of the blind contained a high ratio of fearful objects in their dreams when compared with those of sighted subjects. Blank (1958) found that dreams of the blind contained more thought and language than those of sighted subjects, and Von Schumann (1959) related that intellectual activity, dynamic body movement, and falling were characteristic traits of dreams of the visually impaired.

Hall (1966, 1972) proposed that dreams, including those of the blind, must be continuous with waking behavior in that they must reflect actions or conscious thoughts or attitudes. The studies discounted the compensation theory that contends that dreams can embody complete reversals of waking tendencies.

Findings from separate investigations by Kirtley and Cannistraci (1973) and Kirtley and Hall (1975) agreed that the dreams of blind or visually impaired persons differed significantly from those of sighted persons in regard to the activities and objects found in the dreams. The investigators concluded that these differences are caused by the physical limitations and "special reality problems" of the blind that exist in their waking life.

Kirtley and Cannistraci created five categories—mobility, aggressive behavior, friendly interactions, self-perception, and perception of the physical environment—to describe the differences between the dreams of sighted and visually impaired persons. In their dreams, the visually impaired were more restricted in physical movement, and settings tended to be indoors rather than outdoors.

The dreams of the blind were lower in incidence of physical aggression, yet when incidents did occur, they were unusually extreme. There were few incidents of self-aggression. Verbal aggression incidents were much more frequent than those of sighted subjects. The study showed that the dreams of the blind contained more incidents of friendly speech and thoughts but fewer of friendly acts involving long-term relationships, physical contact, and gift giving.

The study cited more references to body parts and extremities, including the head, and fewer to clothing. Concerning the environment, the study concluded that blind subjects cited fewer incidents of building materials and descriptions of size, including thinness, narrowness, lowness, crookedness, crowding, and vacancy.

Kirtley and Sabo (1979) compared the dreams of visually impaired students, including partially blind, congenitally blind, and adventitiously blind individuals, with those of normally sighted students. The findings revealed that the dreams of the visually impaired group as a whole contained less symbolism than those of the sighted subjects. They concluded that the concreteness of the dreams was a result of the fact that blindness is an internalized stress condition that creates more waking-hour reality problems.

Sabo and Kirtley (1982) discovered that blind subjects tended to dream more often about food and drink; parts of the torso; land areas limited by boundaries such as cities, parking lots, yards, and swimming pools; and construction materials such as bricks, lumber, and boards. They concluded that this is a result of how the blind learn their environment and the limitations surrounding their handicap. The study revealed a significant number of active physical activities such as running, walking, and climbing but the activities tended to take place in a limited area or space.

Kirtley and Sabo (1983) compared the aggression content of dreams of visually impaired females and normally sighted females and found that the visually impaired women exhibited more verbal and covert aggression. These findings agreed with the Kirtley and Cannistraci (1973) report that found less physical aggression in the dreams of visually impaired persons (both male and female) but a higher incidence of verbal and covert aggression. Rainville (1994) concluded that dreams are extremely important in the rehabilitation of people who are newly blind. They are vital to a person's adjustment to blindness, he says.

Helen Keller described her dreams in her book *The World I Live In* and in the article "My Dreams." Although edited for print, they reflect the images of the visually impaired.

Keller related that her dreams were filled with sensations, odors, tastes, and ideas. She described seeing but not with her eyes and hearing but not with her ears. She explained that she did not often talk with her fingers or read with her fingers in dreams and that she possessed greater freedom of mobility.

She recounted seeing a brilliant light of "flash and glory." Keller mentioned colors such as the "velvety green of moss," "the soft whiteness of lilies," and the "distilled hues and sweetness of a thousand roses."

Keller, Helen. "My Dreams," *Century Magazine,* vol. 77, no. 1 (1908): pp. 134–165.

Keller, Helen. *The World I Live In.* New York: Century Company, 1908.

Kirtley, Donald, and Katherine Cannistraci. "Dreams of the Visually Handicapped: Toward a Normative Approach." *AFB Research Bulletin #27* (April 1974): 111–133.

Kirtley, Donald. *The Psychology of Blindness.* Chicago: Nelson-Hall, 1975.

Kirtley, Donald, and Kenneth Sabo. "Aggression in the Dreams of Blind Women." *Journal of Visual Impairment and Blindness,* vol. 77, no. 6 (June 1984): 269–270.

Kirtley, Donald, and Kenneth Sabo. "Symbolism in the Dreams of the Blind." *International Journal of Rehabilitation Research* vol. 2, no. 2 (1979): 225–232.

Rainville, Raymond E. "The Role of Dreams in the Rehabilitation of the Adventitiously Blind." *Dreaming* (1994): pp. 155–164.

Sabo, Kenneth, and Donald Kirtley. "Objects and Activities in the Dreams of the Blind." *International Journal of Rehabilitation Research,* vol. 5, no. 2, (1982): 241–242.

drugs Topical and systemic drugs are used in ophthalmology to treat eye diseases and disorders, to prepare eyes of examination or surgery, to treat or prevent inflammation, and to diagnose disease or disorders.

Mydriatics are drugs that dilate the pupils. They are generally either sympathomimetics or parasympatholytics. Sympathomimetics imitate or initiate the release of adrenaline and direct the action to the dilator muscle of the iris. Parasympatholytics dilate the pupil and retain it in position so that the pupil cannot accommodate its size to changes in light.

Generic sympathomimetics include phenylephrine HCl, hydroxyamphetamine HBr, and cocaine; trade names include Ak-Dilate, Efricel, Mydfrin, Neo-Synephrine HCl, Penoptic, and Paredrine. Generic parasympatholytics include atropine sulfate, cyclopentolate HCl, homatropine HBr, scopolamine, and tropicamide; trade names include Ak-Pentolate, Cyclogyl, Homatrocel, Isopto Homatropine, Isopto Hyoscine, Mydramide, Mydriacyl, and Topicacyl.

Miotics are parasympathomimetics that are used to treat glaucoma and ESOTROPIA. Cholinergic (direct-acting) miotics include the generic carbachol, pilocarpine hydrochloride, and pilocarpine nitrate, and the trade names Carbacel, Isopto Carbachol, Adsobocarpine, Akarpine, Almocarpine, Isopto Carpine, Pilocar, Pilocel, Pilomiotin, Pilopine gel hs 4 percent, Ocusert Pilo, Piloptic, and P.V. Carpine. Anticholinesterasic (indirect acting) miotics include the generic physostigmine sulfate, physostigmine salicylate, demecarium bromide, echothiophate iodide and isoflurophate (DFP), and the trade names Eserine Sulfate, Isopto Eserine, Humorsol, Echodide, Phospholine Iodide and Floropryl.

Ocular infections are treated according whether the infecting agent is bacterial, fungal, viral, or protozoal. Antibiotics are used to treat corneal ulcers and intraocular infections. Antibiotics may be topical or systemic and include the generic ampicillin, bacitracin, carbenicillin, cefazolin, cephalothin, chloramphenicol, clindamycin, colistin sulfate, erythromycin, gentamycin sulfate, lincomycin, methicillin, neomycin, penicillin, polymyxin B sulfate, silver nitrate, streptomycin, sulfacetamide sodium, sulfisoxazole diolamine, tetracycline, tobramycin, and vancomycin. They are known by numerous trade names, including Baciquent, Ak-Lor, Antibiopto, Coly-Mycin S. Ilotycin, Garamycin, Genoptic, Aerosporin, Ak-Sulf, Gantrisin, Achromycin, and Tobrex.

Antifungal drugs are used to treat infections such as fungal KERATITIS and fungal endophthalmitis. Generic antifungal agents include amphotericin B, nystatin, flucytosine, natamycin, miconazole, and ketoconazole.

Antiviral drugs are used to treat infections such as HERPES SIMPLEX. Generic antiviral drugs include idoxuridine, trifluridine, vidarabine (ARA), and acyclovir; trade names for these drugs include Dendrid, Herplex Liquifilm, Stoxil, Viroptic, Vira-A, and Zovirax. Two antiviral drugs, ganciclovir and foscarnet, are used to treat cytomegalovirus retinitis, an infection of the retina associated with AIDS.

Antiprotozoal drugs are used to treat some types of UVEITIS. These drugs include Pyrimethamine, Sulfadiazine, Clindamycin, and corticosteroid preparations.

Anti-inflammatory drugs are used to treat inflammatory disorders such as BLEPHARITIS, CONJUNCTIVITIS, KERATITIS, SCLERITIS, uveitis, and optic neuritis. Corticosteroids are often prescribed under the generic names hydrocortisone, prednisolone, dexamethasone, and progesteronelike compounds. Trade names for these drugs include Hydrocortone acetate, Optef drops, Pred Mild/Pred Forte, Inflamase, Ak-Dex, Decadron, Maxidex, HMS, and FML.

Anesthetic drugs may be topical or regional. They allow the physician to perform procedures on the eye. Topical anesthesia includes the generic cocaine hydrochloride, proparacaine hydrochloride and tetracaine hydrochloride, and the trade names Ak-taine, Alcaine, Ophthaine, Ophthetic, Anacel, and Pontocaine. Regional anesthetics include Tetracaine, Procaine, Hexylcaine, Bupivacaine, Lidocaine, Mepivacaine, Prilocaine, and Etidocaine.

Drugs used to treat glaucoma include sympathomimetics and parasympathomimetics, which increase the flow of AQUEOUS FLUID from the eye;

adrenergic antagonists and carbonic anhydrase inhibitors, which decrease the aqueous fluid supply; and hyperosmotic agents, which decrease intraocular pressure.

Adrenergic agents include the generic epinephrine bitartrate, epinephrine hydrochloride, epinephrine borate, dipivefrin hydrochloride, timolol maleate, levobunolol, and betaxolol. Trade names include E, Epitrate, Mytrate, Murocoll, Epifrin, Glaucon, Epinal, Eppy/N, Propine, Timoptic, Betagan, and Betoptic.

Carbonic anhydrase inhibitors include the generic acetazolamide, acetazolamide sodium, dichlorphenamide, and methazolamide, and trade names Ak-Zol, Cetazol, Diamox, Daranide, Oratrol, and Neptazane. Hyperosmotic agents include the generic glycerin, isosorbide, mannitol, and urea and the trade names Glyrol, Osmoglyn, Ismotic, Osmitrol, and Ureaphil.

Artificial tears are used to treat dry eye conditions. These drugs are known by the generic hydroxyethylcellulose, hydroxyproplycellulose, hydroxypropl methylcellulose, methylcellulose, polyvinyl alcohol, and other polymeric solutions. Numerous trade names include Clerz, Lacrisert, Isopto Alkaline, Muro Tears, Methopto, Methulose, Aqua Tears, Liquifilm Tears, aqua-FLOW, Refresh, Adapettes, Comfort Drops, and Hypotears.

Drugs are used in procedures to examine or test the eyes and diagnose disorders. Small strips of paper impregnated with fluorescein dye are used to test the CONJUNCTIVA and corneal epithelium. Sodium fluorescein is injected intravenously to study the circulation of blood in the retina and CHOROID.

Rose bengal is a solution used to test the conjunctiva and corneal epithelium for unhealthy cells.

Doctors and scientists are working hard to find new drugs to treat vision disorders, and new uses for existing drugs. One of these promising drugs is Visudyne, approved by the U.S. Food and Drug Administration in April 2000 and used in the treatment of the wet form of age-related macular degeneration. Representatives of the American Academy of Ophthalmology said they are hopeful that Visudyne will be the start of a new era in treating a leading cause of blindness among older people.

American Academy of Ophthalmology Medical Library. *American Academy of Ophthalmology Says Newly Approved Drug, Visudyne, Is Promising.* 2000.
Henkind, Paul, Martin Mayers and Arthur Berger, eds. *Physicians' Desk Reference for Ophthalmology 1987.* Oradell, N.J.: Medical Economics Company Inc., 1987.

dry eye   Dry eye is a condition in which the eye lacks the necessary amount or quality of tears. Tears protect, nourish, and moisturize the eye. Without proper tear function, the cornea and CONJUNCTIVA may become dry and develop disorders.

In the normal eye, the tear film is made up of three layers that are produced by the lacrimal gland and accessory lacrimal glands and cells. The lacrimal glands are located in the orbit and inner eyelid. The accessory glands and cells are located in the conjunctiva.

The top layer of tears is formed by the secretion of the meibomian glands and is oily in nature. The second layer is composed of watery tears from the lacrimal glands, and the third layer, which lies next to the cornea, is of mucuslike consistency and is produced by accessory glands. The layers are maintained by constant blinking and are all necessary for proper health of the eye.

Dry eye may occur as a result of poor tear production (called keratoconjunctivitis sicca), poor tear quality, or inadequate blinking, which leaves the eye open to the drying elements or does not properly wet the entire surface of the eye. Conditions that can cause dry eye include sarcoidosis, rheumatoid arthritis, vitamin A deficiency, pemphigoid, trachoma, Stevens-Johnson syndrome, chemical burns, neuroparalytic and exposure keratitis, and aging.

Dry eye may lead to corneal damage, permanent corneal scarring, and opacification. Once the cornea has opacified, vision is lost. Symptoms of dry eye include redness, discomfort or irritation, decreased corneal luster, and loss of visual acuity. Dry eyes can become extremely sensitive to wind, low humidity, heating, air conditioning, and so forth. Excess tearing may occur if the tears produced are inadequate in quality.

Dry eye is diagnosed through a thorough eye examination, including a slit-lamp examination, a Schirmer's test, and a tear film break-up test. The slit lamp is used to examine the tear film for the presence of extraneous microscopic filaments, epithelial cells, and corneal erosion that are apparent and will stain when exposed to rose bengal.

The Schirmer's test involves inserting one end of of a narrow strip of paper into the lower lid. The strip is left in place for five minutes during which time it absorbs tears. At the end of the time, the strip is removed and measured for the amount of tears present. Dry eye may be indicated if the measurement is less than 10 millimeters.

During the tear-film break-up test, the tear film is watched to determine the time needed to break the film once the blinking has stopped. The tears are stained with fluorescein dye and the eye is held open. In cases of dry eye, the tear film may break in less than 10 seconds.

Treatment of dry eye includes treating the underlying cause or disease and the administration of artificial tears. In some cases, antibiotics may be prescribed and the use of home vaporizers or humidifiers advised.

Surgery may be performed to close the tear drainage ducts to ensure better utilization of reduced tear production. If the cornea is severely scarred and vision is lost, a CORNEAL TRANSPLANT or keratoplasty may be indicated. However, those with dry-eye conditions are generally poor candidates for a successful corneal transplantation. Some medications that stimulate tear production are being investigated.

E

early intervention   A term used to describe programs and services offered to families of visually impaired children and preschools for visually impaired children. They provide information on home management and educational child-development skills and opportunities for children to develop skills and participate in socialization. The programs work closely with parents to maximize the potential for growth and development among these children. Services vary and may include home visitations, small group instruction, and community facilities programs.

The Individuals with Disabilities Education Act was signed into law in 1997. Formerly known as the Education of the Handicapped Act, the law mandates that services, such as early intervention programs, vision services, assistive technology and services, and transportation be provided for three- to five-year-old children with disabilities, including visual impairment.

The intent of the act is to provide appropriate public education to all eligible children. Schools must comply with the regulations of the act in order to receive certain funding.

echolocation   See SENSES.

ectropion   A disorder of the eyelids in which the lower lid turns outward. Ectropion is generally caused by aging but may result from scarring of the eyelids or nerve palsy. The exposure of the inner lid may cause tearing, irritation, and conjunctivitis.

Ectropion can be corrected with minor outpatient surgery using a local anesthetic. During the procedure, a portion of the sagging lid or scar tissue may be removed. Skin grafting may be required. Corrective surgery for ectropion may result in an over- or undercorrection of the problem. Complications may include bleeding, infection, or recurrence.

education   Formal education of the visually impaired prior to the middle 1700s was a private matter, lacking in systematic programs or educational formats. Many who lacked educated advocates or resources were not educated at all.

The first school for blind children, the Institution des Jeunes Aveugles (Institute for Blind Youth), was established in 1784 in Paris by Valentin Haüy. The residential school presented a curriculum orally and through embossed print or enlarged raised letters, read tactually.

In 1824, Louis Braille, one of the school's students, developed the BRAILLE method of communication. Braille is a tactually read language involving a series of configurations of raised dots based on a six-dot cell. The braille method made writing possible and reading more accessible to those with vision impairments and revolutionized the ability of blind students to obtain an education.

In the early 1800s, the first three schools for the blind were founded in the United States. In 1829, the New England Asylum for the Blind, later renamed the Perkins School for the Blind, was incorporated and opened in 1832 under the direction of Samuel Gridley Howe. In 1831, the New York Institution for the Blind, later renamed the New York Institute for the Blind, opened under the direction of Dr. John Dennison Russ. The Pennsylvania Institution for the Instruction of the Blind, now named the Overbrook School for the Blind, was started by Quakers in 1833 under the directorship of Julius R. Friedlander.

The schools were residential, privately financed, and based on the programs offered by the Institute for Blind Youth in Paris. The first students were children of families who could afford to pay the tuition and boarding fees.

The first tuition-free, state-supported school was established in 1837 in Ohio. In the next 45 years, over 30 additional public and private residential schools were established and constituted the sole source of education for visually impaired students.

Most of the current residential schools were established before 1900, and there is now at least one in nearly all of the 50 states. Those states without schools for the blind or visually impaired pay the tuition for students to attend residential schools in other states.

In 1871 at a convention of the American Association of Instructors of the Blind (AAIB), Howe, of the Perkins School, described and advocated a cottage-family-based system of education adopted in 1911 by John Bledsoe at the Maryland School for the Blind.

In Chicago in 1900, in reaction to demands from parents of visually impaired students for education with nondisabled children, Frank H. Hall, superintendent of the Illinois School for the Blind, directed one of his teachers to conduct an integrated program. The teacher, John Curtis, instituted a plan in which the city was divided geographically into grids. One school in each grid taught visually impaired students who attended regular classes and received services from special teachers in typing and braille skills. The grid program was widely adopted throughout the United States in following years.

The education system was altered in the years between 1949 and 1966 by two epidemics, RETINOPATHY OF PREMATURITY and RUBELLA. Retinopathy of prematurity (ROP), or retrolental fibroplasia (RLF), increased the population of visually impaired children by nearly 40 percent. The vision-destroying disorder was caused by overexposure to oxygen in incubation cradles. Low-weight, premature infants were primarily affected. Rubella epidemics in the mid-1960s caused disabilities to an additional 30,000 children, up to 20 percent of which included visual impairments. Both epidemics created a generation of students with special needs who outnumbered the facilities established to provide them.

The American Foundation for the Blind, the National Society for the Prevention of Blindness and other organizations sponsored conferences, service programs, scholarships for teacher training, and original educational objectives to meet future needs. As a result, day schools grew and expanded to serve over 80 percent of visually impaired students. Residential schools reevaluated their purposes and extended their programs to include multi-handicapped children.

Education of visually impaired children includes all the goals of general education for nondisabled children and encompasses teaching competencies skills to live, work, and play satisfactorily and successfully in society.

Special education is a supplement to general education that meets the needs and provides the skills necessary to achieve general educational goals for disabled students. It supplies adaptations or modifications to the general education curriculum, materials, learning methods, task skills, environmental factors, and teaching techniques.

Education of a visually impaired student is implemented by four major organizational bodies: the federal government, the state department of education, the local education agency, and organizations that serve the visually impaired.

The federal government, through the executive and judicial branches, enacts laws that shape and control education for all students in the United States. One such law, the Education of the Handicapped Act (EHA), also known as the Education of All Handicapped Children Act, ensures all disabled students, including those with visual impairments, the right to a free and appropriate elementary and secondary education in the least restrictive setting from ages six through 21. The law further ensures the right of parent participation in the educational and decision-making process, protects the rights of disabled students and their parents, and ensures the student of an individualized educational program.

The State Department of Education fulfills the requirements mandated by the laws and implements the EHA. A state consultant from the department acts as an advocate and facilitator for quality education for visually handicapped students. The consultant serves as a liaison to the public, the medical community, the U.S. Office of Education, teacher preparation schools, national organizations, and consumer groups.

The Local Education Agency (LEA), such as the school district or residential school, acts to provide the basic curriculum and special education according to the needs of the student. The teacher serves as the primary advocate for the visually impaired student within the school. The district or school program administrator is responsible to obtain services of a qualified teacher, to secure necessary resources to provide the needed services and to evaluate program effectiveness. The residential school in a state or district acts as an additional resource to all districts in the state.

Organizations that serve the visually impaired supply support services, resources, equipment, or materials to visually impaired students. They may supplement or enhance the program offered by the federal government. General or special education begins before the child formally enters school at age five or six. It begins at birth or as soon as possible after the visual handicap has been diagnosed.

Early intervention programs, services to families and preschools for blind and partially sighted children provide information on home management and educational child-development skills and opportunities for skills development and socialization. The programs maximize the potential for growth and development among these children.

Once a child has reached six years of age and is ready to enroll in kindergarten, he must be assured of a free and appropriate educational program. In order to ensure appropriateness, the school may request a formal student assessment to determine whether the student is eligible for special education services.

The assessment is conducted by a professional staff of educational, psychological, and medical experts. It must be complete, nondiscriminatory, and given with consent of the parent. Assessment may follow a regular periodic schedule of once a month to once a year and not less than once every three years.

Once the need for special education has been assessed and determined, an individualized educational plan (IEP) is developed. This written plan is a blueprint for the child's education. It lists the student's present level of educational performance, a statement of annual goals, a list of special educational services to be supplied, the dates the services will begin and end and the evaluation which will be used to determine whether the goals were met.

The needs and goals stipulated in the IEP will determine the setting where the education will be delivered. The student may have a choice of either a residential setting or a public school.

Those who attend public school are sometimes referred to as "mainstreamed" students. *Mainstreaming* is a term used to describe the practice of educating disabled students, including those with visual impairments, in a standard, public classroom for nondisabled children. Today, although residential schools still provide vital education and training services, the American Foundation for the Blind estimates that nearly 90 percent of disabled students receive all or part of their education in local public schools.

Students may be mainstreamed into a public school program through several models of delivery including the itinerant-teacher model, the teacher-consultant model and the resource-room model. These are three of five basic models or educational plans for the education of visually impaired students that also include the self-contained classroom model and the residential school model.

An itinerant teacher is one who travels to public schools to provide special education modifications to the instructional program of visually impaired children. The visually impaired student lives at home and spends most of the instructional day in a regular classroom.

The itinerant teacher visits every two or three days to work with the student in a section of the classroom, the library, the hall, the office, or any available space. The itinerant teacher provides special equipment, training, and materials adapted to the student's learning needs and consultation services to the regular classroom teacher.

The teacher-consultant is a special educator who advises regular classroom teachers, teacher aides, administrators, and other school personnel in methods that will meet the visually impaired student's needs. The greatest proportion of the work is consultative, rather than instructive.

The teacher-consultant travels from school to school, and often from county to county, to work with personnel. Since traveling time is significant, little time remains for direct instruction with the student.

The teacher-consultant model works best for students who work independently and require minimal skills training. The program is least effective for students who require intensive skills training or lack coping behaviors for study in a regular classroom.

The resource room is a specially equipped room staffed with special education personnel trained to work with blind or visually impaired students. The students live at home and attend public school in regular classrooms and are taught by teachers who provide general curriculum instruction. Students visit the resource room at regularly scheduled intervals or when needed. The resource-room teacher provides specialized skills instruction and counseling relating to vision loss and academic remediation. Special instruction may take place individually or in small groups.

The resource-room model has an advantage over the teacher-consultant and itinerant-teacher models in that it provides instruction or assistance immediately and according to the needs of the student. However, because of its availability, it may foster dependence and restrict growth toward independent working within a self-contained classroom.

The self-contained classroom is a classroom in a public school that is specially equipped and staffed with special-education teachers for the visually impaired. All the students in the class have visual impairments or other disabilities. The teacher of the class provides general curriculum instruction and special education. The program is designed to fit the unique needs of each individual.

Although one-fifth of all programs for visually impaired students centered on self-contained classrooms in the early 1960s, the model has since lost popularity except in large metropolitan areas serving multihandicapped blind students.

In order to achieve maximum enrollment, self-contained classrooms are centered in one or a few schools within a district. This often necessitates busing the visually impaired student to a school outside his neighborhood.

Residential schools are those in which visually impaired students live and receive educational instruction. It is the oldest form of education for the visually impaired and is offered in nearly every state. Many residential schools for the visually impaired share a campus or facilities with schools for the deaf and are referred to as "dual" schools. Residential schools may be either state operated or private. State operated residential schools are funded by state legislatures, are tuition free, and do not charge for room, board, or transportation. Private residential schools charge fees that may be paid by the public school district of the student.

The campus, schoolrooms, and educational program of residential schools are designed and equipped to meet the needs of visually impaired students. The educational materials and curriculum can be designed, or the students may be grouped, to meet each individual's instructional requirements. Trained staff, including houseparents, are on duty 24 hours a day to provide general curriculum instruction, academic remediation, compensatory learning-skills instruction, personal management and independence-skills training, and information counseling concerning blindness.

The residential-school model is superior to many other models in its attempts to meet all levels of student educational needs on an immediate basis. However, because students may return home only on a weekly or monthly basis, some students may suffer from a lack of familial contact or interaction with sighted peers.

The basic curriculum for the visually impaired student is identical to that of the nondisabled student. However, special education may include instruction or counseling in the areas of social-emotional development, living skills, orientation and mobility, communication, and vocational counseling.

Barraga, Natalie C. *Visual Handicaps and Learning.* Belmont, CA: Wadsworth Publishing Company Inc., 1976.

ERIC Clearinghouse on Handicapped and Gifted Children. *Research and Resources on Special Education: Abstract 13.* Reston, VA: ERIC, 1987.

ERIC Clearinghouse on Handicapped and Gifted Children. *Research and Resources on Special Education: Abstract 14.* Reston, VA: ERIC, 1987.

ERIC Clearinghouse on Handicapped and Gifted Children. *Research and Resources on Special Education: Abstract 19.* Reston, VA: ERIC, 1988.

Mitchell, Joyce Slayton. *See Me More Clearly.* New York: Harcourt, Brace, Jovanovich, 1980.

Scholl, Geraldine, ed. *Foundations of Education for Blind and Visually Handicapped Children and Youth.* New York: American Foundation for the Blind Inc., 1986.

Scott, Eileen P. *Your Visually Impaired Student.* Baltimore: University Park Press, 1982.

Education of the Handicapped Act **(EHA)** See INDIVIDUALS WITH DISABILITIES EDUCATION ACT.

electroretinography **(ERG)** The study of the function of the retina when stimulated by light. An electroretinogram is a test often performed to diagnose RETINITIS PIGMENTOSA and other eye diseases.

Retinitis pigmentosa (RP) is a group of progressive, hereditary diseases that cause retinal dystrophy or degeneration. First the rods, and then the cones, of the retina stop functioning. Early symptoms include night blindness and progressive loss of peripheral vision.

The electroretinogram may be necessary to confirm the diagnosis of RP. The test measures the electrical activity of the retina when exposed to light stimulus. Each eye is tested separately. One eye is first patched to exclude all light. Next, drops are administered to dilate the pupil of the other eye. Anesthetic drops are administered and a contact lens attached to electrodes is placed on the cornea of the eye. The chin is placed on a chin rest, and the patient looks into the test machine. Lights that stimulate the retina are flashed into the eye in both dark and light environmental conditions. The electrodes on the contact lens record the responses of the retina and produce a graph that is interpreted by the ophthalmologist.

employment The American Foundation for the Blind estimates that there are approximately 4 million working-age, adult Americans who report some type of vision loss that cannot be corrected. Fewer than 50 percent of visually impaired adults are successfully employed. And of those who are employed, one-third feels that they are underemployed and have a monthly pay that is 37 percent less than that of nondisabled workers. Blind and visually impaired people have the highest unemployment rate of any social or economic group in the country. This disparity of unemployment rates between disabled and nondisabled persons may be due to prejudice and misunderstandings concerning the abilities of disabled workers. Disabled workers may be perceived by management as high in absenteeism, difficult to supervise, and a safety risk; however, studies show that this is not true.

Because of inequities in the public labor market, some visually impaired employees may work in a protected or sheltered workshop or business enterprise. A sheltered workshop is any protected employment. Many are highly industrialized, produce a variety of goods and pay competitive wages. Sheltered workshops sell the goods to governmental agencies, including the military, through programs outlined and enforced by the Javits-Wagner-O'Day Act.

A business in the Business Enterprise Program (BEP) consists of a vending stand or short order, cafeteria-style stand. These businesses are given a priority for placement in federal buildings and are administered by the State Vocational Rehabilitation Agency under the Randolph-Sheppard Act.

With the advent of new technology that adapts job tasks to the needs of those with limited sight, and in response to recent legislation, visually impaired employees are increasingly seeking work in the competitive marketplace. As stated in federal law, discrimination in hiring due to disability is prohibited in companies that receive federal funds.

Blind prospective employees can get help from the National Federation of the Blind, which operates a program called Job Opportunities for the Blind (JOB) Targeted Jobs Initiative. The program is run in conjunction with major national employers to provide pathways for blind people to find jobs with good salaries and benefits.

Other agencies, such as the Lighthouse for the Blind and the National Industries for the Blind, also provide training programs designed to help blind people find and succeed at employment. (See VOCATIONAL REHABILITATION.)

American Foundation for the Blind. *Employment: An Introduction.* www.afb.org/info_document_view, 2001.

National Federation of the Blind. *Job Opportunities for the Blind: Targeted Jobs Initiative.* www.nfb.org/states/newjob.htm, 2000.

employment disincentives   Disincentives to employment exist within the disabled community as a result of the structure of federal benefits systems. Many disabled American workers receive federal benefits from the Social Security Disability Insurance (SSDI) program and, of them, a majority do not rejoin the workforce for fear of penalties associated with self-sufficiency.

Reforms, however, are under way to encourage disabled workers to rejoin the workforce. In 1986, revisions to the SSDI program allowed the recipients of SSI benefits to work and continue to receive limited benefits. In 1989, the Social Security Work Incentive Act was instituted, which provided greater opportunities for disabled people to work and still receive some benefits.

In December 1999, the Ticket-to-Work and Self-Sufficiency Program was established with the aim of providing SSI recipients more choices of employment services. The program calls for SSI beneficiaries to receive tickets, which they can then use to obtain vocational rehabilitation services, employment services, or other support necessary to find and keep a job.

The Ticket-to-Work program is being phased in over a three-year period. The first states in which disabled workers received tickets are: Arizona, Colorado, Delaware, Florida, Illinois, Iowa, Massachusetts, New York, Oklahoma, Oregon, South Carolina, Vermont, and Wisconsin.

More information about the Ticket-to-Work program is available from Maximus, Inc., a private firm that has been contracted by the Social Security Administration to serve as the program manager.

Contact:

Maximus, Inc.
866-968-7842 (toll free)
866-833-2967 (TTY) (toll free)

Johnson, Kurt L. *Incentives and Disincentives in the Vocational Rehabilitation Process.* Washington, D.C.: National Rehabilitation Information Center, 1983.
National Institute of Handicapped Research. *Rehab Brief: Work Disincentives.* Washington, D.C.: NIHR, 1980.
Roth, Wendy Carol. "Let Us Work!" *Parade Magazine,* 17 September 1989, pp. 16.
Social Security Administration, Office of Employment Support Programs. *The Work Site,* www.ssa.gov/work/index2.html, 2001.

endothelial cell count   An endothelial cell count is a measurement of the number of endothelial cells remaining in the cornea. An endothelial cell count is often performed prior to cataract surgery to determine the health of the cornea.

Endothelial cells line the inside of the cornea and protect it from the AQUEOUS FLUID of the eye. Loss of endothelial cells through aging or cataract surgery could cause a clouded cornea. The cornea requires enough endothelial cells prior to surgery to allow for cell loss during the procedure.

A presurgical cornea requires approximately 1,000 endothelial cells to function properly after surgery. The cells are counted by an endothelial cell camera, which is similar to a slit lamp or biomicroscope. The test is painless and accurate.

A low endothelial cell count may require surgical techniques to minimize cell loss. In addition, it may prohibit the possibility of an intraocular lens implantation, a procedure that causes some cell loss.

endothelium   The protective inner lining of the cornea. It is made up of a single layer of endothelial cells. The cells prevent the AQUEOUS FLUID of the anterior chamber from penetrating the cornea. A reduction of endothelial cells could allow seepage into the cornea resulting in swelling, loss of transparency and loss of vision. Endothelial cells are lost through the natural process of aging and through cataract surgery procedures. The cells are generally not regenerated by the eye.

The cornea requires a minimum of approximately 1,000 endothelial cells to maintain adequate vision. The cells can be accurately counted by an endothelial cell camera during an ENDOTHELIAL CELL COUNT. (See FUCH'S ENDOTHELIAL DYSTROPHY.)

enophthalmos   An inward displacement of the eye within the orbit. The condition appears as sunken or deep-seated eyeballs. The opposite condition is exophthalmos or proptosis (bulging eyes).

Enophthalmos may be unilateral or bilateral. It may be caused by injuries, tumors, or aging. Injuries may cause orbital fractures that result in enophthalmos. Aging may cause enophthalmos as fatty tissue within the orbit is absorbed and fails to support the eyeball at the former level. In cases that involve continuous DIPLOPIA (double vision) and cosmetic deformity, surgery may be required.

Tumors that cause enophthalmos are usually metastatic, or malignant tumors that originate in other places in the body but spread to the orbit through the blood stream. Metastatic scirrhous carcinomas are a common cause of enophthalmos. These fibrous tumors often originate from breast carcinoma in women and bronchogenic carcinoma in men. Such tumors may be treated with radiation or chemotherapy.

Degrees of enophthalmos may be measured with an exophthalmometer. As the instrument is held up to the eyes, mirrors on the device superimpose a millimeter scale over a side view of the eye. This enables the examiner to measure the distance from the lateral orbital rims to the corneal apices.

Measurement differences between the eyes are often given most importance since general measurements of exophthalmos vary greatly due to individual anatomy. A variance of 2 millimeters between the eyes is considered serious and worthy of further investigation.

entropion   A disorder of the eyelid in which the lid turns inward. The lashes of the lid scrape against the cornea and irritate it. The condition is generally associated with aging but may occur as the result of an injury, burn, conjunctival scarring, or TRACHOMA.

Entropion usually affects only the lower lid and is most common in those over 50. The disorder may be seen in newborns, but this condition often rectifies itself without treatment during the first few months of infancy. Entropion can be temporary or chronic. In temporary cases, it usually begins in response to something else, such as itchy eyes due to an allergy. The sufferer blinks hard to get rid of whatever is causing the irritation, causing it to become worse.

The condition sometimes respond to a treatment as simple as a piece of adhesive tape placed on the skin of the lower eyelid to prevent it from turning in. Eyelid surgery is performed to correct entropion. The surgery may be performed on an outpatient basis with a local anesthetic. The procedure may involve the removal of sections of the lid or excision of scar tissue with accompanying skin grafts. A TARSORRHAPHY, the placement of stitches to keep the lid in a permanent position, may be performed to hold the lid in an outward position.

enucleation   Enucleation is the surgical removal of the eyeball. Enucleation is performed when the eye contains a malignant tumor such as a melanoma, when the eye is blind and causes pain, and when the eye is nearly blind and sympathetic ophthalmia (an inflammation that occurs in both eyes as a result of injury to one eye) is a risk.

Enucleation is performed under general anesthetic. An incision is made in the limbus, the place where the SCLERA meets the cornea, and the CON-

JUNCTIVA is opened. The eye is severed and removed from the optic nerve and the six extrinsic muscles that hold it in place. The vessels are cauterized to stop internal bleeding. The membrane and muscles are tied together and the conjunctiva is stitched closed.

After a period of two or more days, the conjunctiva-lined socket of the eye is fitted with a plastic shell in preparation for an artificial eye or prosthesis. The prosthetic eye is fitted three to four weeks later. A prosthetic eye is generally undetectable from a natural eye.

esophoria   A condition of strabismus, or misaligned eyes. Often termed squint or crossed-eyes, strabismus may cause visual problems or loss of vision. Esophoria is a type of convergent strabismus in which the eyes tend to turn toward each other. *Esotropia* is a condition in which one eye turns inward.

As in all strabismus, the eyes view two differing subjects. The brain received the two images and double vision results. Often, in an effort to reconcile the two pictures, the brain may suppress the message received from one eye, reducing the vision of that eye. This results in a condition called amblyopia.

Strabismus is associated with high amounts of myopia (nearsightedness), hyperopia (farsightedness), and astigmatism. It can develop after a major illness or injury, and some forms of strabismus may also be hereditary.

Treatment may include the prescription of eyedrops, eyeglasses or bifocals, or exercises. Exercises or eye patching may be prescribed if amblyopia is present. Surgery may be necessary to completely align the eyes.

esotropia   See ESOPHORIA.

Eustis, Dorothy   Dorothy Eustis, born Dorothy Leib Harrison in 1886, founded the first dog-guide training school in the United States. The daughter of a prosperous owner of a sugar refinery, she was educated in Philadelphia and Eastbourne, England. In 1906, she married Walter Abbott Wood Jr., who died in 1915.

In 1923, she married George Eustis and moved to Switzerland to establish a breeding and training kennel to improve the working qualities of the German shepherd breed. She was joined in her work in 1924 by Elliot S. ("Jack") Humphrey, an authority on breeding and genetics.

Dog-guide schools had been established in Germany in answer to the need for German shepherd guides for blinded World War I veterans. Eustis became interested in dog-guide training and wrote an article about it for a 1927 edition of the *Saturday Evening Post.*

The article elicited interest in the project, and in 1929 Eustis returned to the United States to found the Seeing Eye, a dog-guide training facility in Nashville, Tennessee. At the time, attitudes in the United States were generally negative toward dog guides but changed toward acceptance as news spread of successful use of the dogs. Today, Seeing Eye Inc. is located in Morristown, New Jersey.

Everest Expedition   An event held in 2001 to promote the attempt of blind mountaineer Erik Weihenmayer to reach the top of Mount Everest, the highest spot on Earth. Sponsored by the National Federation of the Blind, the NFB 2001 Everest Expedition is intended to let the public know that blind people can overcome limits, and should never be considered helpless or dependent. The expedition began in March and the team of climbers reached the summit of Mount Everest on May 25.

exophoria   Exophoria is a condition of strabismus, or misaligned eyes. Often termed squint or crossed-eyes, strabismus may cause visual problems or loss of vision. Exophoria is a type of latent strabismus in which the eyes tend to turn outward, away from each other. Exophoria occurs when binocular vision is lost due to patching of one eye or when the individual is tired. *Exotropia* is condition in which either eye turns outward constantly.

As in all strabismus, the eyes may fail to converge on an object and view two differing subjects. The brain receives the two images, and double vision results. Often, in an effort to reconcile the two pictures, the brain may suppress one completely. This negation may result in a condition called amblyopia.

Strabismus can be associated with high amounts of myopia (nearsightedness) hyperopia (farsightedness), and astigmatism. It can develop after a major illness or injury, and some forms of strabismus may also be hereditary.

Treatment may include the prescription of eyedrops, eyeglasses or bifocals, or exercises. Exercises or eye patching may be prescribed if amblyopia is present. Surgery may be necessary to completely align the eyes.

exophthalmos   Exophthalmos, or proptosis, refers to a protruding forward of the eyeballs. The condition is usually accompanied by a retraction of the eyelids and infrequent blinking. The condition may be unilateral, involving only one eye, or bilateral, affecting both eyes. Unilateral exophthalmos may be the result of muscle palsy, a vascular condition, tumors, cysts, edema, or trauma and its accompanying hemorrhage and infection.

Bilateral exophthalmos is usually caused by hyperthyroidism, or Graves's disease. This disease is a disorder of the autoimmune system. It causes the thyroid to overproduce hormones that overstimulate the body's metabolism. Over half of those who develop Graves's disease develop Graves's ophthalmopathy, a condition in which the tissues and muscles of the eye are affected.

Pseudoproptosis (the false appearance of exophthalmos) occurs when the other eye has become sunken due to a fracture or trauma. The normal eye appears to bulge forward in comparison. An overly large eye, as in the case of unilateral high MYOPIA (near-sightedness) may also appear to be exophthalmic.

The amount of exophthalmos can be measured with an exophthalmometer. This instrument determines the degree of protrusion and symmetry between both eyes. Readings beyond the normal range of 12–20 millimeters may indicate exophthalmos.

Other tests may determine the underlying cause. X rays may illuminate a tumor, fracture, or erosion within the orbit. A CAT scan or biopsy may detect a pathology within the eye or orbit, and a culture of any discharge may identify an infection.

Treatment of exophthalmos must include therapy for the underlying cause. This may include antibiotics, steroids, radiation, chemotherapy, radiation iodine treatments, or surgery such as TARSORRHAPHY, a stitching of the eyelid, or removal of the mass causing the proptosis.

exotropia   See EXOPHORIA.

eye bank   Eye banks are organizations that acquire, evaluate, and distribute eyes from eye donors. The eyes are used for CORNEAL TRANSPLANTS, medical research, and educational purposes.

Donated eyes are necessary for corneal transplantation, or keratoplasty. According to the Eye Bank Association of America, more than 46,000 corneas were replaced by transplants in 2000, 90 percent of which successfully restored vision.

The cornea is the clear, curved portion of the eye over the colored IRIS. The cornea bends or refracts light to focus vision. When the cornea becomes clouded or damaged due to injury or disease, vision is decreased. Cornea transplantation replaces the damaged cornea with a healthy one to restore sight.

Eyes are donated anonymously from people who die. Donors may make their intention to donate their eyes known before death by a donor card or the section about organ donation on some state driver's licenses. The Uniform Anatomical Gift Act allows relatives of the deceased to donate the eyes if the donor has not provide written intention. Eye donors are not limited by age or degree of eyesight and pay no fee to donate their eyes.

The eye is enucleated (removed) from the donor as soon as possible after death. It is usually stored in special solutions or fixatives, or in some cases, it may be quickly frozen and stored at low temperatures. Tissue deterioration may occur if the eye is not treated within six to eight hours after death.

The eye bank evaluates the donor's general health, medical history, and the health of the eyes according to strict medical standards. After this evaluation, the cornea is distributed to the corneal surgeon who makes the final determination as to whether the cornea is suitable for transplantation. Tissue and blood typing and matching normally are not necessary in corneal transplantation, except in rare instances, such as cases of major chemical burns or graft rejection.

Corneas that qualify for transplantation are distributed to recipients according to fair, just, and equitable standards. Distribution is made without regard to age, sex, religion, race, creed, color, or national origin.

If the corneas are not suitable for transplantation, or the sight-restoring procedure of epiketophakia, the eyes are used for research and education. Because many sight disorders can not be simulated, donated eyes are valuable in the research of glaucoma, diabetes, retinal diseases, and other eye disorders and conditions.

eyeglasses   Eyeglasses, or spectacles, are devices that improve sight. They correct the refracting errors of the eye's lens and enable the wearer to see more clearly.

Eyeglasses contain a frame and a pair of lenses. The plastic or metal frame holds the lenses in place in front of the eyes. Side pieces of the frame that fit along the sides of the head and over the tops of the ears are called temples. The section of the frame between the two lenses that rests on the nose is called the bridge.

The lenses are specifically prescribed to correct the individual needs of the wearer. They can improve nearsightedness, farsightedness, astigmatism, and presbyopia. Lenses to correct nearsightedness, or MYOPIA, are concave in shape. Those prescribed for farsightedness, or hyperopia, are convex. Cylindrical lenses are incorporated into the concave or convex lenses to correct an astigmatism, a nonspherical shape in the eye's lens that causes distortions.

Presbyopia (aging of the eye) results in the inability of the eye's lens to change shape to focus on near objects. Bifocals are eyeglasses that correct this problem. They contain two lenses within each lens frame so that the wearer can adjust to near and distant objects without changing glasses. Trifocals add a third lens designed to help see distances of two to three feet.

Another type of lens, called progressive addition lenses, also contain different prescriptions within the same lens. They do not, however, have seams, as bifocals and trifocals do, which allow your eye to make a smooth movement from one part of the lens to another.

Lenses may be made of glass or plastic and are required by federal law to be shatter resistant. Additional coatings or filters may be added to the lens to screen out light or reduce unwanted glare and reflection.

Eyeglasses are prescribed by an ophthalmologist or an optometrist. The type of lenses needed are determined by an eye examination and vision test. The shape and width of the lenses is set by the shape and size of the frame, the length of the bridge, the weight of the lenses, and the shape of the head.

The eyeglass frame must be carefully fitted to the wearer to ensure optimal correction by the lenses. The center of the lenses must be directly in front of the eye, which may not necessarily be in the center of each lens frame. To center each lens, the distance between the pupils of the eyes is measured and recorded. The distance is also measured from the top of the ear to the place where each temple is attached to the frame. This measurement plus two inches is the amount needed for each temple.

New eyeglasses often require adjustment time. Nearsighted wearers may find that things look sharper but smaller with the new lenses. Farsighted wearers may notice that objects seem sharper but larger. Those with an astigmatism may feel off balance because the world looks temporarily slanted or curved. Bifocal wearers may need to develop additional head or eye movements to accommodate the needs of two lenses.

eyelids   Eyelids are the eyes' protection from environmental injuries. They shut automatically when an object threatens to enter the eye and provide protection from unwanted light. They blink to produce cleansing tears and have lashes that filter out dust and small debris.

The eyelids are subject to several conditions. BLEPHARITIS is an inflammation of the margin of the lid. The disorder is associated with allergies or dandruff. The lids become red, swollen, and crusty at the base of the lashes. In less severe forms of the disorder, temporary loss of lashes may occur. Severe blepharitis destroys the lash follicles and results in permanent lash loss and deformity of the lid margin.

A HORDEOLUM or sty is an infection of a lash follicle. A spot on the lid margin becomes red, painful, and swollen with pus. The sty eventually ruptures, drains, and heals itself if not treated.

CHALAZION is a swelling of the lid glands. The enlargement grows slowly and painlessly. It may be associated with an inflammation and can become a chronic condition.

PTOSIS is a sagging of the upper eyelid. It may occur as a result of aging or a neurological problem, such as lid muscle paralysis.

ENTROPION is a turning inward of the margin of the eyelid. As a result, the lashes often scrape against the cornea and inflame it. Entropion may occur after an injury or burn or as a result of aging.

ECTROPION is a turning outward of the margin of the eyelid. The inner lid is exposed to the elements, which results in tearing and irritation. Ectropion is commonly caused by aging.

Tumorous growths may develop anywhere in the eyelids. Benign cysts and tumors include papilloma, a viral tumor, "strawberry nevus," a reddish tumor, cyst of gland of Moll, a watery, clear cyst, and xanthelasma, a fatty tumor. Malignant tumors most often develop on the lower lid but may be found elsewhere on the lids. These include basal cell carcinoma, squamous cell carcinoma, keratoacanthoma and malignant melanoma.

TRACHOMA is a viral disease that infects the inside of the eyelids, causing scarring of this area, and eventually of the cornea. It is a common cause of blindness in developing countries with limited eye care and sanitation.

TRICHIASIS occurs when the eyelashes grow inward. This may cause a corneal irritation.

DACRYOCYSTITIS is an inflammation of the tear drainage sac caused by an infection. Symptoms include redness, swelling, and pain.

facial expressions   See NONVERBAL COMMUNICATION.

facial vision   See SENSES.

federal resources   A myriad of federal agencies exist for the purpose of providing services to individuals with disabilities. These agencies are administered under the U.S. Departments of Education, Health and Human Services, and Labor, plus the Veterans Administration and other agencies. (See Appendix for addresses.)

The U.S. Department of Education encompasses the Center for Libraries and Educational Improvement, which grants funds to states for library services for the blind and physically disabled and administers the Library Services and Construction Act. The Clearinghouse on the Handicapped provides information to the public concerning disabilities.

The Division of Blind and Visually Impaired administers the Randolph-Sheppard Act and aids state rehabilitation agencies in development of methods, standards and procedures. The National Council on the Handicapped develops policy and plans for the National Institute on Disability and Rehabilitation Research. The National Institute on Disability and Rehabilitation Research awards contracts and grants for research and demonstration projects concerning disabilities and directs training and research centers.

The Office of Special Education and Rehabilitative Services supervises the offices of Rehabilitation Services Administration, Special Education Programs and National Institute on Disability and Rehabilitation Research. The Office of Special Education Programs administers the Education of the Handicapped Act, provides funding to the states for the education of disabled students and funds personnel training, research, special program grants, demonstration grants, and scholarships.

The Rehabilitation Services Administration assists state agencies in vocational rehabilitation programs by providing leadership, grants, and demonstration and training programs. It awards independent-living grants for the disabled.

The Department of Health and Human Services contains the Administration for Children, Youth and Families, which operates the Head Start program and advises the secretary of Health and Human Services on issues and programs concerning early childhood education. The Administration on Aging aids states in developing programs for aging citizens and administers the Older Americans Act of 1965.

The Health Care Financing Administration is responsible for the Medicare program and awards state grants for Medicaid. The Health

Services Administration/Division for Maternal and Child Health Bureau of Health Care Delivery and Assistance controls state block grants for disabled children's services and maternal and child health services. The National Institutes of Health/National Eye Institute funds eye disease and disorder research and training of researchers.

The Office of Human Development Services administers the social services programs of the Social Security Act and supervises various agencies, including the President's Committee on Mental Retardation and the Administration on Developmental Disabilities. The Social Security Administration dispenses Social Security benefits, including disability insurance and Supplemental Security Income (SSI).

The Department of Labor controls the Employment Standards Administration Branch of Special Employment, which enforces laws concerning disabled workers in sheltered workshops and industry. The Office of Federal Contract Compliance monitors affirmative action as legislated by the Rehabilitation Act of 1973. The U.S. Employment Service controls the federal-state service program.

The Veterans Administration operates the Blind Rehabilitation Service, which administers programs for blinded veterans at Rehabilitation Centers and Clinics. The Department of Medicine and Surgery furnishes outpatient and hospital treatment and nursing-home care in Veterans Administration facilities. The Department of Veterans Benefits administers compensation and pension programs and provides vocational rehabilitation services and counseling.

Other agencies outside these departments include the Office of Civil Rights, which enforces laws prohibiting discrimination on the basis of race, color, national origin, sex, age and disability. It protects the rights of disabled individuals and investigates cases of discrimination due to disability.

The Library of Congress administers the National Library Service for the Blind and Physically Handicapped, which provides free library service to those unable to use standard print materials. The service provides braille and recorded magazines and books, talking book players, and cassette players.

The President's Committee on Employment of People with Disabilities is a partnership of national and state organizations and individuals that work to increase opportunities for the employment of disabled persons.

The Architectural and Transportation Barriers Compliance Board enforces the Architectural Barriers Act of 1968. The Committee for Purchase from the Blind and Other Severely Handicapped administers the purchase of products and services from nonprofit workshops as legislated under the Javits-Wagner-O'Day Act.

The Equal Employment Opportunity Commission monitors and enforces laws that prohibit discrimination on the basis of disability in the federal government. The U.S. Office of Personnel Management Governmentwide Selective Placement Programs Division sets policy for the employment of disabled individuals within the federal government. The Small Business Administration makes loans to small businesses owned and operated by disabled individuals as legislated by the Small Business Act. Contact information for these agencies can be found in an appendix in the back of this book.

fluorescein angiography   Fluorescein angiography is a type of ophthalmologic photography used to examine the retina and CHOROID inside the back section of the eye. The procedure, which is also called fundus photography, allows a more detailed examination than the ophthalmoscope.

In the procedure, fluorescein dye is injected into a vein in the patient's arm. As the dye passes through the retinal vessels and capillaries a specially filtered camera takes photographs every few seconds to record the flow. Analysis of the resulting angiogram can determine the presence of tumors or clogged or leaking blood vessels, diabetic retinopathy, or macular edema. Fluorescein angiography may be used after photocoagulation (sealing of blood vessels with laser treatments) to determine the results of the procedure.

fluorescein eye staining   Fluorescein eye staining is a procedure performed to examine the cornea, the transparent covering of the eye. The test allows the examiner to look for suspected scratches, irritations, or infections.

The examiner applies fluorescein dye into the eye by touching the lower eyelid with a fluorescein-laden paper strip. The dye covers the cornea and settles into any cuts or scratches of the surface. The excess dye is washed from the cornea with the natural tearing process.

The examiner observes the eye under an ultraviolet light. The fluorescein dye glows bright green, illuminating any irregularities such as cornea abrasions, ulcers, burns, or overexposure to light.

fovea   A small hollow or indentation in the macular section of the retina. The retina is an inner layer of the eye behind the vitreous. The retina contains millions of light-sensitive cells, including rods and cones. These cells give the retina image information that it sends to the brain.

The macula is the central section of the retina, which is packed with cones, the cells that distinguish detail and color. The fovea is in the center of the macula. It contains the highest concentration of cones. Light is focused directly on the fovea, making it the site of greatest perception.

free matter for the blind and handicapped   See MAILING PRIVILEGES.

freezing method   See CRYOSURGERY.

Fresnel prism   See PRISMS.

Fuch's endothelial dystrophy   Fuch's endothelial dystrophy is a hereditary disease in which the corneal endothelium is destroyed. It is a leading cause of corneal transplantation in the United States.

The endothelium is the protective inner lining of the cornea made up of a single layer of endothelial cells. The cells prevent the AQUEOUS FLUID of the ANTERIOR CHAMBER from penetrating the cornea. A reduction of endothelial cells allows seepage into the cornea, resulting in swelling, loss of transparency, and loss of vision.

The disease usually becomes apparent when a person is in his or her 40s or 50s. It is more common in women than in men. It is diagnosed from a slit-lamp examination by dystrophic spots in the endothelium. As the condition progresses, CORNEAL EDEMA or fluid retention and swelling develops, the cornea thickens and vision is lost. In later stages, blisters form on the epithelium, resulting in painful ruptures.

Early treatment of Fuch's endothelium dystrophy may include CORNEAL TRANSPLANTATION (keratoplasty), or replacement of a disk of healthy cornea for a disk of diseased cornea. Keratoplasty is not effective for later-stage dystrophy. Severe, painful forms of this disease are treated with cryotherapy; a cryoprobe is applied to the sclera of the CILIARY BODY to alleviate the pain.

Washington Academy of Eye Physicians and Surgeons. Fuch's Corneal Endothelial Dystrophy. On the Internet at: www.wa-eyemd.org, 2001.

fundus   The term for the back section of the inner eye. It contains the retina, the CHOROID, and the optic nerve.

The retina is the section of the eye where light information is processed and sent to the brain where it is transformed into an image. The choroid is the pigmented layer behind the retina that supplies the eye with blood. The optic nerve is the cord of nerve fibers that acts as a conduit to transmit information from the eye to the brain.

The fundus can be viewed with an instrument called an ophthalmoscope. This handheld instrument lights and magnifies the fundus for examination. Examination of the fundus, called funduscopy or ophthalmoscopy, allows the examiner to detect disorders within the eye and to determine other diseases of the body, such as hypertension, diabetes, and arteriosclerosis.

fundus photography   See FLUORESCEIN ANGIOGRAPHY.

G

galactosemia   A rare, congenital disease that prevents infants from metabolizing galactose, a sugar found in milk. Galactosemia occurs in about two of every 100,000 births. As a result of the inability to process the galactose, it accumulates in the blood and lens of the eye. The galactose in the lens absorbs water and disrupts the lens fibers forming vacuoles, or pockets of liquid in the tissue. Bilateral cataracts form from these vacuoles.

Cataracts may be avoided or reduced in severity by early removal of milk and milk products from the diet. Dense opacities may be surgically removed within the first month. Early extraction limits the possibility of developing amblyopia.

genetics   the study of genes, segments of DNA located on the chromosomes that carry information for all inherited characteristics. Genetics explores the heredity and variation of organisms and the conditions that affect them. Genetic disorders are diseases caused by gene abnormalities or irregularities. Genetic disorders may be evidenced at birth as congenital diseases or may surface as a disease or disorder later in life.

Over 3,000 major and minor hereditary disorders have been identified, 30 percent of which affect the eye. Hereditary and congenital diseases cause one in every five cases of blindness in the United States. Thousands more are affected by these visual disorders to a less severe degree. Genetic factors are the major cause of blindness for children from birth to six years. The cost of health care, aid to disabled persons, and lost income due to visual disorders, many of which are genetic diseases, is in the billions of dollars.

RETINITIS PIGMENTOSA (RP), a retinal degenerative disease, is the most common of all inherited retinal disorders. It affects approximately 100,000 persons and roughly one of every 80 persons carries the recessive gene for RP. The disease most often is diagnosed during childhood or young adulthood and may lead to blindness or severe visual impairment.

USHER'S SYNDROME occurs when those with RP are also born deaf. Usher's syndrome is the leading cause of deaf-blindness and accounts for more than half of all adults seeking rehabilitative services for deaf-blindness.

There is no treatment or cure for RP or Usher's syndrome. Low-vision aids may be helpful, and genetic counseling may help define the risks to relatives and future offspring.

Inherited macular disease, also called macular dystrophy, is almost always a genetic disorder that appears at birth or up to age six. This disorder destroys the macula, or center of sharpest vision of the retina. Although the disorder blurs and eventually may eliminate central vision, most patients retain some peripheral vision. There is no medication or

129

cure for macular degeneration but a small number of patients may benefit from laser treatments.

Genetic cataracts appear at birth or later in childhood as infantile or juvenile cataracts. The lens may be partially or completely opaque at birth. Surgery to remove dense cataracts may occur following the neonatal period, but it is often postponed until the density threatens to affect the child's performance at school or home. After surgery, patients may develop amblyopia or retinal detachments.

Some corneal dystrophies are genetic and may appear early in life or in middle age. Corneal dystrophies lead to the formation of opacities and may result in blindness or vision impairment. Treatment may include corneal transplantation.

SICKLE-CELL DISEASE is a single cell disorder that affects one in every 400 Americans of African descent. The trait is present in one of every 10 Americans of African descent. Sickle-cell disease may cause blockage of the blood vessels in the CONJUNCTIVA, CHOROID, or retina. Sickle-cell retinopathy and vision loss may result. There is no cure for sickle-cell disease. Visual complications are treated with varying results using scleral buckling and photocoagulation therapy.

Tumors may be genetic and congenital. RETINOBLASTOMA is the most common intraocular tumor in children. The malignancy is usually present at birth and may be inherited. It may occur in one or both eyes. Treatment often involves enucleation, or removal of the eye, but in less severe cases may include radiation, chemotherapy, or cryotherapy treatments.

Color blindness is a single gene disorder predominant in males. The inherited characteristic is transmitted by the male chromosome. The disorder does not affect the visual field or visual acuity.

Other diseases and conditions that result in visual impairments or blindness are genetic in nature. These include albinism, galactosemia, Marfan's syndrome, and Down's syndrome. Diabetes may also be linked to genetic defects that react to environmental or other factors.

Genetic research with an emphasis on the eye and vision continues. Recombinant DNA technology is producing new knowledge about gene function, diseases and treatments of the eye. The research strives to identify and confine the underlying genetic defects in cataracts, retinal degenerations, color vision disorders, and inherited ocular tumors.

Genetic counseling may determine the risk of disease for future children by determining the chances for recurrence. Genetic counselors also describe methods of diagnosis (such as amniocentesis) and recommend reproductive options.

Galloway, N. R. *Common Eye Diseases and Their Management.* Berlin: Springer-Verlag, 1985.

Kaiser-Kupfer, Muriel I., and Julian Morris. "Advances in Human Genetics—The Long Range Impact on Blindness and the Visually Impaired." *Yearbook of Association for Education and Rehabilitation of the Blind and Visually Impaired.* Vol. 2

Alexandria, VA: Association for Education and Rehabilitation of the Blind and Visually Impaired, (1984, 1985): pp. 46–49.

Maumenee, Irene. "Discoveries in Genetic Eye Disease." *Sight-saving* vol. 53, no. 4 (1984–85): 14–15.

gonioscopy Gonioscopy is a test to determine the width of the angle of the eye's ANTERIOR CHAMBER. This angle, formed by the cornea and the iris, is the place where fluid drains from the eye. If the angle becomes narrow or blocked, the fluid cannot drain effectively, pressure builds up within the eye and glaucoma may develop.

The angle of the chamber is examined with a *gonioscope,* sometimes called a gonioprism. This instrument is a mirrored lens, which the examiner holds up to the patient's eye. Gonioscopy is performed during glaucoma screening and the routine eye examination of a person with glaucoma. The procedure detects abnormalities or changes in the angle of the chamber and assists the examiner in prescribing treatment.

Gonioscopy is a routine part of a presurgical eye examination for those undergoing cataract surgery. The surgeon may administer cycloplegic or dilating drops prior to surgery, which could further restrict a narrow angle and cause complications. In addition, if an anterior chamber INTRAOCULAR LENS (IOL) implant is planned, the gonioscopy could indicate the amount of space, or lack of space, available to accommodate the implant.

Gonioscopy may be performed on any patient prior to the application of cycloplegic drops. During an examination or other procedure, cycloplegic drops may be used in a patient with a narrow angle if care is taken to ensure that the pupil has returned to normal size after the procedure.

gonorrhea A type of venereal or sexually transmitted disease. It is the most frequently reported communicable disease in the United States. Approximately 1 million cases of gonorrhea are reported each year, a figure that the Centers for Disease Control estimates to be roughly only half of all cases contracted in the United States annually.

Gonorrhea is caused by the gonococcus bacteria and may result in blindness when contracted congenitally. The disease is passed from mother to child during birth. As the child moves through the birth canal the eyes come into contact with the gonococcus bacteria growing in or near the cervix and become infected.

The infection, called gonococcal ophthalmia, or ophthalmia neonatorum in the case of newborns, causes severe conjunctivitis. Early symptoms include swelling and redness of the cornea, CONJUNCTIVA, and eyelids. Without treatment, the condition may progress to damage the cornea and result in blindness.

Adults may contract gonococcal ophthalmia by exposing the eyes to anything carrying the bacteria. Adults exhibit more severe signs and symptoms than newborns, including a copious pus-like discharge. Blindness can result from untreated cases. Gonorrhea in adults may be diagnosed from a Gram's stain or a cervical culture.

Treatment for gonococcal ophthalmia involves use of local antibiotic drops or ointments such as penicillin or tetracycline. Systemic or injected antibiotics may also be prescribed.

At one time, congenital gonorrhea was the leading cause of blindness in children. The passage of laws in all states requiring the administration of silver nitrate drops, or comparable antibiotics, to the eyes of all newborn infants has drastically reduced its incidence. Many doctors also recommend that pregnant women be tested for gonorrhea before giving birth.

grants Grants are available from the federal government to disabled individuals and agencies serving the visually impaired. The grants may be in the form of formula grants, block grants, or discretionary grants.

Formula grants are funds allocated to local and state governmental agencies rather than individuals or institutions. They provide support for established major state programs concerning the disabled. The amounts of the grants are determined by criteria such as population, per capita income, unemployment rate, and percent of population made up of disabled individuals or disabled veterans.

Block grants also provide ongoing support for programs for the disabled but are specially designed to fund programs that have been consolidated into another program and were formerly separately funded. Although states are allowed great discretion in dividing the block grant funds among the various consolidated programs, general guidelines of percentages are usually set.

Discretionary grants are distributed to state and local governments and dispersed to other institutions, including universities and private organizations. Unlike formula or block grants, discretionary grants fund small, undiversified programs. They are administered by a federal agency and often include grants for training, research, experimentation, demonstration, evaluation, planning, construction, fellowships, and scholarships.

The Office of Management and Budget publishes the *Catalog of Federal Domestic Assistance,* which describes federal programs, projects, and services that provide public assistance or benefits. The catalog lists goals, guidelines, eligibility requirements, application process, and specific interest location indices. The catalog is available from the Superintendent of Documents, U.S. Government Printing Office, Washington, DC 20402 (202-783-3238). It can also be accessed on the Internet at the Catalog of Federal Domestic Assistance website at www.cdfa.gov.

The *Federal Register* is a daily periodical that informs the public of all federal agency regulations, funding information, and policy changes. It provides information concerning federal grant background data, eligibility requirements, and funding information.

The *Federal Register* is available in public libraries and in many organizations that serve the disabled. It can be obtained through the Superintendent of Documents for subscription and is available on DIALOG Information Services and System Development Corporation. It can also be found online at the National Archives and Records Administration website at www.access.gpo.gov/su_docs/aces/aces.

Graves's disease   Graves's disease or hyperthyroidism is a disorder of the immune system. The Irish doctor Robert Graves first described the disease in 1835.

The disease is hereditary and affects approximately one of every 1,000 people. It is often diagnosed among young women and teenage girls or among late-middle-aged persons of either sex.

The disease was once thought to be caused by stress but is now recognized as a disorder of the autoimmune system. In this disorder, the immune system produces antibodies against cells in the thyroid gland causing it to overproduce hormones. The hormones, which regulate the body's metabolism, increase the metabolism in many of the body's tissues causing the symptoms of nervousness, weight loss, sensitivity to heat, and tremors.

Graves's disease is treated with medication or radioactive iodine treatments. Drugs such as methimazole, pills that block thyroid hormone production, may be prescribed. As a side effect, they may rapidly destroy the body's white cells and are therefore generally used for short periods only.

Radioactive iodine treatments involve drinking a liquid solution containing radioactive iodine. The iodine treatments destroy the thyroid gland after two to three months. After the thyroid gland ceases to function, a daily hormone supplement pill is taken to sustain appropriate hormone levels. The radioactive iodine treatments have been used successfully for 40 years and have relatively few side effects. In some cases, surgery to remove most of the thyroid gland is performed.

In some cases, Graves's disease may also develop into Graves's dermopathy or Graves's ophthalmopathy. Graves's dermopathy is a rare condition in which the skin becomes inflamed due to a dysfunction in the immune system.

Over half of all patients with Graves's disease develop Graves's ophthalmopathy. It is a condition in which the immune system attacks the muscles and tissues of the eyes.

Symptoms of Graves's ophthalmopathy may include mild conjunctivitis, tearing, eyelid retraction, protruding eyeballs, and impaired or constricted vision. Eyelid retraction and protrusion of the eyeballs may lead to exposure keratitis, an inflammation of the cornea and corneal ulceration.

Symptoms of Graves's ophthalmopathy may be exhibited in the absence of other symptoms of Graves's disease. It may be seen in patients previously treated with radioactive iodine or in those who are without thyroid dysfunction. The condition is serious, and although it may spontaneously resolve itself after three or four years, it can cause blindness before resolution if the condition is not treated.

If the symptoms are mild, the disease may be treated with antibiotic ointments for keratitis and tarsorrhaphy, a stitching of the lids, to improve lid retraction. In more severe cases, steroids may be prescribed to reduce swelling. Muscle surgery and surgery for decompression of the orbits may become necessary.

It is recommended that people with Graves's ophthalmopathy care for their eyes by applying cool compresses to sooth them. Also, wearing sunglasses protects vulnerable eyes from ultraviolet light and bright light, which can be uncomfortable. Lubricating eyedrops may relieve dry, scratchy sensations on the eyes. And elevating the head to keep the head higher than the body reduces the blood flow to the head and may relieve pressure on the eyes.

guide horses   Used in much the same way as guide dogs, guide horses are a mobility alternative for visually impaired people. They typically are small horses, known as dwarfed or pigmy horses. Although horses have been recognized for their ability to guide and lead for many years, they only recently have been trained to assist visually impaired people.

The Guide Horse Foundation, located in North Carolina, trains horses that meet the criteria to be a guide horse and provides the animals free of charge to visually impaired people who qualify. The horses must pass a physical examination by an equine veterinarian and are tested for intelligence. They must be no more than 26 inches high at the withers, must have structurally sound legs, and demonstrate good stamina.

Guide horses are recommended for rural or suburban use. They are popular among blind people who are allergic to dogs or afraid of dogs, those who love horses, and those who want an animal with a longer life span than a dog has. Dwarfed horses typically live to be between 25 and 35 years old and have been known to live to be 50. Advocates say that horses are easier for people who have physical disabilities to use than dogs are, due to the docile nature of the dwarfed animals. And, some people prefer using horses because they can be housed outside. Horses are natural guide animals, have good memories, and remain calm in difficult situations when trained to do so. Because their eyes are located on the sides of their heads, they have a very wide range of vision. They also have very good night vision. They are trained to wear special sneakers so they do not skid on smooth surfaces.

The Guide Horse Foundation reports that dwarfed horses are very clean and can be housebroken. They do not get fleas, and horses shed only twice a year. Although the organization recognizes that guide horses are not right for everyone, it claims that many people do extremely well with the small animals and are able to move very confidently with them. More information about guide horses can be obtained by contacting:

Guide Horse Foundation
2729 Rocky Ford Road
Kittrell, NC 27544
252-433-4755

H

handicap   There is no complete consensus on terms concerning the topic of blindness and vision impairment, since experts in the field (educators, rehabilitation specialists, doctors) define the TERMINOLOGY according to their own preferences and viewpoints. In recent years, those involved in the field of blindness and vision impairment have made efforts to standardize terms such as handicap to eliminate confusion or misinterpretation.

The word *handicap* stems from "cap in hand," a reference to beggars. Because of this negative connotation, the word *disability* is often the preferred term. When the term *visually handicapped* is applied to a child it usually refers to the requirement for special educational provisions due to the sight loss.

haptic sense   The haptic sense refers to the sense of touch. It is used extensively by blind and visually impaired individuals to gather information. The other senses of hearing, taste, smell, and sight are associated with a central organ to receive the information and transmit it to the brain. The haptic sense is not centrally located but receives information throughout the body via the skin.

The haptic sense defines temperature, shape, size, texture, moisture and consistency, movement, and presence. It is used as a compensation for sight, as in the performance of tasks, or perceptually, as in reading braille or using an abacus. Early stimulation of the haptic sense is especially important to blind infants and children. It helps to link the infant to the surrounding world and indicate the presence of a protective or loving person.

Blind infants and children rely heavily on the haptic sense for developmental progress. Since the lips and hands of the body have large concentrations of sensitive haptic receptors, blind children tend to mouth and handle objects longer than sighted children in an effort to gain information. Blind and visually impaired children rely on the haptic sense for aid in movement and exploration, essential developmental activities. Tactual experiences such as fondling a stuffed animal may be stimulating for a blind child and alleviate the need to develop self-stimulating behaviors such as rocking.

Factors such as the ability to move the hands, finger dexterity, wrist flexibility, and motor control may affect the effectiveness of the haptic sense. If the haptic sense itself is impaired, information gathering may be impaired. Those who have lost sensitivity of touch in the fingertips due to diabetic neuropathy may be unable to feel the detail necessary to read braille, and those with motor-control problems may be unable to direct the hands in place to gather information.

heat cautery   See PHOTOCOAGULATION.

hemianopsia   A loss of vision in one-half of the eye. This results in a loss of the right or left half of the field of vision. Objects or people in the field of vision may appear to be cut in half.

Hemianopsia is a common symptom of migraine headaches. It occurs during the preheadache or prodrome stage. The loss of vision may be accompanied by shimmering zigzag light patterns and blind spots called scotomas. Hemianopsia accompanying migraines usually lasts from five minutes to one hour. The lost vision generally returns with the onset of the headache.

Retinal migraine occurs when a spasm occurs in the blood vessels in the retina of one eye. One half of the vision of the affected eye is lost but the unaffected eye retains full vision. The condition is temporary and abates with the migraine.

Hemianopsia is also associated with strokes. As a result of a stroke, vision may be blurred or lost in one half of the field of vision, or the entire vision in one eye may be lost. Recovery of this visual loss depends on the damage done during the stroke and the progress made during recovery.

As a result of a focal transient ischemic attack, a temporary disruption of the flow of blood to the brain and eye, the vision may be lost and then may suddenly return in a matter of minutes. Usually, the vision lost due to these attacks is completely recovered within 24 hours.

herpes simplex   A virus that causes most corneal blindness due to infection in the United States. According to the National Institutes of Health, 500,000 cases of ocular herpes simplex are diagnosed each year. Herpes simplex is the most common virus found in humans.

Herpes simplex is one of four types of herpes virus that also include HER-PES ZOSTER, cytomegalovirus, and Epstein-Barr virus. Herpes simplex may infect the genitals, skin, brain, and eyes. All herpes viruses contain a central core of DNA, the genetic code of the organism, enveloped by a layer of protein. The organism cannot reproduce itself but must obtain reproduction molecules from a healthy host human cell. The virus invades a healthy cell and uses its molecular properties to reproduce. After prolific reproduction, the host cell may burst.

Herpes simplex virus cells usually enter the body through the mouth, genitals, or eyes. In the past, those infections that occurred above the waist were commonly referred to as Type I, and those below the waist

were referred to as Type II. However, the above and below the waist cat-
egorizations are used less commonly since Type I herpes is now frequently
seen below the waist and Type II is increasingly diagnosed above the waist.

Approximately 90 percent of the population has been exposed to and
infected by herpes simplex. Most first infections are generally Type I and
usually infect the mouth. The symptoms of fatigue and a low-grade fever
may go unnoticed. Others may have a more severe infection that is called
primary herpes. In each case, the infection appears to run its course, and
the symptoms disappear.

After the symptoms subside, the virus has not been killed. Herpes simplex Type I passes through nerves in the mouth or skin to deep nerve tissue centers, called ganglia, located the base of the brain and upper spinal
cord. Herpes Type II travels through nerves to the ganglia at the base of
the spinal cord. Here the virus lies dormant. The virus may remain dormant or reactivate and reinfect the body. During latency, healthy host cells
are not infected, and the virus cannot be passed to others.

Herpes simplex may infect the eyes in one of three ways: congenitally,
primarily, or recurrently. Congenital herpes is contracted by infants during
birth. If the mother has active genital herpes, the infant may become
exposed to the virus when the water breaks or when traveling through the
birth canal. It is estimated that 1 of every 7,000 births involves infection
of the newborn from the maternal reproductive system.

Congenital herpes is a serious disease that carries a fatality rate of 50
percent. Survivors may retain permanent damage to the eyes, brain, liver,
or kidneys. Damage to the eyes usually concerns the retina but may also
entail the CONJUNCTIVA, optic nerve, lens, and cornea.

If the mother is aware of an active case of genital herpes, a Caesarean
section delivery may avoid newborn infection. However, mothers are
often unaware of the infection when the symptoms are mild or hidden, or
when the virus is a first infection. In these cases, congenital herpes may be
unpreventable.

Primary herpes infection of the eyes is rare in adults and generally
occurs only in children or adolescents. The symptoms include fever,
fatigue, swollen eyelids, CONJUNCTIVITIS, and a blistering rash around the
eyes. The infection is usually mild and short-lived. It can be treated with
antiviral eye drops or ointments.

Recurrent ocular herpes is an eye infection, usually involving only one
eye, which happen as a result of a reawakening of the herpes virus. The
virus, which may have first infected the mouth, travels to the fifth nerve
ganglion, the trigeminal, where it remains dormant. The fifth ganglion has
connecting fibers to the upper part of the face, including the eyes. On reac-
tivation, the virus travels back up these fibers and infects the eye.

A recurrent infection is typified by redness, pain and a watery discharge
of the eye. Herpes keratitis, or corneal infection, iritis, an infection of the
iris, glaucoma, and cataracts may result from this infection. As the eye

attempts to heal itself, corneal scarring may develop, followed by loss of vision. Each recurrence increases the possibility of scarring and vision loss.

Most patients do not experience a recurrence after an initial recurrent attack. A patient has a 25 percent chance of a new recurrence within five years of the first and the possibility of additional recurrences increases with each attack. However, the virus is unpredictable, and the recurrences may suddenly discontinue for no known reason.

Herpes keratitis is treated with the drugs vidarabine, trifluridine, idoxuridine, acyclovir, and antiviral eye drops or ointments. These drugs are not a cure for herpes. They stop the reproduction of viral cells but cannot rid the body of the virus. During periods of dormancy, the drugs are ineffective in fighting the virus.

Severe scarring is treated with cortisone eye drops. Cortisone is a steroid that may actually worsen the herpes infection and is therefore used only for short periods of time. Severe vision loss due to scarring may in some cases be corrected with a CORNEAL TRANSPLANT, or keratoplasty.

U.S. Department of Health and Human Services. *Vision Research: Report of the Corneal Diseases Panel.* vol. 2, part 2, NIH Publication No. 83-2472 (1987) Washington, D.C.: USDHHS.

Review of Optometry Online. "Handbook of Ocular Disease Management, Herpes Simplex Keratitis." www.revoptom.com/handbook/sect3m: 2001.

herpes zoster   Herpes zoster, or shingles, is a painful skin disease that may involve the eye. It is caused by the same virus that causes chicken pox or varicella. According to the National Institutes of Health, it is responsible for roughly 7 percent of all skin disorders, a substantial amount of which affect the eye. If you have shingles on your face to any extent, it is extremely important to see your eye doctor promptly.

Generally, only one eye is affected. Complications may include corneal ulcers, scarring and cataracts, which can cause loss of vision. Additional conditions may include recurrent KERATITIS (corneal inflammation), increased eye pressure resulting in glaucoma, UVEITIS, secondary infections, and eye-muscle paralysis.

Treatment of eye disease caused by zoster is problematic. Corneal ulcers are often treated with soft contact lenses that remain on the affected eye for a period of months until the ulcers heal.

Keratitis is treated with antiviral drops or ointments. These drugs are effective only when the virus is active. During periods of latency, they are impotent. Since the virus is not destroyed, it may become active again and the keratitis may recur.

Glaucoma is treated with medication or eye drops and cataracts may eventually be removed. Eye muscle paralysis is not treatable with medication or therapy but usually heals itself in time.

Zoster scarring causes unique problems. Vision loss caused by zoster scarring cannot be corrected by corneal transplantation. The scarred cornea becomes vascularized, a condition in which blood vessels invade the cornea and interfere with post-transplantation healing. In addition, there may be lid abnormalities and epithelial or tear function disorders as a result of the scarring, which further complicate a transplant. An unsuccessful cornea transplant may develop complications during healing that could result in the loss of the eye.

U.S. Department of Health and Human Services. *Vision Research: Report of the Corneal Diseases Panel,* vol. 2, part 2, NIH Publication No. 83-2472 (1987). Washington, D.C.: USDHHS.

Hoover, Richard E.   Richard E. Hoover is credited with developing the long cane foot travel system, a method of independent traveling using a long cane as an aid.

Born in 1915, Hoover began as a teacher and physical training coach at Maryland School for the Blind. At the time, there was no comprehensive system for teaching blind people how to use the existing cane of the time, the white cane. Hoover found the white cane too short, heavy, and awkward for efficient mobility use.

As an army sergeant (and later lieutenant) in World War II, he was transferred to the Valley Forge General Hospital in Phoenixville, Pennsylvania, to work as the eye center's director of physical reconditioning, orientation, and recreation. Convinced that the men needed a lighter, longer cane, he experimented with several adaptations of the white cane until he developed the prototype for the long cane. The new cane was made of metal with a plastic tip and a crook at the top. It was up to 10 inches longer than the white cane, half the diameter, and weighed only seven ounces.

Hoover developed a series of techniques for using the long cane in sweeping arc movements, low, in front of the body, rather than by the side. The techniques were incorporated into the orientation and mobility program that was then transferred to the Veterans Administration Hospital at Hines, Illinois, where word of its achievements spread.

Today, the Hoover methods and the long cane are universal components of orientation and mobility programs. Hoover entered medical school after World War II and became a distinguished ophthalmologist. He died in 1986.

hordeolum   An infection on the outside or inside of the eyelid, also called a sty. An external hordeolum is an infection of an eyelash follicle. As the sty begins to form, the entire lid swells and becomes painful. A localized area on the lid margin then becomes red and swollen with pus. If untreated, the sty eventually bursts, drains, and heals itself.

An internal hordeolum is a sty on the inside of the eyelid. It is the result of an infection of a gland. If untreated, the hordeolum becomes inflamed and swollen, and is called a chalazion. These chalazia normally do not affect vision unless they are located in the middle of the upper eyelid, where they can flatten the central cornea and distort sight. Sties can be treated by holding a warm, damp cloth over the site for 20 minutes, three or four times a day. Most sties and chalazia go away on their own, without medication.

Howe, Samuel Gridley   Samuel Gridley Howe was born in 1801 in Boston. He graduated from Harvard Medical School in 1824 and offered his services for six years as a soldier and surgeon to Greece during the Greek War of Independence against Turkey. He continued to raise money for relief shipments after his return to America in 1831.

In 1829, the New England Asylum for the Blind, the first school for the blind in the United States, was incorporated. In 1831, the state of Massachusetts hired Howe to serve as director. Howe journeyed to Europe to study prototypes and returned in 1832 with two teachers. He opened the school in his home with six pupils. The school was renamed the New England Institution for the Education of the Blind and finally the Perkins School for the Blind after a wealthy philanthropist, Thomas Handasyd Perkins, who donated a mansion to house the school.

Howe developed new methods and devices for instruction of the blind, including a variation of raised-letter printing and textbooks on geography, grammar, and spelling. He became internationally renowned for his successful instruction of Laura Bridgman, a deaf-blind girl who became his student in 1837.

Howe founded a school printing department in 1831 to produce reading materials for the students. In 1879, three years after his death, the printing department was named the Howe Memorial Press in his honor.

Throughout his 44 years as director of Perkins School, he maintained an activism in the abolition of slavery and reform of public schools, prisons, and treatment of the insane. In 1843, he married Julia Ward, author of the words for "The Battle Hymn of the Republic." He died in 1876.

hypertropia   A condition of strabismus, or misaligned eyes. Often termed squint or crossed-eyes, strabismus may cause visual problems or loss of vision. Hypertropia is a type of strabismus in which one eye turns upward. *Hypotropia* is condition in which one eye turns downward. As in all strabismus, the eyes fail to converge on an object and view two differing subjects. The brain receives the two images, and double vision results. Often, in an effort to reconcile the two pictures, the brain may suppress one completely, causing partial vision loss. This results in a condition called amblyopia.

Strabismus is associated with high amounts of MYOPIA (nearsightedness), hyperopia (farsightedness) and astigmatism. It can develop after a major illness or injury, and some forms of strabismus may also be hereditary.

Treatment may include the prescription of eye drops, eyeglasses or bifocals, or exercises. Exercises or eye patching may be prescribed if amblyopia is present. Surgery may be necessary to completely align the eyes.

hyphema   A bleeding into the ANTERIOR CHAMBER of the eye. Hyphemas may occur as a result of an injury or following intraocular surgery such as cataract removal. Hyphemas may appear spontaneously due to diabetes-related neovascularization, tumor, juvenile xanthogranulomatosis, or previous vascular occlusions.

Hyphemas due to injury are caused by damage to blood vessels in the iris or CILIARY BODY. In most cases, the bleeding slows and then ceases, and the blood is reabsorbed within the eye over a period of a week. Secondary bleeding that starts one to five days following the injury may fill the anterior chamber and elevate intraocular pressure.

The raised intraocular pressure of secondary bleeding may cause secondary glaucoma, a serious result for which children are particularly at risk. The cornea may also become permanently bloodstained, causing an opacity or clouded area.

Hyphemas due to surgery are common but much less likely to result in secondary bleeding. The bleeding generally recedes within days, and no further treatment of hyphema is necessary.

Hyphemas are treated initially to prevent secondary bleeding and its consequences. Treatment varies according to the practitioner. Patients may be admitted into the hospital, confined to bed rest for several days, treated with cycloplegics, which widen the pupil, or with steroids or undergo patching of the eyes.

Secondary bleeding may be treated surgically. Medication is given to reduce intraocular pressure. The hyphema may be removed or flushed out of the eye with a saline solution.

hypotropia   See HYPERTROPIA.

hysterical blindness   An emotionally caused condition of blindness. The blindness occurs as a result of the need to physically resolve an emotional upset or shock. It also is called psychogenic or psychic blindness.

The blindness is usually bilateral and often occurs suddenly. Often the blindness is not total and is restricted to a particular field. Additional symptoms of hysterical blindness include lack of regard for the loss of sight, ability to travel within surroundings, and normal blink response.

An eye examination is necessary to diagnose hysterical blindness. The examination reveals that the pupils react normally, and the fundus (back of eye) appears normal, discounting damage to the optic nerve, cortical blindness, chiasmal lesions, or other ocular disease. The condition is usually diagnosed in light of information gathered through the eye examination and study of the patient's psychological history.

Treatment of hysterical blindness may include reassurance to the patient that the condition will right itself, presentation to the patient of ability to see, and placebo medicine therapy. The patient may recover from the hysterical blindness only to replace it with another physical illness. Psychiatric counseling is often recommended to address the underlying emotional problem.

Hysterical blindness is not to be confused with malingering, a condition of feigned blindness often undertaken as an attempt to receive continued compensation for an accident or injury.

idoxuridine   An antimetabolite drug used in the treatment of ocular HER-PES. It is also called IDU, Herplex, Stoxil, and Dendrid. It was one of the first drugs developed for the treatment of herpes keratitis, a disorder involving corneal inflammation.

Idoxuridine is activated by enzymes contained in healthy human cells and cannot differentiate between viral and healthy cells. Therefore, while it is effective in destroying viral cells, it unfortunately may attack and destroy healthy cells. Because of the toxicity, idoxuridine cannot be taken intravenously; possible side effects could cause potentially dangerous disorders.

Idoxuridine is available in ointment or eye-drop form. Normal dosing for the ointment is to apply it five times per day. The eye drops normally are administered every hour during the day and every two hours during the night. The period of use for either form is roughly two to three weeks. Dosing varies from patient to patient, however, so the doctor's instructions should be followed.

Idoxuridine is not a cure for herpes keratitis. It is only effective once the virus is active. During periods of latency, the drug is ineffective against the virus. Its ocular side effects include redness and swelling of the conjunctiva and possible irritation of the cornea.

illumination   The density of light falling on a surface. Illumination is a factor in visibility, and control of illumination may result in improved vision for those with impairments.

To properly control illumination, type of light source, intensity of the light source, distance from the light source, surface the light falls on, diffuseness, the amount of glare, and environmental changes must be considered. The best lighting situations involve properly intense, diffuse light from overhead (or the side of usable vision if reading with one eye only) that causes the least amount of shadows and glare.

Light sources commonly include daylight, incandescent light, and fluorescent light. Daylight varies according to time of day and weather conditions. Incandescent lights simulate daylight but in a constant, steady flow. Fluorescent lights may flicker but can be linked and adjusted to eliminate the flicker.

Specially designed lights may be used to maximize residual vision. The BLBS (Better Light Better Sight) lamp is a study lamp constructed according to requirements of the Illuminating Engineering Society of America and incorporates ideal lighting components.

Tensor-type lamps are intense lights that can be adjusted for maximum illumination with limited glare. Small clip-on lamps are available that attach to the sides of spectacle frames.

The intensity of light is measured in footcandles. One footcandle equals the intensity of light that falls on one square foot of a surface located one foot from one international candle.

The intensity of light on an object is controlled by the distance from the light to the object. A lamp two feet from the reading page has four times the light intensity as a lamp four feet away.

The surface the light falls on affects the visibility. An uneven surface may contribute to uneven diffuseness of light, and a smooth, reflective surface may increase glare.

Diffuseness is the distribution of light. Shadows and spotlights may decrease visibility. Glare results from an excess of light, a concentration of light, or an uneven distribution of light, and may decrease visibility.

Illumination may be controlled or manipulated by making changes in the environment as well as the light source. Light transmission, reflection control, and contrast enhancement may be used to maximize available illumination.

Light transmission is improved through lenses, filters, and absorptive lenses that reduce glare and highlight contrast for those with light sensitivity, or photophobia. Lenses, filters, and absorptive lenses are available in a wide range of degrees of protection from simple filters that reduce glare to photochromic lenses that use gray, green, and amber filters to block all ultraviolet light.

Reflection is controlled by visors, side shields, specially treated lenses, and typoscopes. Visors may be supplied by the brim of a hat or can be a filtering visor lens attached to the spectacle frame. Sideshields are filters that attach to the sides of spectacle lenses to control the light on the sides of the eyes.

A typoscope is a slit reading device that isolates one line of type at a time, thus reducing glare from the light reflected from the page. Typoscopes are especially helpful for those with cataracts.

Contrast is enhanced by using highly contrasting colors near one another such as black ink on white or yellow paper or fluorescent strips on stair risers. Contrast for reading pale or bluish print may be improved by using pale yellow tinted lenses or by placing a clear yellow or amber sheet over the page.

Lighting requirements vary according to the age of the individual and the cause of the visual impairment. As the eyes age, they need greater amounts of illumination to function properly. Sixty-year-old eyes need twice as much light to complete a task as 20-year-old eyes.

Eye disorders and conditions may create a need for either reduced or increased light. Those who function best in low light include persons with ALBINISM, ANIRIDIA (lack of iris), cataract, and corneal opacities. Those who function best in maximum light include those with glaucoma, OPTIC ATROPHY, surgical aphakia (lack of natural lens), MYOPIA, COLOBOMA, and macular disease.

impairment   There is no complete consensus on terms concerning the topic of blindness and vision impairment. Educators, doctors, rehabilitation specialists, and other leaders in the field define TERMINOLOGY according to their own preferences but have recently made efforts to standardize terms such as impairment to eliminate confusion or misinterpretation.

An impairment refers to a recognizable defect or malfunctioning of an organ or any part of the body, such as an eye. The defect or malfunction can be diagnosed and defined by a medical doctor. A visually impaired person may include an individual with no sight as well as someone with low vision.

independent living aids   See ADAPTIVE AIDS.

independent-living center   A program of services or a facility that provides a variety of independent living services for persons with disabilities. The services are directed to provide resources, training, counseling, and assistance to promote the independence, productivity, and quality of life of persons with disabilities. They may be supported by federal, state, local, or private funds.

Individuals with Disabilities Education Act   (IDEA)   Formerly known as Public Law 94–142, this law guarantees that all children between the ages of three and 21 who need special education and services due to a disability will have access to a free and appropriate public education. The law provides money to assist states in providing an individualized education program (IEP) for each student. The IDEA was formerly known as the Education of the Handicapped Act (EHA). The original act—EHA—was implemented in 1975 and changed to IDEA in 1991. IDEA was amended in 1997.

Before 1975, about 1 million disabled children did not have access to public schools, and thousands more did not receive appropriate education in the schools. Ninety percent of children with serious disabilities used to be housed in state institutions and did not attend public schools.

IDEA states that school administrators, teachers, and parents should be involved with developing an individualized education program for each student who needs one. The 1997 amendments to the act, signed into law by President Bill Clinton on June 4, include the following:

• Changes in the formula for distributing federal money to states

• Instruction in braille and the use of braille for visually impaired students, unless braille is not considered by the IEP team to be in the best interests of the child

• More freedom for school districts to serve disabled children who attend private schools

- Requirement for a state to set performance goals for disabled children and a means for mapping progress
- More flexible, but more frequent re-evaluations of children with individualized programs
- Changes in the way in which disputes between the parents of a disabled child and the local education agency are handled
- Changes in the way in which discipline problems involving disabled students are to be handled
- Children with disabilities must be included in statewide and district-wide assessments
- Regular education teachers must be included in IEP teams if there is any possibility that a disabled child will participate in regular class
- Children with disabilities must be given access to the regular curriculum

Office of Special Education and Rehabilitative Services, the U.S. Department of Education. *IDEA '97 Amendments, Final Regulations.* www.ed.gov/offices/OSERS, 2001.

injuries   According to the National Society to Prevent Blindness, nearly 1.3 million people suffer eye injuries each year in the United States. Injuries are responsible for 4 percent of all cases of blindness and 3 percent of all new cases of blindness in the United States each year. Currently, approximately 1 million people have sustained some vision loss due to injuries. Nearly half of these injuries occurred in or around the home in product-related incidences.

Four product groups—construction materials, home products, personal products, and workshop tools—account for more than half of these injuries. Construction materials include nails, metal parts, lumber, and any other building matter. Home products are those used to maintain a household and include bleaches, chemicals, glues, and acids. Personal products consist of items such as contact lenses, sun lamps, combs, and brushes. Home workshop materials encompass tools and machinery, wet cell batteries, and welding gear.

In order of severity, the most hazardous materials are metal debris, contact lenses, and automobiles, followed by batteries, sun lamps, and adhesives or glue. Among children aged five to 14, most accidents involve metal debris, baseball gear, workshop apparatus, and adhesives. Injuries for those aged 15–24 most often involve contact lenses, metal debris, sun lamps, automobiles and batteries. Injuries for those 25–64 generally include metal debris, automobiles, and contact lenses.

Sports or recreational injuries are responsible for nearly 40,000 eye treatments in hospital emergency rooms each year according to the National Society to prevent blindness. The society estimates as many as 100,000 such injuries each year, although not all are reported. Nearly one third of those treated are children five to 14 years of age. Generally, baseball and basketball account for most injuries, followed by racquet sports and football.

It is estimated that 90 percent of all injuries can be prevented if proper precautions are taken to wear protective safety goggles and to store harmful chemicals and spray cans. When a chemical or acid injury occurs, the National Society to Prevent Blindness suggests gently flushing the eyes with water for 15 minutes and immediately obtaining a medical examination. Do not use an eye cup or bandage the eye.

When specks or debris enter the eye, lift the upper eyelid outward and down over the lower lid. If the tears do not wash out the particle, do not rub the eye, keep it closed, bandage it lightly and see a doctor.

When an impact to the eye occurs, apply cold compresses for 15 minutes and each successive hour until pain and swelling are reduced. If the eye becomes discolored, see a doctor.

In the case of a puncture or cut to the eye, do not wash with water or try to remove a foreign body. Bandage the eye lightly and see a doctor immediately.

National Society to Prevent Blindness. *Vision Problems in the U.S.: Facts and Figures.* New York: NSPB, 1998.

Internal Revenue Service   See TAX BENEFITS.

intraocular lens   See IOL SURGERY.

IOL surgery   Intraocular lens implants, or IOL surgery, is the implantation of a small, clear plastic lens in the eye to replace the section of natural lens lost in cataract removal surgery. As a permanent substitute for the lens, it enables the cornea to focus light onto the retina and produce a distinct image.

The intraocular lens is made up of two parts. The optic is the center portion of the lens that does the job of focusing. It is approximately one-quarter of an inch long and is made of PMMA plastic. The portion called the haptic holds the lens in place.

The power of the IOL is determined by two tests. KERATOMETRY is a test that determines the curvature of the cornea. More curved corneas require incrementally weaker implants. An ultrasonic A-scan determines the length of the eye. The longer (more nearsighted) the eye, the weaker the implant needed. An A-scan may determine that an IOL is unnecessary.

Intraocular lens implantation can be performed in either intracapsular or extracapsular cataract removal. Significant advances have been made in the technology of IOLs. They are smaller than they used to be and can be folded and placed into the eye through a tiny incision. There are three implantation methods: ANTERIOR CHAMBER, POSTERIOR CHAMBER, and iris supported. The lens is placed in front of the iris in the anterior method behind the iris in the posterior method and is clipped or sewn to the iris in the almost obsolete iris-supported method. Most ophthalmologists prefer the posterior method, claiming the lenses are more secure there and in a better position to help restore eyesight. IOLs provide constant, immediate improvement in vision and require no ongoing care. Patients may require normal glasses or bifocals as a supplement.

IOL surgery is often restricted to older patients since long-term side effects are unknown. It is recommended that the surgery not be repeated if an implant was unsuccessful in one eye or in the presence of other serious eye problems.

iridectomy   The surgical removal of part of the eye's iris. The procedure is often performed as treatment for narrow-angle glaucoma, a condition in which AQUEOUS FLUID builds within the eye due to a pupillary block and causes a rise in intraocular pressure.

The removal of the section of iris creates a passageway between the posterior and anterior chambers of the eye and eliminates an iris bombe, a condition in which the iris is abnormally bowed forward due to the increased intraocular pressure. The procedure allows aqueous fluid to pass from the posterior to ANTERIOR CHAMBER and thus reduces intraocular pressure.

The surgery is performed under general or local anesthetic. Traditionally, a small incision is made at the limbus through the cornea and SCLERA, into the anterior chamber of the eye. Since the iris is malleable, the incision allows a peripheral portion of the iris to prolapse out of the eye. The prolapsed section is held with forceps and excised with scissors. The iris bombe sinks backward into the eye. Often, the condition or blockage requires only a cut to be made rather than a removal of the iris. The cut is called an iridotomy. The cut or incision may be made surgically or with an argon laser, which burns a hole in the iris through the closed eye. Iridectomy or iridotomy is usually performed at the initial attack of narrow-angle glaucoma after treatment with medication has begun. It is used as a treatment and as a prophylactic measure to prevent recurrent attacks of narrow-angle glaucoma.

iridocyclitis   A condition of the iris and ciliary body in which these two portions of the eye become inflamed. Because of the close proximity of the CILIARY BODY to the iris, inflammation and infection pass easily from one body to the other. Since the iris and ciliary body are located in the front portion of the uveal tract, which also includes the CHOROID, the condition is also called anterior UVEITIS, or inflammation of the uveal tract.

Symptoms of iridocyclitis may include pain, especially when focusing on near objects, redness, light sensitivity, and changes in the appearance of the pupil. The inflammation irritates the sphincter muscle of the pupil, which causes it to constrict, appear misshapen, or develop spasms. As a result of iridocyclitis, posterior SYNECHIAE may occur. This is a condition in which the pupil adheres to the underlying lens.

Iridocyclitis may be caused by IRITIS, which in turn is caused by injuries, viruses, HERPES ZOSTER, funguses, parasites, arthritis, and sinus or tooth infections. The condition may be treated with cycloplegic, or dilating, drops, local steroids, and medications for underlying causes. The condition may last for two weeks or more and carries a tendency to recur. Several recurrences may raise the possibility of cataract development.

iridodonesis   A trembling of the iris. This condition is frequently seen with a subluxated (displaced) lens or following cataract surgery. It also is associated with MARFAN'S SYNDROME.

iritis   An inflammation of the iris. Symptoms of iritis may include pain, especially when focusing on near objects, redness, light sensitivity, and changes in the appearance of the pupil. While the cornea remains clear, the pupil may appear constricted or misshapen and develop spasms.

Because the iris is part of the uveal tract, iritis may be present in UVEITIS. Other causes may include injuries, viruses, HERPES ZOSTER, funguses, parasites, arthritis, and sinus or tooth infections. When the inflammation of iritis spreads to the adjoining CILIARY BODY, the condition is termed IRIDOCYCLITIS, or anterior uveitis.

Iritis is most often treated with cycloplegic, or dilating, drops and local steroids. The condition may last for two weeks or more and carries a tendency to recur. Several recurrences may increase the possibility of cataract development.

Ishihara Test   See COLOR BLINDNESS.

Isopto Carpine   An ophthalmic solution used in the treatment of glaucoma. The main ingredient, pilocarpine hydrochloride, is also contained in the equivalent products known as Adsorbocarpine, Adarpine, Almocarpine, Akarpine, Ocusert Pilo-20, Ocusert Pilo 40, Pilocar and Pilopine HS. The medicine causes the pupils to constrict and lowers pressure within the eye.

The dosage is administered in drops. Some patients may suffer side effects. Minor side effects may include headache or aching in the brow, loss of night vision, blurred vision, and twitching eyelids. Major side effects may include diarrhea, nausea, difficulty urinating, stomach cramps, sweating, palpitations, shortness of breath, muscle tremor, nearsightedness, or other changes in vision.

Isopto Carpine should not be taken by those with a pilocarpine allergy. It should be used with caution by those with a history of heart disease, asthma, thyroid disease, peptic ulcer, gastrointestinal spasms, urinary tract blockage, Parkinson's disease, or seizures.

J

Javits-Wagner-O'Day Act   The Javits-Wagner-O'Day Act of 1971 was enacted as an amendment to the Wagner-O'Day Act of 1938. The Wagner-O'Day Act mandated a program in which federal agencies may buy specific products from qualified workshops for the blind in an effort to improve employment opportunities.

In 1971, the Wagner-O'Day Act was renamed the Javits-Wagner-O'Day Act and amended to include severely disabled workers and add services as well as products. The products for sale to the federal government are approved by the Committee for Purchase from the Blind and other Severely Handicapped, a presidentially appointed committee that oversees the act.

A study in 1998 concluded that the Javits-Wagner-O'Day Act contracts have the potential to provide significant cost savings to the federal government.

The committee is composed of 15 members; 11 are representatives of federal agencies, three are representatives of the general public, and one is a private citizen representative of the disabled community. The committee determines and lists the products and services reasonable for purchase from qualified workshops, decides the fair market price for such products and services and sets the rules and regulations to execute the act.

U.S. Department of Education. *Summary of Existing Legislation Affecting Persons with Disabilities.* Washington, D.C.: USDE, 1988.

juvenile retinoschisis   An inherited disease that causes progressive loss of central and side vision due to degeneration of the retina. Loss of sight usually occurs at about age 13. The condition, which also is known as X-linked retinoschisis, almost always occurs in males.

The condition begins at birth, but there usually are no symptoms until about the age of 10, when a decline in vision begins. Other early signs of the disease include involuntary eye movements and the loss of ability to focus both eyes on an object. Blindness sometimes occurs within three years of diagnosis, while other people with the disease retain some vision into adulthood.

Juvenile retinoschisis is genetically passed along by the X-linked pattern of inheritance, because the gene for the disease is located on the X chromosome. There is no treatment or cure at this time for juvenile retinoschisis, but surgery can be performed to repair retinal detachments, which often occur as part of the disease. People with the disease may benefit from the use of low-vision aids, orientation and mobility training, and so forth.

K

Keller, Helen   Helen Keller is perhaps the best-known figure in history associated with blindness. Born sighted in 1880 in Alabama, she contracted a fever at 18 months, which left her deaf and blind. The infant grew into a wild and unruly child with few methods for communication with others. Her father, Captain Arthur Keller, editor of the *North Alabamian*, sought advice from Alexander Graham Bell in his search for help for his daughter. Bell suggested that Captain Keller write to the Perkins Institution for the Blind to request a teacher for Helen.

In 1887, Anne Mansfield Sullivan arrived to teach the child. Sullivan taught her to fingerspell the words for objects, but Keller showed no understanding of the connection between the spelling and the object. The breakthrough came one day at the well when water gushed onto Keller's hand as Sullivan spelled W-A-T-E-R. Keller continued to study with Sullivan, mastering the alphabet in both manual and raised print.

Keller entered the Cambridge School for Young Ladies in 1898 in preparation for Radcliffe College. She enrolled in Radcliffe in 1900 and graduated with a bachelor of arts degree cum laude in 1904. Sullivan remained at Keller's side throughout Keller's studies, translating lectures and textbooks.

Keller began a writing career while studying at Radcliffe. In 1902, her autobiography, *The Story of My Life,* was published. The book was written with the assistance of John Macy, a critic and socialist reformer. When Sullivan married John Macy in 1905, Keller went to live with the couple.

Keller worked for the interests of blind and deaf-blind individuals throughout her life by appearing before legislatures, writing articles and books, and lecturing. She became a member of the first board of directors of the Permanent Blind Relief War Fund (later named the American Braille Press, the American Foundation for Overseas Blind and Helen Keller International) in 1915.

She was a member of the staff for the Foundation of the Blind from 1924 until her death in 1968, serving as an adviser on national and international relations. In 1924, she founded the Helen Keller Endowment Fund to benefit the foundation. She established the foundation's special-service program for deaf-blind individuals in 1946.

In 1946, when the American Braille Press became the American Foundation for Overseas Blind, she became a counselor on international relations for the organization. She embarked on speaking tours that covered 35 countries on five continents between 1946 and 1957. Her last speaking tour, at age 75, covered over 40,000 miles in Asia.

Keller received honors during her lifetime for her work benefiting blind persons. Honorary degrees include those from Temple University, Harvard

University, and the Universities of Glasgow, Berlin, Delhi, and Johannesburg. Awards bestowed on her include the Presidential Medal of Freedom, Brazil's Order of the Southern Cross, Japan's Sacred Treasure and the Philippines' Golden Heart. She was elected to the National Institute of Arts and Letters and named a Chevalier of the French Legion of Honor.

Versions of Keller's life have been the subject of stage and film productions. The documentary *Helen Keller in Her Story* and the play and movie *The Miracle Worker* all chronicle the events of her life.

Sullivan, long separated from Macy, died in 1936. Polly Thomson, who joined the two in 1914 when Sullivan's eyesight deteriorated, continued to serve as Keller's interpreter and companion. In 1961, Keller retired from public life to her home, Arcan Ridge, in Westport, Connecticut. She died in 1968 at the age of 87.

keratitis   An inflammation of the cornea caused by viruses, bacteria or, infrequently, fungi. Keratitis can occur as a result of a corneal abrasion caused by CONTACT LENSES or by an injury. Elderly persons, diabetics, those with poor tear functions, and those treated with corticosteroid drugs may be more likely to develop keratitis after an abrasion.

Keratitis is a serious infection and should be treated by a physician. Symptoms of keratitis include redness, sharp pain, tearing, impaired vision, light sensitivity, and dulled or milky corneal surface.

Simple viral keratitis is generally the least serious type. Patients are usually treated with medication on an outpatient basis. However, herpes keratitis is a very serious viral infection that can result in scarring and permanent visual impairment.

Bacterial keratitis is more dangerous than viral types and often must be treated in a hospital. The infection is treated with antibiotics and cortisone-based steroid drugs. Bacterial keratitis can permanently scar the cornea and cause vision loss. Bacterial keratitis may be contracted congenitally as in syphilis.

The most common forms of fungal keratitis are caused by yeasts. Fungal keratitis may require hospitalization and treatment with antibiotics. Scarring frequently results, despite treatment, and causes vision impairment. Another type of keratitis is exposure keratitis. This sometimes occurs when the eyelid cannot cover the eye because of bulging, as found in some thyroid conditions. Exposure keratitis can vary from mild dry spots to ulcers on the cornea.

keratoconus   A degenerative disorder of the cornea in which the central part of the cornea thins and bulges forward into a cone shape. As the cornea thins, vision becomes distorted. As a result of further stretching, the cornea may break at the peak. The cornea will heal itself, but scar tissue will form at the break, causing vision loss.

It is a chronic, progressive disease. The exact cause of kertatoconus is not known, but it is thought that there is a genetic predisposition to the disorder. Most researchers agree that there probably is more than one factor involved in the cause in the disorder, and there is a "trigger" that sets off a series of events in the tissues of the eye that eventually result in keratoconus. It is most often diagnosed in children or adolescents and usually presents symptoms when they are near 10 years of age. The National Keratoconus Foundation estimates that one of every 2,000 people will develop the disorder.

Keratoconus may be diagnosed during the routine ophthalmologic exam. Examination with the BIOMICROSCOPE, or slit lamp, will reveal thinning of the central cornea or presence of the Fleischer ring, a narrow, greenish-brown ring in the cornea. Later stages of keratoconus, in which the cornea has markedly bulged forward, can be seen without benefit of examination instruments.

This disorder progresses slowly and affects both eyes. Milder forms of the condition are often corrected with spectacles or special CONTACT LENSES that cover the cornea and part of the SCLERA. More serious and advanced forms are corrected surgically or by a CORNEAL TRANSPLANT, called keratoplasty.

Keratoconus is a prime reason for keratoplasty in the United States. It is a highly successful procedure since, in cases of keratoconus, the cornea remains vessel free.

keratometer   See KERATOMETRY.

keratometry   Measurement of the curvature of the cornea with an instrument called a keratometer. The exact keratometer measurement is used to determine the power of an INTRAOCULAR LENS to be implanted during cataract surgery.

The greater the degree of corneal curvature, the more nearsighted is the eye. Higher degrees of nearsightedness require weaker implants. The curvature measurement and the length of the eye, measured with an ultrasonic A-scan, are analyzed by a computer that determines and prescribes the precise power of the implant.

keratoplasty   See CORNEAL TRANSPLANT.

keratotomy   A procedure in which incisions are made in the cornea to change its curvature over the pupil. There are two kinds or keratotomies: radial and astigmatic. Radial keratotomy, done to reduce myopia (nearsightedness), was introduced in North America in 1978. During the procedure, the surgeon makes several deep incisions in the cornea to change the curvature of the cornea over the pupil. The incisions are made in a spokelike, or radial, pattern. No cuts are made in the optical zone, which is the portion of the eye that you see through. The surgeon measures the thickness of the cornea to determine how deep to make the incisions, then, under a microscope and using a calibrated diamond blade, the surgeon will make the precise cuts.

Normal pressure within the eye causes the areas around the incisions to bow, which results in a flattening of the center of the cornea. The flattened area reduces the refractive power of the cornea and allows light rays to focus on the retina, thus reducing nearsightedness. Radial keratotomy is an outpatient procedure that normally takes no more than 30 minutes to perform. Approximately 85 percent of people who have this type of surgery can pass a standard driver's license exam that requires 20/40 vision without corrective lenses.

Astigmatic keratotomy is a similar procedure that is used to reduce astigmatism. The incisions used in astigmatic keratotomy are made in a curved, rather than a radial, pattern. Astigmatic keratotomy sometimes is used in combination with radial keratotomy to reduce myopia with astigmatism.

The cornea heals slowly after keratotomy is performed, and there may be side effects such as fluctuating vision, a weakened cornea, infection, temporary pain, or difficulty in getting contact lenses to fit. Rarely, patients develop cataract, serious infection, or experience rupture of an incision. In extreme cases, loss of vision may occur.

American Academy of Ophthalmology. *Radial and Astigmatic Keratotomy.* www.eye-net.org, 1997.

large print   Large print is a low-vision aid that benefits visually impaired individuals who have some usable vision but cannot read conventional print. Large print, 18-point type is roughly 3/16 of an inch high and therefore easier to read than standard print.

In the United States, large print originated in 1913 in sight-saving classes. In order to help their students who could not read conventional print, teachers began to hand-print enlarged text. In 1914, the early large-type books were printed, and by 1935 the American Printing House for the Blind began to publish large-print textbooks for children.

Today, large-print books, magazines, and literature are available through publishers, visual-aids catalogs, and public libraries. There also is computer software available to get large print on a computer screen.

laser cane   An electronic traveling device. It is prescribed by an ophthalmologist or optometrist, and it requires specialized training from an orientation and mobility instructor.

The laser cane is a long cane that sends out three thin beams of invisible infrared light. The beams detect objects within 20 feet at face level, waist level, and ground level. It can detect changes in the terrain of the path, including drops down to five inches below surface, such as curbs and potholes. When the laser light hits an obstacle, it sets vibrating pins into motion and/or sends out an auditory signal.

The signal is pitched according to the height of the obstacle. When the beam touches an obstacle at face level, the auditory signal is a high-pitched beep. When it hits a center or waist-high obstacle, the beep is pitched lower. When it hits a ground-level obstacle, the pitch is low.

The laser cane requires from 30 to 40 hours of training with a qualified instructor to operate.

leprosy   A disease with complications that causes between 50,000 to 100,000 cases of blindness throughout the world. In 1997 there were estimated to be 1.2 million leprosy patients in the world, as reported by 91 countries. About half a million new cases are detected each year.

Leprosy is widespread in 60 countries. The 16 rated "most endemic," which account for 90 percent of all leprosy cases throughout the world, are Bangladesh, Brazil, Cambodia, Ethiopia, Guinea, India, Indonesia, Madagascar, Mozambique, Myanmar (Burma), Nepal, Nigeria, Philippines, Sudan, Tanzania, and Democratic Republic of the Congo (formerly Zaire). India, and Nepal account for nearly 70 percent of all cases.

Leprosy is a chronic infectious disease caused by *Mycobacterium leprae,* a bacillus that reproduces very slowly and mainly affects the skin, nerves, and mucous membranes. If untreated, it leads to progressive damage of the skin, eyes, and limbs. Visible symptoms might not appear for five to 20 years after a person has contacted the disease.

Advances are being made in controlling leprosy, and public health officials are hopeful that the disease will soon be eliminated. A combination of drugs has been found to be effective in treating leprosy.

World Health Organization. *A World Without Leprosy.* www.who.int/lep/index.html, 2000.

Library Services and Technology Act   (LSTA)   An act passed by Congress on September 30, 1996, to replace the Library Services and Construction Act. The act provides federal funding for libraries in the United States and guidelines for library programs and services.

The goal of the LSTA is to enhance technology in America's libraries, including that which will benefit people who are blind or visually impaired. Some of the aims of the LSTA are to establish or enhance electronic link-ups among or between libraries; link libraries electronically with educational, social, or information services; help libraries access information from electronic networks; buy computers and telecommunications equipment for libraries that do not have them; provide library services in areas that do not have them; and provide services for everyone who wishes to use them, including blind, visually impaired, and learning impaired persons.

The original act to fund libraries in the United States was the Library Services Act, which went into effect in 1956. It was replaced by the Library Services and Construction Act in 1964. In 1966, the act was amended to authorize special library-access programs and services, including those that benefit blind or visually impaired people.

Contact:

The American Library Association. Highlights of the Library Services and Technology Act.
www.ala.org.washoff/lstahigh.html, 2000

low-vision clinics   Low-vision clinics provide special services to people with low vision. They may be located in clinics or hospitals or medical, rehabilitation or optometric centers. Many ophthalmologists and optometrists specialize in low-vision services and offer them through private practice.

Low-vision services vary. Most offer vision assessment, low-vision eye examinations, training in techniques to help maximize remaining vision, and prescription of aids or devices to enhance vision.

Some low-vision clinics extend this basic program and offer pediatric low-vision exams, genetic counseling, and contact lens evaluation and disbursement. Others add rehabilitation experts to train patients in orientation and mobility instruction and counsel them in vocational and financial matters.

A standard low-vision eye exam includes an assessment interview, specialized examination of the eyes, assessment of remaining vision use, evaluation of vision needed to complete daily tasks at work and home, counseling, and prescription for and training in the use of adaptive devices or aids.

The assessment interview may be conducted by a social worker, rehabilitation or mobility instructor, psychologist, counselor, nurse, or other professional worker in the low-vision field. The oral-assessment interview consists of questions that determine how the patient feels about loss of vision and how it interferes with daily living. The patient may be asked about general health, living conditions, traveling needs, and job tasks.

Next, the eye examination is performed by an optometrist or an ophthalmologist. The examiner uses specifically designed eye charts and carefully monitored light levels to assess the patient's distance vision. Powerful lenses and magnifiers are used to evaluate the patient's near vision and reading skills. The examination may take many sessions to complete, and each session may last up to an hour in length.

After the eye examination, the patient receives training in visual techniques and/or the use of low-vision aids. The instruction is given by a rehabilitation counselor or professional low-vision clinician. During the lesson, the patient is taught skills for using his vision efficiently and is introduced to appropriate devices or aids. These may include optical lenses such as magnifiers, clip-on loupes, and telescopic devices or nonoptical aids such as lamps, reading stands, filters, or large print. The patient may take the aids home for a trial period. The half-hour lesson may be repeated until the proper prescription can be made. An additional recheck examination is usually scheduled after six months.

A patient may be referred to other professionals in the field such as an orientation and mobility instructor or a vocational rehabilitation counselor for additional training. These specialists may direct the patient back to the low-vision clinic at any time during training to reevaluate the patient's vision or aids.

lupus   Lupus or lupus erythematosus (LE) is the name for a series of chronic autoimmune diseases in which the body's immune system attacks its own tissues. The Lupus Foundation of America estimates that between 500,000 and 1.5 million Americans have been diagnosed with the disease. Lupus occurs more frequently in women than in men, and its more prevalent in people of African-American, Indian, or Asian origin. It is a lifelong illness but is not considered life threatening.

Lupus attacks collagen, the support material for tissue. As a result, it can affect the kidneys, skin, joints, blood, heart, eyes, and virtually any other organ in the body. Since its symptoms of skin rash, painful swelling of the joints, fever, headache, and exhaustion mirror those of other disorders, lupus can be difficult to detect immediately.

The cause of lupus is unknown, but heredity, viruses, exposure to ultraviolet or sunlight, extreme stress, and various drugs may play a role. There is no cure for lupus, but treatment can control and relieve symptoms and often result in a remission.

Since collagen is found in every part of the eye, many eye disorders can result as a complication of lupus or its treatment. Hypertension associated with lupus can swell the blood vessels of the optic nerve, causing hemorrhaging. When this occurs, the blood vessels of the brain and eye become protectively constrictive, shutting off necessary oxygen to the eye and causing permanent damage.

Vasculitis, swelling of the blood vessels, can center in the eye, causing blockage of the eye's main artery. Sudden, severe vision loss may occur.

Optic neuritis, swelling of the optic nerve, can cause retinitis and an accompanying vision loss. Cortisone treatment may reverse the damage caused by optic neuritis.

UVEITIS, an infection in the eye's iris, can be caused by lupus. It is treated with cortisone drugs.

Unfortunately, the drug therapy of lupus patients may contribute to their eye disorders. Many lupus patients are treated with cortisone and other steroids, which may cause cataracts or glaucoma in those predisposed to glaucoma.

Plaquinil, an antimalarial drug used in the treatment of lupus, can cause glaucomalike symptoms, such as the loss of peripheral vision. This drug may also be damaging to the eye's macula.

lutein   A nutrient in the carotenoid family that is thought by some people to reduce the risk of developing age-related macular degeneration. While most researchers and doctors agree that good nutrition is important to overall eye health, there is little scientific evidence to support the theory that lutein can prevent macular degeneration, despite recent publicity to the contrary. The National Eye Institute (NEI) in March 2000 issued a statement concerning the value of taking lutein supplements. The NEI advised that claims concerning lutein and eye health should be regarded cautiously and stated that the possible benefits of lutein are uncertain.

Foods that are rich in carotenoids include green, leafy vegetables such as kale and cabbage. While the NEI recognizes that these lutein-rich foods are beneficial to overall health, it questions that direct relationship between lutein and eye health.

Lyme disease   An infection caused by *Borrelia burgdorferi,* a spirochete bacteria spread by the bite of an infected tick carried by deer, mice, birds, raccoons, chipmunks, and domestic animals. Lyme disease has a worldwide prevalence and has been recorded in six continents, 20 countries and 48 of the United States. More than 100,000 U.S. cases have been reported to the Centers for Disease Control and Prevention. States most affected by Lyme disease are New York, Connecticut, Pennsylvania, and New Jersey.

Symptoms of Lyme disease include a circular or oblong rash, headache, stiff neck, fever, muscle aches, fatigue, and other flulike discomforts. The symptoms usually subside, only to reappear later or give way to more serious problems such as infections of the eye, muscles and joints, brain, heart, skin, liver and lung, skin tumors, gastrointestinal disorders, birth defects, and loss of nerve conduction.

Early stages of Lyme disease are manifested in the eyes as conjunctivitis, episcleritis, and photophobia. Later, cranial nerve palsies may result and cause exposure keratitis and corneal abrasion. Lyme disease may cause papilledema, optic neuritis, and loss of vision. Ocular disorders may be transmitted from an infected mother to the fetus.

Diagnosis of the disease is problematic. A blood test can measure the immune system response to the infecting spirochete but is not completely reliable. Those who test negative to the disease may be infected.

Lyme disease is treated with oral antibiotics in the early stages and with intravenous antibiotic treatments in later stages. The antibiotic treatment is not a cure. Although some individuals remain symptom free, others experience recurrences and require long-term antibiotic treatment. There is a vaccine against Lyme disease called Lymerix, but it is not always effective. Scientists and doctors are working to improve the vaccine.

M

macular edema   A condition of the macula stemming from retinal edema. The macula is an indentation of the retina that contains an abundance of cones, light-sensitive cells that are responsible for discerning color and detail. Light is focused directly on the macula by the eye, making it the center of sharpest sight.

Retinal edema occurs when the capillaries of the retina bleed, filling the spaces between retinal cells with fluid. Retinal edema may be present throughout the retina and involve the macula, or it may contained in a general area that spares the macula. If the macula is spared, vision may be relatively unaffected at first. However, the macula tends to accumulate the fluid. In this case, macular edema occurs. The condition is characterized by inflammation of the macula and blurred or impaired vision. If untreated, macular fluid collects in small pockets of space and forms cysts, a condition called cystic macular edema. The condition leads to degeneration of the macula in which central vision may be permanently lost.

Macular edema is caused by diabetic retinopathy, hypertension, retinal vein obstruction, traction of the vitreous, inflammations such as UVEITIS and retinitis, and cataract surgery. It is diagnosed with fluorescein angiography, a procedure in which fluorescein dye is injected into a vein in the arm and monitored as it passes through the veins of the retina. Macular edema may right itself spontaneously or persist. Treatment of the condition varies according to the cause. Cases due to inflammation are treated with corticosteroids.

Those conditions of edema caused by vascular problems and diabetes may be treated with photocoagulation, a treatment that uses a laser to seal leaking blood vessels. There is no treatment for edema due to traction or cataract surgery.

mailing privileges   Materials may be mailed free of postage by legally blind individuals or those unable to read or use conventionally printed materials as a result of a physical disability. The program is entitled "Free Matter for the Blind or Handicapped."

In order to become eligible, the individual must present written certification by a competent authority to the post office where mailings will be sent and received. An authority may include a licensed doctor, ophthalmologist, optometrist, registered nurse, or professional staff member of a hospital or other agency or institution.

Material eligible for mailing includes books, magazines, musical scores, braille material, 14-point Sightsaving Type, records, or cassette tapes. Equipment and parts of equipment used for writing or educational purposes, sound play-back equipment for use by the visually impaired, and equipment designed or adapted for use by visually impaired persons, such as braille watches and white canes are also eligible.

The material must be free of advertising and must be specifically designed for and used by visually or physically disabled individuals. The mail is subject to inspection by the Postal Service.

Noncommercial agencies or organizations, individuals, and libraries serving eligible persons may mail the material to an eligible person or organization free of charge. The eligible person may exchange or return material postage free to other eligible persons or organizations. Commercial producers of this material may mail it free of postage to an eligible individual or organization so long as the fee, charge, or rental does not exceed the cost of the material.

Eligible persons may send letters in braille, large print, or recorded form. Handwritten or typed letters are subject to postage when mailed to or from an eligible person. Letters must remain unsealed to allow inspection by the Postal Service. All mailed material must be stamped, printed, or handwritten with the words. "Free Matter for the Blind or Handicapped" in the space reserved for postage. Free international delivery of some materials also is included. Special services, however, such as Express Mail or Certified Mail, are not included.

malignant melanoma   A tumor of the eye that grows from melanin-laden cells in the CHOROID, iris, or CILIARY BODY. Also called an intraocular melanoma. According to the U.S. Department of Health and Human Services, malignant melanomas account for up to 80 percent of all eye malignancies, making them the most common primary (originating in the eye) inner-eye tumor. The tumor may develop from a mole or spontaneously and is usually slow to grow and spread. It generally affects one eye only (unilateral), may appear at any age and is more common in whites than blacks. Symptoms include redness of the eye, inflammation, vision loss, and the presence or development of glaucoma. Melanomas of the iris may distort the shape of pupil.

A melanoma can be detected in the ophthalmologic examination. It may first appear to be a choroidal hemorrhage, but can be identified further by FLUORESCEIN ANGIOGRAPHY or ULTRASONOGRAPHY.

Three types of treatment are commonly used for intraocular melanomas. They are: surgery, radiation therapy, and photocoagulation. Surgery is the most common treatment. It can involve removing a portion of the diseased eye, or enucleation, which is the removal of the entire eye. Radiation uses X rays and other high-energy rays to kill cancer cells and shrink tumors. It can be used by itself, or in combination with surgery. Photocoagulation treats the melanoma by destroying blood vessels with a tiny beam of light, usually from a laser. Destroying the blood vessels kills the tumor.

Clinical trials to test other treatment methods are ongoing. More information about the trials can be obtained by calling (toll free) the National Cancer Institute's Cancer Information Service at 800-422-6237. If the diagnosis is uncertain, a period of observation may be prescribed, possibly including chemotherapy or radiation treatments.

Little is known concerning the cause of malignant melanomas. Unlike skin or conjunctiva melanomas, sunlight exposure is not related to these tumors. Limited data exists concerning metastatic rates (growth or spread of tumor) and spontaneous regression rates

National Cancer Institute. "What is Intraocular Melanoma?" NCI website: www.cancernet.nci.nih.gov, 2000.

Marfan's syndrome   Marfan's syndrome (arachnodactyly) is a rare genetic disease. It is characterized by long, thin bones, elongated limbs, especially of the extremities, tall slender figure, lack of subcutaneous fat, nonelastic ligaments, congenital heart disorders, high infant-mortality rate, malformations of the spine, joints, and ears, and ocular disorders.

Ocular disorders include dislocation or subluxation of the lens, serious refractive errors (nearsightedness, far-sightedness, etc.), glaucoma, cataract, and uveal COLOBOMAS. IRIDONESIS, or a trembling of the iris, also associated with Marfan's syndrome. The most common symptom, subluxated lens, is a condition in which the lens becomes displaced in an up and out direction.

The subluxated lens may increase myopia and cause astigmatism or cataracts. Often, the displaced lens blocks or narrows the angle of the ANTERIOR CHAMBER and causes secondary glaucoma. If glaucoma cannot be treated successfully with medications or surgical procedures, the lens may be removed. In some cases, aphakic (without lens) patients may experience corrected vision with aphakic spectacles or contact lenses.

For more information contact:

The National Marfan Foundation
382 Main Street
Port Washington, NY 11050
800-8-MARFAN (ph)
516-883-8040 (fax)
www.marfan.org

Maternal and Child Health Services Program   The Maternal and Child Health block-grant program evolved from the original Sheppard-Tower Act of 1921. Also known as the Maternity and Infant Act, it was the first national health services grant program. In 1935, the act was amended and revised by Title V of the Social Security Act to include services for disabled children.

Amendments to Title V in 1963 authorized a grant program to improve health and prenatal care for low-income women. The effort was designed to reduce preventable mental retarda-tion and birth defects. The legislation provided funding for research studies and additional grant funds for states under the Maternal and Child Health program and the Crippled Children's program.

The Social Security Act Amendments of 1965 extended and improved health-care services for mothers and children. Project grants were established to develop maternal and children's health-care programs and comprehensive training services for specialists working with disabled children. Project grants were authorized to support and improve health-care services to low-income school-age and preschool-age children.

In 1967, amendments to the Social Security Act combined the separate Crippled Children's Service grants and Maternal and Child Health Services grants into one authorization. One-half of the funding was allotted to formula grants; the other half was divided 40 percent for project grants and 10 percent for training and research. In 1981, this grant authority was consolidated with those for all the programs established in Title V into one state block-grant authority by the Omnibus Budget Reconciliation Act.

The words "crippled children" were removed from the wording of the Act in 1985 and the words, "children with special health-care needs" was substituted. In 1986 and 1987, appropriations were raised for the Maternal and Child Health program.

Block grants awarded to the states may be used to provide health-care services, and fund development, administration, training, education and evaluation of the programs. According to the Office of Special Education and Rehabilitative Services, the law authorizes the states to use MCH block-grant funds to:

- Assure mothers and children access to quality health services
- Reduce infant mortality, preventable diseases, and disability conditions among children
- Reduce the need for in-patient and long-term care services
- Increase appropriate child immunization
- Increase health assessments and follow-up diagnostic and treatment services for low-income children
- Provide preventative and primary-care services for children and prenatal, delivery, and postpartum services for low-income mothers
- Provide rehabilitation services for blind or disabled children under 16 who receive Supplemental Security Income benefits
- Provide information services regarding diagnosis, hospitalization, and after-care for children who have disabilities or conditions that may lead to disabilities

- Provide for Special Projects of Regional and National Significance (SPRANS), research and training for genetic disease testing, counseling, and information dissemination
- Provide grants relating to hemophilia and sudden infant death syndrome

U.S. Department of Education. *Summary of Existing Legislation Affecting Persons with Disabilities.* Washington, D.C.: USDE, 1988.

Medicaid legislation   In 1965, amendments to the Social Security Act added Title XIX, a grants program that allowed states to establish medical-assistance systems. Title XIX extended the Kerr-Mills medical-aid program for low-income blind and disabled individuals and dependent children.

The new program became known as Medicaid. Unlike Medicare, it allowed states to offer coverage not only to those who receive public assistance, but also to eligible needy people who did not qualify for welfare or Medicare. The program varies from state to state.

Although the original legislation of 1965 made no specific reference to disabilities, Medicaid has become the main source of medical services funding to severely disabled individuals. In 1992, U.S. federal and state budgets included $118 billion in Medicaid benefits. This may be because later amendments added specific benefits for mentally ill and mentally retarded institutionalized individuals, and because the funding targets low-income groups where the incidence of disability is greater.

Medicaid eligibility is determined by financial need. Recipients generally fall into one or more of the three qualifying categories: categorically needy, medically needy, or qualified severely impaired.

The categorically needy receive Aid to Families with Dependent Children (AFDC) benefits or Supplemental Security Income (SSI) benefits or qualify under specific regulations for their state.

Medically needy persons may have incomes too high to qualify for AFDC or SSI benefits yet cannot afford to pay for necessary medical treatment. States determine a different qualifying income level for those who are medically needy.

Qualified severely impaired individuals are those under 65 who receive federal SSI benefits because of blindness or disability and are able to be employed but do not have incomes that allow them to pay for health-care coverage.

Medicaid provides hospital services, both inpatient and outpatient, as well as laboratory tests or X-ray services. Special nursing facility services and, for those over 21 years old, home health services are also provided.

The benefits cover the recipient's doctor services and diagnostic tests such as those classified as EPSDT, or early periodic screening, diagnosis and treatment services, for those under 21. Additionally, some rural health-clinic care and family-planning services are also provided under the plan.

States must arrange to transport recipients to and from medical services if needed; they must allow the recipient to choose the medical caregivers and must provide health-care services statewide. If adequate medical care is provided, states may limit the quantity, extent, and range of these services.

If listed in the state plan, the state may provide any optional services that are allowed under state law and permitted by the Secretary of Health and Human Services. Since each state designs a program to meet the specific needs of its citizens, coverage differs greatly from state to state.

The optional services may include private nursing, health-clinic, and dental services. Physical and occupational therapy and rehabilitation services may be covered, as well as hearing, speech, and language therapy or treatment.

The plan may include prescriptions such as drugs, eyeglasses, dentures, prosthetics, and prosthetic aids. Other services may include those not covered specifically under federal law in such areas as diagnostic screening, inpatient hospital procedures, nursing or intermediate-care facility services, in-patient psychiatric treatment for those under 21 or over 65, and case-management services for specific categories of eligible people.

U.S. Department of Education. *Summary of Existing Legislation Affecting Persons with Disabilities.* Washington, D.C.: USDE, 1988.

Medicare legislation   Title XVIII of the Social Security Act authorizes the Health Care Financing Administration, a division of the Department of Health and Human Services, to offer Medicare health-insurance benefits to qualified handicapped and elderly individuals. Generally, eligible individuals are those 65 years or older who qualify for Social Security benefits. Disabled individuals may qualify for Medicare after a two-year waiting period if they are:

- No longer able to work and their pre-disability contributions to the Social Security FICA meet the required limit
- People with severe childhood disabilities who are dependents of eligible Social Security recipients who are retired or have died
- People with childhood disabilities who qualify for Social Security benefits
- Disabled widowed persons, 50 years of age or older
- Diagnosed as having an end-stage renal condition

In 2001, nearly 40 million people in America were eligible for some Medicare health coverage. Medicare has two parts: Part A is hospital insurance and Part B is medical insurance. Part A helps pay for necessary in-patient and limited home services including hospital or emergency-room care, nursing facilities, hospice services, and some home-health care.

Part B of the insurance plan helps pay for doctors, services, outpatient hospital care, and other medical treatment not covered by Part A. Services covered by the plan are paid according to reasonable costs and fee schedules. Any eligible individual may register for Part B benefits. Although the individual is required to pay a monthly premium, some states or other agencies may pay the premium for a disabled person.

At the end of March 2001, a bill was pending in Congress that would make orientation and mobility specialists, rehabilitation teachers, and low-vision therapists eligible providers under Medicare.

U.S. Department of Education. *Summary of Existing Legislation Affecting Persons with Disabilities.* Washington, D.C.: USDE, 1988.

Health Care Financing Administration. "Medicare Basics." www.medicare.gov, 2001.

migraine   A migraine is a type of recurrent headache. It differs from the normal tension headache in that it usually affects one side of the head only and is often accompanied by visual disturbances, nausea, and vomiting.

Migraines are thought to be caused by a sudden dilation of the arteries in the brain and scalp following a period of spasm or narrowing. The sudden expansion of the arteries causes the blood to surge against the artery walls and surrounding tissues. The dilation and constriction may occur when the body over-produces serotonin and norepinephrine, amines or biological substances that dilate and constrict blood vessels of the body and brain.

Migraine attacks tend to run in families and may be triggered by a variety of causes. It is estimated that between 11 and 18 million Americans suffer from migraines, most of them women. In addition, it is estimated that up to 38 million Americans have the genetic propensity for migraines. The following have been linked to migraine attacks: intense direct, reflected, or flickering lights; rapidly changing images, sudden or persistent noises; reaction to stress; strong odors; allergies; hypertension; hormonal changes; nitroglycerin; anesthetic; drugs; alcohol; cheese; chocolate; cured foods; MSG; poor ventilation; change in barometric pressure; exercise; tight clothing; steam; motion; dental problems; a shock or blow to the head; and too little or too much sleep.

The two major categories of migraine headaches are common and classic. Each is preceded by a preheadache state, called the prodrome stage, which may last from five minutes to an hour. During this stage, symptoms of the oncoming migraine may be noted. They include nausea, vomiting, weakness or tingling on one side or section of the body, mental confusion, fatigue, irritability, dizziness, pallor, euphoria, water retention, and lack of coordination.

Common migraines are associated with light, noise or odor sensitivity, and vomiting or nausea. Classic migraines may include these symptoms but are further characterized by visual disturbances. Patients may experience blurred vision, tunnel vision, double vision, SCOTOMAS, scintillating scotomas, fortification spectra (angled, shimmering lines), HEMIANOPSIA, or distorted vision.

Blurred vision is common to migraine attacks and may be accompanied by tunnel vision, the loss of peripheral or side vision. Tunnel vision has been described as vision seen when looking through a straw. Double vision, or DIPLOPIA, may result during a migraine if ophthalmoplegia, paralysis of the eye muscles, occurs. When a muscle is paralyzed, one eye moves out of alignment and the brain receives two images instead of one, or double vision.

Scotomas are blind spots in the field of vision of one or both eyes. The vision in the scotoma may be blurred or completely obliterated. Scintillating scotomas are blind spots that shimmer with bright light to block out vision. Scotomas may appear anywhere in the field of vision and may move during the course of the prodrome stage or during the headache stage.

Fortification spectra is a shimmering, glittering pattern of bright or colored lights in the field of vision. The lights form shapes such as auras or semicircles and appear in zigzag formations much like a prism. They may block vision or lie atop it.

Hemianopsia is a decrease or loss of vision in one half of each eye. The entire right or left half of the field of vision may be obliterated or may be blocked by fortification spectra.

Distorted vision may result from migraine. Objects or people may appear elongated or stretched out of shape as by a funhouse mirror. This phenomenon is sometimes called the Alice in Wonderland syndrome in reference to the distorted figures pictured in *Alice's Adventures in Wonderland*. The author, Lewis Carroll, was said to have suffered migraines and collaborated closely with the illustrator to produce illustrations that captured the visual effects he experienced.

The visual effects of the prodrome stage may disappear with the onset of the headache or my overlap. When the visual symptoms occur, but a headache does not follow, the condition is known as a migraine equivalent.

The migraine headache itself is often severe. It usually affects only one side of the head and may include the face, extending as far as the jaw. Patients may experience light sensitivity, head, neck, and scalp sensitivity or tenderness, nausea and vomit-ing. The headache may last from one to 24 hours. In rare cases, the headache may last for days.

Migraines can occur at any time of life. They may appear in children as recurring attacks of headache and vomiting or as migraine equivalents. The attacks may disappear or return later in middle life. Migraines can occur for the first time in middle age and may decrease in regularity as time goes on. Women are more likely to suffer from migraines, but the problem tends to improve with menopause.

At present, there is no cure for migraines. Analgesics such as aspirin and acetaminophen or either compound with codeine may be taken to ease pain at the first sign of the headache. Severe pain is often treated with vasoconstricting agents such as ergotamine. These drugs constrict the blood vessels of the scalp to reduce the flow of blood. Ergotamine must be taken during the early stages of the headache and cannot be taken in conjunction with drugs for hypertension.

Migraines may recur. Patients may reduce recurrences by avoiding triggering factors and managing stress and tension. Drugs to prevent migraine attacks may be prescribed in cases in which the severity or frequency of migraine attacks has not been affected by the elimination of triggering factors. The drugs, such as Bellergal, Pizotyline, Propranolol, Elavil, and Sansert, have varying degrees of effectiveness, side effects, and safety. New treatments for migraines are being developed and tested.

Migraines can be very upsetting and distressing to those who suffer from them and to their families and friends. Also, there are many misconceptions about migraines, including the theory that a migraine is not a bona fide physical illness.

Joel R. Saper, M.D., director of the Michigan Head-Pain & Neurological Institute, explained the problem of misconception as it relates to migraines. "There is no condition of such magnitude that is shrouded in myth, misinformation, and mistreatment as is this condition, and there are few conditions which are as disabling during the acute attack," Saper said.

There is a support group for migraine sufferers called Migraine Awareness Group: A National Understanding for Migraineurs, or M.A.G.N.U.M. Contact:

M.A.G.N.U.M., Inc.
113 South Saint Asaph, Suite 300
Alexandria, VA 22314
703-739-9384
www.migraines.org

mobility   See ORIENTATION AND MOBILITY.

Mowat Sensor   The Mowat Sensor is a mobility aid designed for use by visually impaired persons and developed by Humanware. The device uses high-frequency sound waves to detect objects in the user's path. The sensor vibrates if an object is present and increases the vibration rate as the user nears the object. The sensor has a short range for objects less than one meter away and a longer range for objects up to four meters away.

Approximately the size of a flashlight, the device may be hand held or carried in a pocket or purse. A model for those with poor tactual sensation produces an audible signal heard through an earphone attachment. Other similar devices are manufactured under various names, including the Bliss Passive Detector.

The device is designed to be used with a long cane or dog guide. Several hours of practice and/or training with a qualified instructor are required for proficient use.

multiple sclerosis   (MS)   A chronic disease of the central nervous system. According to the National Multiple Sclerosis Society, approximately 333,000 Americans have been diagnosed with MS or MS-related diseases, and approximately 200 new cases are diagnosed each week.

The disease attacks the body's myelin, a fatty substance that coats and insulates nerve fibers of the brain and spinal cord. As the myelin is damaged, sclerosed or hardened tissue, called plaques, form. The plaques interrupt or obstruct the impulses transmitted along the nerves.

Symptoms of MS include tingling in the limbs or extremities, numbness, blurred or double vision, nystagmus, impaired sensation, fatigue, weakness, dizziness, slurred speech, tremor, spasticity, and bladder, bowel, or sexual function problems.

Half of all those who are diagnosed with MS may experience visual disturbances. The three most common disorders are optic neuritis, DIPLOPIA, and NYSTAGMUS.

Optic neuritis, or inflammation of the optic nerve, often results in a condition termed retrobulbar neuritis. It may first appear as a loss of vision in one eye, blurring of vision, color blindness, or blind spots. The disruption of vision usually first occurs in the central field of vision and progresses to peripheral fields.

Optic neuritis may be treated with steroids or the drug ACTH. Recurrence is possible, but remission of the visual impairment is good. Most cases respond to treatment in three months.

Diplopia, or double vision, may occur if the eyes do not move together to focus on an object. Diplopia occurs when the myelin along nerve fibers controlling coordination of the eye movement is damaged. Diplopia is treated with steroids and ACTH or by patching one eye. The condition usually improves within several weeks but may recur.

Nystagmus is an involuntary, jerky movement of the eyes that makes focusing difficult. It may cause dizziness and blurred vision. The condition is treated with steroids, ACTH, and Meclizine for symptoms of dizziness. Within a few weeks the symptoms may subside, although recurrences are possible.

The symptoms and progression of MS are unique to the individual. Although an initial attack may never be followed by a recurring incident, most people experience periods of exacerbation, in which symptoms of the disease are most pronounced, and remission, symptom-free periods.

The degree of disability varies by individual but two thirds of all those with MS remain ambulatory over their lifetimes. The disease is rarely fatal and studies indicate that life expectancy is only reduced by 15 percent or less.

MS usually first appears between the ages of 20 and 40. Women, whites, and those who live in colder climates are more likely to develop the disease. Twice as many women as men have MS. Studies suggest that where one was born and lived for the first 15 years of life affect the risk of developing the disease more than later places of residence.

The cause of MS is unknown. It is not contagious or inherited, although certain genetic conditions within individuals may make them more receptive to MS. These factors include exogenous (outside the environment) factors such as viruses and endogenous (inside the environment) factors such as body immunity.

Because families tend to share similar exogenous and endogenous factors, susceptibility to the disease may run in families. Four percent of all families with an incidence of MS have an additional case of MS.

Although there is no cure for MS, it may be treated with medications to reduce the symptoms. Muscle relaxants may reduce spasticity and medications may be prescribed to reduce pain, tension, bowel and urinary distress.

The drug ACTH or steroids such as prednisone may shorten the duration and lessen the intensity of exacerbations. ACTH is usually administered by injection and monitored for effects on the body in the hospital. Steroids are given orally or by injection but also require monitoring. Side effects of these medications may include weight increase, fluid retention, mood alteration, and tendency toward the development of ulcers. Since 1993, three new medications to treat relapsing forms of MS have been approved by the Food and Drug Administration. They are: Betaserona, Copaxonea, and Avonexa. These medicines have been shown to lessen the severity and frequency of MS attacks. They also help to reduce accumulations of lesions on the brain and to slow the progression of disability.

Since increasing evidence links MS to disorders within the body's immune system stemming from a viral infection, current areas of research include virology and immunology. Some researchers believe that MS is associated with physical trauma, but that theory is controversial.

Frames, Robin. "Insight into Eyesight." *MS: Facts and Issues*. New York: National Multiple Sclerosis Society, 1985.

National Multiple Sclerosis Society. *Living with MS*. HealthNet Library, CompuServe, 1988.

National Multiple Sclerosis Society. *What Is Multiple Sclerosis?* New York: NMSS, 2001.

myasthenia gravis   Myasthenia gravis is an autoimmune disease in which abnormal antibodies in the blood disrupt transmission of impulses from the nerve endings to muscle tissue. This condition results in severe or fatal (in the case of respiratory failure) fatigue of the muscle. It is estimated that there are about 36,000 cases of the disease in the United States, with a prevalence of 14 in every 100,000 people. Women are affected more often and earlier in life than men.

The disease may affect one group of muscles or those of the entire body. Approximately 75 percent of all initial myasthenia cases involve the ocular muscles, and nearly 90 percent develop some ocular involvement over time. Those cases that involve only the ocular muscles for a period of two years will probably be limited to the ocular muscles and not progress systemically. Ocular myasthenia cases account for approximately 20 percent of all cases.

Ocular symptoms of the disease include PTOSIS (drooping eyelid), lid twitch or quiver, and NYSTAGMUS (uncontrollable movement of the eyes). Ptosis may be absent at the start of the day but becomes more pronounced as the day progresses.

Myasthenia gravis is diagnosed with a Tensilon test. The drug Tensilon is injected to stimulate nerve transmission. Muscle strength is measured before and after the injection. Those who show a temporary gain in strength or improvement of symptoms after the injection test positively for myasthenia gravis.

Myasthenia gravis is generally treated by a neurologist. Treatment may consist of oral drugs and corticosteroids. Removal of the thymus gland may produce an improvement in symptoms.

myopia   Nearsightedness, occurring when the refractive power of the eyes is too great in relation to the length of the eyes. Myopic eyes are too "long" for their refracting capabilities. Myopic people see close objects more clearly than distant objects. Corrective concave lenses in the form of contacts or eyeglasses are prescribed to correct the problem.

High myopia is a condition in which the eye is extremely long or large, producing extreme nearsightedness. In very large eyes, the structures within them are stretched, causing the retina to become thin and weak. Tears or detachments that impair vision can develop as a result.

Myopia usually occurs from the preteen to teenage years. As the child grows, the myopia may worsen with each growth spurt. Once the child reaches maturity, it generally levels off and stabilizes for many years.

myths   Myths about blindness have existed for centuries and grew from ignorance about the condition and nature of blindness. Myths are perpetuated by modern attitudes toward, and stereotypes of, blindness.

Some commonly held myths surrounding blindness include the concept of all forms of blindness as darkness, the concept of blind as dependent, the connection between blindness and punishment as in the Oedipal legend, the belief that the other senses compensate for a loss of sight, and that people who have a vision loss have ESP or musical talent.

Being blind does not necessarily mean seeing nothing, or being in darkness. Of the half million people who are legally blind in the United States, most retain some usable vision. Only a fraction have no light perception or usable vision. Because darkness is so closely associated in society with ignorance, evil, and fear, the concept of blindness as darkness also links it to these negative traits.

The lack of understanding about visual abilities of the blind fosters the perception of blind persons as dependent. Throughout history, blind persons have been seen as liabilities to the social group, wards of society, or beggars. This myth disregards the abilities of blind individuals to work and be self-supporting and exists today in the unwillingness of employers to hire blind persons.

The evil-eye myth stems from ancient times when blindness was perceived as a sign of evil or a punishment from God for some evil-doing or sin. Those with the evil eye were thought to be able to kill with it, and were therefore shunned.

The Oedipal legend supports the myth that blindness is equated with evil. Oedipus blinded himself as a punishment for wrong-doing. The legend supports blindness as a just punishment for sins and suggests that blind persons may have brought the condition on themselves.

A commonly held myth about blindness concerns the compensation of senses. It is falsely believed that once eyesight is gone, nature heightens the other senses to compensate for the lack of sight. In reality, the blind person may learn to use the other senses in more efficient ways to gather information, but the senses remain unchanged.

Blind persons are often believed to have extraordinary abilities or talents, as well. It is commonly held that blind individuals develop extrasensory powers, or ESP, as a compensation for the sight loss. Perhaps because of some popular blind performers, the myth exists that blind persons are innately musically talented.

Curiously, the reverse situation is also widely believed. It is held that blind persons lose sense abilities, especially hearing, with the loss of sight. This myth prompts people to shout questions to a blind person with normal hearing.

As blind and visually impaired persons become more widely integrated into social, vocational, and education situations, myths may dissipate. Through personal experiences, society can discover that blind persons are not condemned or blessed as a group, but rather, are individual members of society who happen to lack some degree of sight. (See EMPLOYMENT.)

Carroll, Thomas J. *Blindness, What It Is, What It Does, and How to Live With It.* Boston: Little, Brown, 1961.

Goldberg, Maxwell H., and John R. Swinton. *Blindness Research: The Expanding Frontiers.* University Park: Pennsylvania State University Press, 1969.

Haskins, James. *Who Are the Handicapped?* New York: Doubleday, 1978.

Jernigan, Kenneth. *Disability and Visibility: Uncle Tom, Blind Tom, and Tiny Tim.* Baltimore: National Federation of the Blind, 1970.

Mitchell, Joyce Slayton. *See Me More Clearly.* New York: Harcourt, Brace, Jovanovich, 1980.

National School Lunch Act As amended, the National School Lunch Act of 1946 offers assistance to public and private institutions, schools, camps, and day-care centers, including those that serve handicapped or mentally retarded students, to provide meals to eligible children. The assistance outlined in the act includes grants, reimbursements, and commodity donations.

The School Lunch Program, as authorized under Section 4 of the act, provides institutions with the funding and food donations necessary to serve free or reduced fee lunches to eligible children. Children qualify according to their family income and the number of children participating in the program.

The participating schools, child-care centers and residential-care centers are reimbursed for the lunches that must meet nutritional guidelines determined by the Department of Agriculture. The rate of reimbursement is set by the states according to figures in the Consumer Price Index.

The Commodity Distribution Program, as outlined in Section 6 of the act, allows donations of food bought by the federal government under price-support or surplus-removal programs. Formula grants to state agencies are used to distribute the food to eligible schools, institutions, child and elderly nutrition programs, nonprofit summer camps, families, and individuals.

Section 13 of the act provides for the Summer Food Service Program, a nonprofit summer meal program for children in summer camps or institutions, including those that serve the disabled. The program awards formula grants to states that introduce, support, or extend the program and pay according to the number of meals served. The meals must meet nutritional criteria set by the Department of Agriculture.

The Child-Care Food Program, Section 17 of the Act, provides grants-in-aid to states maintaining nonprofit meal programs for children in nonresidential day care. The programs serve meals, including breakfast, lunch, snack, and dinner, to eligible children. Qualified nondisabled children under 12 years of age or disabled children of any age are entitled to two meals and one snack per day under the program. The meals must meet the Department of Agriculture's nutritional requirements.

The states distribute the funds to facilities such as public or private nonprofit institutions or organizations, day-care and recreation centers, and other day-care services. Grants are awarded according to how many meals are served based on reimbursement rates set by the federal government.

U.S. Department of Education. *Summary of Existing Legislation Affecting Persons with Disabilities.* Washington, D.C.: USDE, 1988.

night blindness   The inability to see clearly at night or in low light. The condition results from damage or defect in the rods of the retina.

The retina receives reflected light from an object. Light-sensitive cells called rods and cones translate the light into electrical impulses that the retina sends to the brain through the optic nerve. The brain changes the impulses into an image.

The cones, packed into the center (or macular section) of the retina, discern detail and color and require bright light to work effectively. The rods function in dim light and are responsible for detecting movement and shape. Any dysfunction of the rods may cause damage to night vision. Any peripheral vision loss that restricts the field to 5 degrees central vision results in night blindness because the usable foveal area contains no rods.

Damage to the rods may occur as a result of nutritional deficiency or disease. Vitamin-A deficiency may cause night blindness since the presence of vitamin A is necessary for proper rod functioning. Vision impairment due to vitamin-A deficiency is common in developing countries. A resulting disease, XEROPHTHALMIA, is the second major cause of blindness in the world.

Xerophthalmia causes changes in the cornea, CONJUNCTIVA and anterior segments of the eye. In acute cases, the cornea can perforate, the iris may adhere to the cornea, and the eyeball may be destroyed. A common and early symptom of xerophthalmia is night blindness. The condition can be detected with an electroretinogram or a thorough corneal examination. The condition is treated with megadoses of vitamin A given orally.

Night blindness is also a first symptom of RETINITIS PIGMENTOSA (RP), a degenerative disease of the rods and cones. RP first affects the rods, decreasing vision in the peripheral fields and causing night blindness. RP is a hereditary condition for which there is no cure or treatment.

nondiscrimination laws   Congress has enacted legislation that entitles individuals with disabilities, including blindness and vision impairment, to freedom from discrimination on the basis of disability. The laws guarantee the right to a free, appropriate education, the right to medical treatment for infants born with disabilities, the right to protection from harm in institutions, the right to protection from discrimination in federally conducted programs, the right to access to federally supported or operated facilities and programs, and the right to access to advocacy and protection programs or services for developmentally disabled or mentally ill individuals.

Eight major bills were passed during the 1970s and 1980s that aimed to ensure these rights. They include the Rehabilitation Act of 1973, the Education of the Handicapped Act, the Architectural Barriers Act, the Civil Rights of Institutionalized Persons Act, the Child Abuse Prevention and Treatment and Adoption Reform Act, The Civil Rights Commission Act Amendments of 1978, the Developmental Disabilities Assistance and Bill of Rights Act, and the Protection and Advocacy of Mentally Ill Individuals Act.

The *Rehabilitation Act of 1973* provides assurances that disabled individuals are protected from discrimination in acceptance to, or benefits from, federally funded or operated programs. Sections of the act protect against employment discrimination by federal agencies or contractors. The act authorizes grants to states to establish systems for protection and advocacy for disabled rights.

The Individuals with Disabilities Education Act, formerly known as the *Education of the Handicapped Act,* ensures the right of all disabled children to a free and appropriate public education. It supplies assistance to states to support this education and offers grants to states that provide appropriate educational programs to disabled students.

The *Architectural Barriers Act of 1968* required all buildings constructed or altered with federal funds after 1969 to be accessible to persons with disabilities, in compliance with accessibility guidelines issued in 1969. The act was amended to include public buildings and government-leased buildings intended for public use.

The *Civil Rights of Institutionalized Persons Act of 1980* granted the right of the U.S. Department of Justice to sue states for violation of rights of institutionalized persons.

The *Child Abuse Prevention and Treatment and Adoption Reform Act of 1978* includes a section prohibiting the withholding of medically indicated therapy or treatment to physically or mentally disabled infants.

The *Civil Rights Commission Act Amendments of 1978* expanded the jurisdiction of the Civil Rights Commission to include protection from discrimination to disabled persons on the basis of disability.

The *Developmental Disabilities Assistance and Bill of Rights Act* ensures the rights of appropriate services, treatment, and rehabilitation to those with developmental disabilities.

The *Protection and Advocacy for Mentally Ill Individuals Act of 1986* establishes a formula-grant program to states to provide mental-health advocacy programs and services. The Fair Housing Act, as amended in 1988, prohibits housing discrimination on the basis of a variety of factors, including disability.

In the spring of 1990, a landmark disability rights bill called the *Americans with Disabilities Act* passed in the United States Senate and House of Representatives. The bill bars employment discrimination for qualified applicants with disabilities and calls for changes in the workplace if needed to accommodate the worker. It requires accessibility to all new businesses, trains, and buses, and requires telephone companies to provide operators to relay messages from deaf to hearing individuals.

The National Voter Registration Act of 1993 is intended to increase the number of registrations of people with disabilities and of minorities. Both groups have historically had very low registration rates.

The Rehabilitation Act prohibits discrimination on the basis of disability in programs conducted by federal agencies or supported by public funds. It also applies to employment in federal jobs and to the employment practices of federal contractors. The standards pertaining to employment discrimination are the same as those used in the Americans with Disabilities Act.

The Rehabilitation Act also sets requirements for electronic and information technology that is developed, maintained, owned, or used by the federal governments. All technology that falls into those categories must be accessible to people with disabilities, whether they are federal employees or members of the public. To be considered accessible, an information technology system must be operable in a variety of ways and not be dependent on a single sense or ability of the user.

The Architectural Barriers Act requires that buildings and facilities that are built with federal money or leased by a federal agency comply with federal accessibility standards. These standards apply to new buildings, and those that have been remodeled or altered. U.S. post offices are included in this act.

U.S. Department of Education. *Summary of Existing Legislation Affecting Persons with Disabilities.* Washington, D.C.: USDE, 1988.
US Department of Justice. *A Guide to Disability Rights Laws.* www.usdoj.gov, 2000.

nongonococcal urethritis (NGU)   Nongonococcal urethritis, NGU, is a venereal disease caused most often by two organisms, *Chlamydia trachomatis* and plasma urealyticum. NGU causes inflammation of the urethra in men and cystitis and pelvic inflammatory disease (PID) in women.

NGU may infect the eyes of adults when the eyes are exposed to the live infection, or congenitally as the infant travels through the birth canal. When the eyes become infected, conjunctivitis results. If left untreated, the infection could lead to corneal scarring and blindness. Symptoms of NGU conjunctivitis are similar to those of gonococcal conjunctivitis and include redness, swelling, and a pus discharge. Those with symptoms of NGU are given a Gram's stain test to rule out gonorrhea. If the culture from the stain is negative for gonorrhea, treatment for NGU is prescribed. Treatment involves local administration of antibiotics such as chlortetracycline ointment and oral antibiotics.

nonverbal communication   Nonverbal communication involves ideas or emotions expressed by the face and body. Components of nonverbal communication include eye contact; facial expressions; head nodding or listing; shrugs; body posture; hand, arm, and foot gestures; touching; and regard for personal space.

A review of literature on communication skills of the blind indicates that blind individuals present different behaviors than sighted individuals. Individuals who become blind after birth (adventitiously) tend to exhibit more standard types of behaviors than do congenitally blind individuals (Bonfanti, 1979).

Nonverbal communication is generally learned through observation. Because blind or severely impaired persons do not have the opportunity to observe these gestures, they often do not form a pattern of appropriate gestures. This lack of knowledge can result in inappropriate behavior or a lack of nonverbal feedback to the other party. The resulting awkwardness or confusion can impede communication with sighted individuals.

Blind people may show a lack of facial expression, inappropriate voluntary or involuntary facial expressions, distracting or unattractive physical behaviors such as rocking or eye rubbing, excessive blinking, lack of eye contact, overuse or underuse of hand or arm gestures, and more intense touching techniques.

Blind individuals can be trained in nonverbal communication skills. The individual is made aware that such gestures or signals are received, translated, and acted on by the receiving party. Instruction includes methods to improve eye contact, form appropriate voluntary facial expressions, improve posture and appearance, develop appropriate, light touching behaviors, and correctly judge personal space or territory.

The training usually involves tactile props and techniques. It may include instruction in the workings of the eye and explanations of clues received visually as opposed to tactually. Although results vary with the individual, training usually results in some improvement of nonverbal skills.

Bonfanti, Barbara H. "Effects of Training on Nonverbal and Verbal Behaviors of Congenially Blind Adults." *Journal of Visual Impairment and Blindness* (January 1979), pp. 1–7.

Scholl, Geraldine, ed. *Foundations of Education for Blind and Visually Handicapped Children and Youth.* New York: American Foundation for the Blind Inc., 1986.

nutritional amblyopia   See TOXIC AMBLYOPIA.

nystagmus   The term for an involuntary movement of the eyes. The eyes may move vertically, horizontally, in circles, or some combination of the three. The condition causes focusing problems and blurred vision. Nystagmus may be congenital or acquired as a result of another disorder.

Jerking nystagmus is the most common form of the disorder. The eyes move faster in one direction than the other. It may be caused by lesions or changes in the brain stem, cerebellum, or vascular system; overstimulation of the systems within the inner ear; hypertension; stroke; multiple sclerosis; Ménière's disease; labyrinthitis; drug or alcohol toxicity; or brain inflammations, including meningitis and encephalitis.

Pendular nystagmus is the less common form of the disorder. The eyes move horizontally and equally quickly in both directions. Pendular nystagmus may be caused congenitally as in congenital cataract or disorder of the OPTIC DISC. It may be acquired after birth as the result of astigmatism, albinism, OPTIC ATROPHY, or corneal opacification or cataracts.

The underlying cause of nystagmus is treated to alleviate the symptom. If the cause is astigmatism, prescription eyeglasses may be helpful. When the cause is a disease or disorder that can be treated, control of the disease usually results in control of the nystagmus. In unmanageable conditions the patient may learn to hold the head or body in accommodating positions or learn to focus with one eye only. A nonprofit agency to serve people affected by nystagmus was formed in 1999. The American Nystagmus Network offers on-line support and discussion groups and provides information concerning the condition.

It does not, however, offer medical advice.

Contact:

American Nystagmus Network
P.O. Box 45
Jenison, MI 49429-0045
www.nystagmus.org

O

object of regard   The object of regard is the object on which the eyes are focused.

Ocusert   The trade name of a medication used in the treatment of glaucoma, a condition in which intraocular pressure builds within the eye. Manufactured by the Alza Corporation, which merged with Johnson & Johnson in the second half of 2001, Ocusert is a thin membrane worn in the eye like a contact lens. The membrane rests in the conjunctival cul-de-sac and continually dispenses pilocarpine into the eye.

Pilocarpine is a parasympathomimetic drug that constricts the pupil and facilitates an increased aqueous humor outflow from the eye, decreasing intraocular pressure. It also is available in drop and gel form.

Ocusert may be prescribed in one of two strengths: Ocusert Pilo-20, which releases 20 micrograms of the drug per hour, or Ocusert Pilo-40, which releases 40 micrograms of the drug per hour. The Ocusert is effective for one week, at the end of which time it must be replaced.

Ocusert may induce MYOPIA (nearsightedness) within the first few hours of insertion because it stimulates the CILIARY BODY. Ocusert should not be used by those with a history of acute inflammatory disease of the anterior segment of the eye because pupil constriction will occur and may exacerbate the problem. It is also contraindicated for those with glaucoma who have had an extracapsular cataract extraction because posterior SYNECHIAE (adherence of the iris to the lens) may occur.

The Ocusert membrane may be placed in the eye by the patient. Recommended insertion time is just before retiring since the myopia induced by the drug will have stabilized by morning. The system must be stored in a refrigerator.

onchocerciasis   One of four major causes of blindness in the world including TRACHOMA, XEROPHTHALMIA and cataract. The disease occurs primarily in developing countries and is found mainly in West Equatorial Africa, Central America, and South America. According to Helen Keller International, it may have infected over 30 million people and blinded an estimated 1.5 million people. It is projected that 20 percent of all those infected will become visually impaired. In Africa, approximately 40,000 people become blind each year due to this disease.

Onchocerciasis, also known as river blindness due to association of the infection with vector breeding sites, is a systemic disease caused by the filarial worm *Onchocerca volvulus,* a parasite transmitted by the blackfly. Humans become infected with the disease when the worm infests the body through tainted water or direct contact. The worm may live up to 15 years within the human skin, kidneys, blood, or cerebrospinal fluid. The disease causes corneal inflammation or KERATITIS, corneal scarring, and vision loss. It may be seen in conjunction with chronic IRIDOCYCLITIS and glaucoma.

A drug called Stromectol, manufactured by Merck & Co., Inc., was approved by the U.S. Food and Drug Administration in 1997. Stromectol is a very effective antiparasite medicine, and can be used to treat onchocerciasis. It is available under the name Mectizab in many parts of the world, including Africa and Central and South America. However, the treatment is very expensive and may not be affordable to all people.

Prevention of the disease may include insecticides to rid the community of the worms, avoidance of breeding sites such as rivers and open water-ways, wearing protective clothing, and excising of skin nodules that contain the worms.

(See WORLD BLINDNESS.)

Bath, Patricia E. "Blindness Prevention Through Programs of Community Oph-
    thalmology in Developing Countries." *Ophthalmology,* vol. 2. K. Shimizu and J.
    Oosterhuis, eds. Amsterdam: Excerpta Medica, 1979.
Center Watch. "Drugs Approved by the FDA."www.centerwatch.com/patient/
    drugs, 2000.
Cupak, K. "The Importance of Eye Camps in Underdeveloped Countries." *Ophthal-
    mology,* vol. 2. K. Shimizu and J. Oosterhuis, eds. Amsterdam: Excerpta Medica,
    1979.
Helen Keller International. *Facts About Helen Keller International.* New York: HKI,
    1988.
Phillips, Calbert I. *Basic Clinical Ophthalmology.* London: Pitman Publishers Limited,
    1984.
World Health Organization. *Available Data On Blindness (Update 1987).* New York:
    WHO, 1987.

opacification   A cloudiness or lack of transparency that blocks the transmission of light. This usually refers to a clouding of the eye's lens, which leads to a cataract.

Opacities in the lens are very common in aging persons and are not termed cataract until the opaque lens fibers significantly interfere with vision. Opacities often progress so gradually that the patient is unaware of the cataract until it becomes large or crosses the center of vision. Opacities that do develop into cataracts can be removed by surgery. Prognosis is excellent, and satisfactory results are achieved in 90 percent of cases.

ophthalmia neonatorum   An inflammation of the eyes of newborn infants. The condition generally affects the cornea and CONJUNCTIVA. Once a common cause of blindness arising from unhygienic conditions at birth, the infection is now successfully treated with antibiotics immediately after birth.

The condition is not hereditary but occurs during birth. Bacteria such as gonococcus, staphylococcus, streptococcus, or pneumococcus and viral infections such as chlamydia are present within the maternal birth canal. The inflammation is transferred from the mother to the infant's eyes as the child passes through the birth canal.

A herpes infection is the most common infection transmitted at birth, affecting approximately 1 in 5,000 births, according to the International Herpes Alliance. Gonococcus or staphylococcus germs and other bacteria may cause ophthalmia neonatorum also. Symptoms of the infection are apparent shortly after birth when the cornea, conjunctiva, and eyelids of the infant begin to inflame. The eyes may be treated with local antibiotics such as penicillin, streptomycin, or tetracycline administered at one hour intervals. Systemic antibiotics may be prescribed if the cornea is involved. If not treated, the condition can cause blindness and spread to other parts of the body.

The standard postbirth therapy to prevent ophthalmia neonatorum consists of the administration of silver nitrate, or comparable antibiotics, in eyedrop or ointment form. In order to prevent blindness from ophthalmic neonatorum, all states have passed laws that require the routine application of silver nitrate drops or antibiotic ointment to all newborn infants' eyes.

ophthalmic technician   A skilled assistant who works with an ophthalmologist. Ophthalmic technicians complete patient medical histories, perform simple vision tests, administer eye drops or ointments, change eye dressings, take optical measurements, and assist in surgery. Under the supervision of an ophthalmologist, the ophthalmic technician may also aid patients in fitting contact lenses, instruct patients in lens care, and perform some treatment procedures.

Ophthalmic technicians must have completed high school before entering the accredited training programs offered by medical schools, hospitals, and colleges. The two-year training program is followed by two years of supervised work experience in a clinical setting. Graduates of the program are required to take the certification exam issued by the Joint Commission on Allied Health Personnel in Ophthalmology. Certification is not, however, a requirement for employment in all cases.

optic atrophy   Optic atrophy is a loss of nerve tissue on the OPTIC DISC, the place where the optic nerve joins the eye. The optic disc is nonseeing and corresponds to the blind spot in vision. Optic atrophy may cause a loss of visual field. Both central and side vision may be lost, although visual acuity may remain unaffected. It can also cause abnormal color vision or blurred vision. Often called pale disc, optic atrophy is characterized by pallor, or whiteness, of the disc. Because nearsighted eyes and those of children also have disc pallor, the condition may be misdiagnosed or confused with other conditions.

Optic atrophy may be caused by glaucoma, an obstruction of a retinal vein or artery, a disorder of the optic nerve such as optic neuritis, a tumor, PAPILLEDEMA (swelling of the disc due to intracranial pressure), RETINITIS PIGMENTOSA, toxic-related causes, such as tobacco amblyopia, or injury. Treatment of optic atrophy consists of therapy for the underlying cause with medication or surgery or withdrawal of toxic substances.

optic disc   The part of the retina where the optic nerve meets the eye and the blood supply enters the eye. The optic disc contains no light-sensitive rods or cones and is therefore unable to "see." It is responsible for the blind spot in the normal field of vision.

Optic atrophy, a condition in which nerve tissue has been lost from the disc, results in loss of visual field. This condition may be caused by glaucoma, retinal vascular occlusion, PAPILLEDEMA, RETINITIS PIGMENTOSA, or injury.

The optic disc is subject to swelling. Papilledema is a condition that occurs when the optic disc becomes swollen due to an obstruction to the circulation of blood within the eye or by increased pressure within the cranium. Swelling may also be caused by optic neuritis (swelling of the optic nerve), blockage of a central retinal vein due to arterial disease, MULTIPLE SCLEROSIS, diabetic retinopathy, and postoperative conditions following intraocular surgery.

optic neuropathy   Optic neuropathy or neuritis is a swelling of the optic nerve. The condition is serious and may result in permanent vision loss.

Optic neuropathy is often associated with MULTIPLE SCLEROSIS. This form of neuritis, called retrobulbar neuritis, involves sudden loss of vision in one eye accompanied by pain associated with eye movement. Blind spots, or SCOTOMAS, may appear within the field of vision as well as COLOR BLINDNESS and difficulty seeing in bright light. Vision may be affected in the entire field or may begin in the center of the field and progress to peripheral areas. The condition is treated with steroids, and the prognosis is excellent. The vision loss may be partially or completely recovered after three months.

Optic neuropathy or neuritis unrelated to multiple sclerosis may be caused by collagen disease such as LUPUS; vascular disease such as arteriosclerosis, arteritis, or arterial hypertension; a viral, fungal or bacterial infection; tumors or cysts; and alcohol or tobacco overuse and other toxic causes. There is also a hereditary form of optic neuropathy that is passed through the mother to her children. It affects males more than females, usually occurring in the mid-20s. This type of optic neuropathy is called leberis hereditary optic neuropathy. Symptoms may include loss of vision in one or both eyes. Treatment may consist of medication for the underlying systemic cause and may include corticosteroids. Vision loss produced by neuritis unrelated to multiple sclerosis may be irreversible.

orbit   The bony socket lined with fatty tissue that cradles and protects the eye. The globe of the eye is held in place in the orbit by six extrinsic muscles.

The orbit is subject to several conditions. The fatty tissue surrounding the globe may become inflamed due to bacterial infection. The infection may spread to the globe. Tumors may also form within the orbit.

Hemangioma, a common tumor of the orbit most often seen in children, is benign and rarely requires surgery. Dermoid cyst is a growth that appears at the level of the eyebrow in the upper portion of the orbit. The cyst may be removed for cosmetic reasons and for biopsy. Pseudotumor is an inflammatory mass of the orbit without known cause. This tumor is treated with steroids to reduce the inflammation.

Other rare tumors include glioma of the optic nerve and rhabdomyosarcoma. Glioma of the optic nerve is a slow growing tumor that causes OPTIC ATROPHY. It may be linked with Von Recklinghausen's disease. Rhabdomyosarcoma is a rare tumor of the orbit seen in children. It is highly malignant and rapid growing but may be controlled by radiation therapy if treated in the earliest stages. Tumors originating from diseases of the body may metastasize to the orbit.

Tumors of the orbit often cause DIPLOPIA (double vision) or EXOPHTHALMOS, bulging of the eyes. Exophthalmos, also known as proptosis, is also caused by thyroid dysfunction, muscle palsy, injury, and infection. ENOPHTHALMOS, the appearance of sunken eyeballs, may occur due to an injury that displaces the fatty tissue lining of the orbit.

Injuries to the orbit may result in vision-limiting conditions. A common injury, the blow-out fracture, occurs when the globe is forced back into the orbit. A fracture forms on the orbital floor and bone is forced downward. Such an injury often causes damage to the rectus muscle and infraorbital nerve. The injury may be treated with placement of a plastic implant in the orbital floor and return of the displaced tissue to its correct position.

Fractures of the skull may extend into the orbit and cause cranial nerve palsy or optic nerve damage. A blow to the eye may result in OPTIC DISC atrophy. Such conditions resulting from injuries may affect vision or result in vision loss.

orbital cellulitis   An inflammation of the orbit. The infection is considered an emergency and must be treated promptly. If untreated, the optic nerve may become damaged and vision permanently lost. If allowed to spread to the brain, the infection could cause meningitis.

Orbital cellulitis may be the result of an infection of the sinuses that spreads to the bony orbit socket. Symptoms include forward displacement of the eye, restricted ocular motility, fever, and red, swollen eyelids. Movement of the eye also may be limited. Treatment involves admission to the hospital where antibiotics are administered in intensive therapy. Surgery may be performed to drain an abscess. If treatment is timely, the prognosis for the eye and vision are excellent.

Organizations for the Visually Impaired   There are many organizations dedicated to serving those who are blind or visually impaired. These organizations may be local, state, national, or international. Some are privately run and funded while others are government sponsored. These types of organizations provide many services, including the following: assistance finding employment; educational programs and activities; counseling and advice; special equipment; informational material, large-print books, texts, and other reading materials; medical advice and/or treatment; advocacy for the visually impaired, scholarships, outreach programs; and referral services. Many of these organizations, including contact information, are listed in Appendixes 4 and 5.

orientation and mobility   The term used to describe methods to navigate safely, gracefully, and confidently in an environment. Orientation and mobility skills are taught as a part of the rehabilitation and education program for the blind and visually impaired.

Formal orientation and mobility programs came into existence after World War II. In response to the need for rehabilitation-skills training for blinded veterans, the United States military established rehabilitation programs at four hospitals. Richard E. Hoover, an ophthalmologist working as a director of physical reconditioning, orientation, and recreation at Valley Forge General Hospital in Phoenixville, Pennsylvania, developed a long cane and a set of methods for using the cane that are the basis of today's orientation and mobility programs.

As word of the benefits of Hoover's program grew, a demand for mobility training developed. In 1959, at a conference cosponsored by the American Foundation for the Blind and the Of-fice of Vocational Rehabilitation, guidelines for mobility instructor criteria were outlined. Training programs were established in universities, and by 1960 Boston College established a graduate Peripatology Program, to be followed in 1961 by the establishment of the Center of Orientation and Mobility in Western Michigan University.

Current programs in universities require course work in education, physical and behavioral sciences, sensory training and awareness, preventive and restorative resources, and field training. Qualified orientation and mobility instructors are certified by the American Association of Workers for the Blind.

Orientation and mobility skills instructors individualize the program to the needs and abilities of the user. It is important for blind children to have orientation and mobility training early, in order to develop confidence in their surrounding and their ability to negotiate their environments. Although programs vary, orientation and mobility courses usually include sensory training, concept development, motor skills, orientation to surroundings, self-protection, long-cane skills, and use of a human guide.

Sensory training involves learning to use and sharpen the SENSES, including remaining vision, to their greatest abilities. The senses are used to determine landmarks, orient oneself to surroundings, and maneuver safely within an environment. The training may include development of echo perception or echo location, listening to the echo of self-emitted sounds to determine objects or surfaces in the environment.

Concept development is essential for those congenitally blind and includes learning spatial concepts such as perpendicular and parallel, and understanding fundamental structures such as compass directions, the layout of a building, or the design of a city block.

Motor skills include proper posture and body movement and the maintenance or improvement of coordination. These skills may be enhanced or developed through exercise, such as walking, skipping rope, jumping, or running.

Orientation training may include skills using landmarks and shorelines, squaring off, and trailing. Landmarks are objects in specific areas used to orient oneself in the environment. Shorelines are places where two different surfaces meet, such as where the floor meets the wall or where the floor meets the rug.

Squaring off uses landmarks as guides for determining direction, such as lining up with the edge of the curb to cross the street. Trailing involves lightly trailing the back of the hand to follow a shoreline such as a table edge, a hedge, or a wall. The back of the hand is used to avoid injuring the fingers.

Self-protection includes teaching protective body techniques. Upper-body protective techniques involve using the arm to protect the upper body and face from obstacles. The user carries one arm horizontally in front of the body with the elbow bent at a 90 degree angle. The arm then comes into contact with impeding objects before the body. If the head or face is the area most likely to come into contact with obstacles (such as when horseback riding) the arm is held up vertically to the side of the body with the hand held slightly ahead, protecting the face. The upper- and lower-body protective technique combines the horizontally held arm with the other arm held in front of the body, below the waist, at a 45-degree angle.

Long-cane skills are taught once the preceding skills are mastered. Training involves correct grip, movement of the cane, and use of the cane while walking to identify and circumvent obstacles.

Although use of a human guide is the least independent form of travel, it is sometimes necessary. The training in use of a human guide includes mastery of the SIGHTED GUIDE TECHNIQUE, a method for traveling with a sighted person.

Visually impaired persons receiving orientation and mobility training may be instructed in the use of optical or electronic travel aids prescribed by an optometrist or ophthalmologist. Optical aids include telescopes, magnifiers, and hand-held or spectacle-mounted devices that improve or enhance remaining vision.

Electronic travel aids include the laser cane, the Pathsounder, the Sonicguide, and the Mowat Sensor, all of which require specialized training to use. Electronic travel aids send out light beams or ultrasound waves that come into contact with objects in the path. When the beam or waves hit an object, the device responds by vibrating or emitting a sound. Electronic travel aids are used by approximately 1 percent of visually impaired persons and often cannot be used with a dog guide.

Dog-guide training is not a part of a standard orientation and mobility program. Only approximately 1 percent of visually impaired persons use dog guides because restrictions of age, health, hearing ability, remaining vision, and temperament limit those who may qualify to receive a dog. Those who do qualify for a dog guide are trained with the dog at the dog-guide school in specifically designed orientation and mobility programs.

American Foundation for the Blind. *How Does a Blind Person Get Around?* New York: American Foundation for the Blind, 1988.

Kelley, Jerry D., ed. *Recreation Programming for Visually Impaired Children and Youth.* New York: American Foundation for the Blind, 1981.

Scott, Eileen P. *Your Visually Impaired Student.* Baltimore: University Park Press, 1982.

Skurzynski, Gloria. *Bionic Parts for People.* New York: Four Winds Press, 1978.

orthokeratology   A procedure that uses contact lenses to reshape the cornea to reduce MYOPIA. The curvature of the cornea is measured, and hard contact lenses are prescribed at a slightly flatter degree. As the cornea is flattened, new lenses are prescribed at increasingly flatter degrees. The process may take up to three years to complete.

The eyes are regularly measured and the visual acuity tested to determine the degree of correction. The goal is to reshape the cornea to allow a visual acuity of 20/20 without correction. As this is achieved, the lens-wearing time is gradually reduced.

After the process, the cornea may maintain its new shape for a period of time but eventually reverts to its original shape. Retainer lenses may be prescribed to discourage regression. The retainer lenses may be worn as little as once every month or as much as eight hours a day.

Objective analysis of the procedure has revealed the dangers of permanent damage to the cornea, unimpressive and transient success rates, discomfort during the procedure and expense. Those with mild myopia stand the best chance of success, but those with severe myopia may benefit only in a reduction of strength needed in the lens prescription.

The procedure, although acclaimed by some doctors, is not widely used.

orthoptist   A skilled health-care worker who diagnoses and treats people who have fused-vision, eye-muscle, and crossed-eye disorders. Orthoptists work under the supervision of an ophthalmologist to teach patients vision exercises that enable the patient to accurately focus and coordinate the movement of both eyes. They may also be trained in glaucoma and vision-field testing.

Orthoptists must complete a minimum of two years of college or registered nurse's training in addition to the two years orthoptist academic program offered by hospitals, medical schools, or eye clinics. They may be certified by the American Orthoptic Council, although this is not a requirement for employment in every case.

P

panophthalmitis   A painful condition in which inflammation or infection affects the entire globe of the eye. This may result from the inflammation of posterior UVEITIS or an infection due to surgery or injury.

Panophthalmitis also occurs when an inflammation or infection that affects the posterior chamber and center of the globe, a condition called endophthalmitis, spreads past the center to involve the ANTERIOR CHAMBER and the SCLERA.

The underlying condition is usually not treatable once it has reached the stage of panophthalmitis. Panophthalmitis usually results in complete, permanent loss of vision in the affected eye. The eye may begin to shrink and it may require surgical removal.

paperless braille   Cassette braille, an information system that is stored on discs and accessed in braille. The system reduces the storage space normally needed for thick braille texts.

To use paperless braille systems such as VersaBraille, the individual runs his fingers over display cells to read the text. The push of a button accesses the next segment of recorded material. The user can produce, edit, and record braille with the system.

Although it consists of several pieces of equipment, the system is portable. It can be adapted for use with computer terminals, calculators, and typewriters.

papilledema   A swelling of the OPTIC DISC due to an increase in intracranial pressure. Intracranial pressure may be the result of cerebral tumor or abscess, hypertension, subdural hematoma, or hydrocephalus, an increase in cerebrospinal fluid within the cranial cavity. It is a symptom of intracranial pressure increase and is often accompanied by vomiting and headache, enlargement of the blind spot, and transient blurring or loss of vision. It almost always is bilateral, and may develop over hours to weeks.

Since papilledema may indicate a tumor, it is a serious condition that requires prompt medical attention. Papilledema may be diagnosed by a visual-field examination, ULTRASONOGRAPHY, computerized TOMOGRAPHY, and FLUORESCEIN ANGIOGRAPHY, a test in which fluorescein dye is injected into the body and observed as it travels through the eye.

Pseudopapilledema is a degeneration or abnormality of the disc that exhibits the same symptoms as those of papilledema. Pseudopapilledema may actually be a misshapen disc or multiple drusen, waste particles of the optic nerve.

Papilledema is treated according to its cause. Hydrocephalus is treated with a shunt to drain the extraneous fluid. Tumors are surgically removed. Medication or surgery may be necessary for hypertension or hematoma.

pathsounder   One of the ultrasonic electronic travel aids designed for use by visually impaired persons. The device is manufactured under several names, including the Russell Pathsounder and the Polaron.

The device consists of a small box that may be hand held or worn at chest height from a strap around the neck. The box sends ultrasonic waves into the path of the user to detect objects up to 16 feet away. The reflected waves are converted into an audible sound to warn the user.

The device is designed to be used in conjunc-tion with a long cane, and some manufacturer's models may be used with a dog guide. Use of the Pathsounder requires training from a qualified instructor.

peripatology   See ORIENTATION AND MOBILITY.

peripheral vision   The side vision of the visual field. It gives information about the area surrounding central vision, where detail is perceived.

Peripheral vision is controlled by the rods, light-sensitive cells of the retina. The retina is the inner layer between the CHOROID and the vitreous gel that contains photosensitive rods and cones. The rods and cones provide information about the shape, color, size, and movement of an object in view. The retina processes the information from the rods and cones and encodes it into electrical impulses. The impulses are sent via the optic nerve to the brain where they are translated into an image.

The rods outnumber the cones by an average of five to one and are scattered throughout the retina. They react to faint light, shape, and movement. Because the rods do not require high levels of light to function, they enable the eye to see at night. Because they are scattered throughout the retina, unlike the cones which are concentrated in the center, they are responsible for peripheral vision.

Diseases of the retina and other disorders of the eye may damage cones or destroy peripheral vision. RETINITIS PIGMENTOSA (RP) is a hereditary group of diseases that attack the retina and cause degeneration of the rods and cones. The rods are affected first. As they are destroyed, night vision deteriorates and peripheral vision is lost. As the disease progresses, ever-increasing tunnel vision results. Currently, there is no treatment for RP.

Retinal detachment may cause a sudden loss of peripheral vision. A retinal detachment occurs when the retina pulls away from the epithelial layer next to the choroid. This may be caused by holes or tears in the retina, by traction or by leakage of the vitreous gel. The tears may result from aging, injury, cataract surgery, or severe myopia (nearsightedness). As the retina detaches, it fails to function in the detached area, and vision is lost. Detached retinas are usually treated surgically.

Glaucoma is a disease that attacks and destroys peripheral vision. It is the leading cause of blindness among adults in the United States. It may be caused by heredity, aging or as a result of another eye condition. As the AQUEOUS FLUID in the ANTERIOR CHAMBER of the eye fails to drain normally, the fluid builds within the eye, forcing the vitreous in the *posterior chamber* against the retina and optic nerve. The pressure cuts off the blood supply to nerve cells in the retina and optic nerve, damaging them and destroying vision. Since glaucoma first affects those cells that determine peripheral vision, a loss of peripheral vision is a major symptom of glaucoma. Other symptoms include pain, blurred vision, the presence of halos around lights, and a loss of night vision. Without treatment, glaucoma causes increasing tunnel vision. Vision lost as a result of glaucoma cannot be restored, but once diagnosed, glaucoma may be effectively treated and controlled with medication or a combination of medication, laser treatments and surgery.

phoroptor   An instrument used in the ophthalmologic examination. The phoroptor determines the refraction errors, or the degree of inability to properly focus.

It is a large butterflylike apparatus that has two round sections affixed to a vertical base. The patient faces the phoroptor, with one round section centered in front of each eye. The patient places his chin on a chin rest and looks through lenses in each round section to read a wall chart.

The phoroptor holds hundreds of lenses of varying degrees in each round section. The examiner uses a dial to change the lenses in front of each eye. The patient is asked to determine which lenses provide the clearest vision or image of the chart.

From the information provided by the patient in response to the phoroptor lenses, the examiner can prescribe the proper corrective lenses.

photocoagulation   A procedure in which light is used to coagulate or congeal hemorrhages. Photocoagulation is used routinely in ophthalmological therapy and as an alternative to surgery.

Light was first used in the 1950s to coagulate retinal detachments. The procedure used a German device that produced a powerful beam of light from a xenon arc. In the 1960s lasers were introduced and became the instrument of choice for photocoagulation because they generate less heat and can be focused more precisely.

The low energy, finely concentrated light of the laser is directed into the eye where it is absorbed by the tissue. The energy converts to heat, which forms a burn. The burn develops into scar tissue, which congeals the hemorrhage.

Photocoagulation is used to treat diabetic retinopathy. An ARGON LASER is directed into the eye where the light is absorbed into the pigmented layer of the retina. The surgeon makes several "burns" around each leaking vessel of the retina. The resulting scar tissue stops the leaking. Unhealthy tissue that is generating neovascularization (new, weak vessel growth) is treated with the laser to destroy it and prevent the cycle of new growth.

In much the same manner, photocoagulation is used to treat subretinal neovascularization, a complication of age-related maculopathy. A break in the pigment epithelial layer beneath the retina causes the underlying vessels to bleed into the retina and cause scarring. The scarring destroys vision in the macula, the central section of the retina responsible for sharpest sight.

This treatment utilizes a laser, which is absorbed only in the deepest layers of the retina where such damage occurs. The light passes through the upper, unaffected layers and treats only the targeted areas below.

Photocoagulation may be used in some instances to treat glaucoma. A laser may be used to create a series of burns that develop into scars and form openings in the meshwork of drainage channels that allow fluid to flow more easily from the eye.

Photocoagulation is generally a painless procedure, usually performed without anesthesia. The patient sits in front of a slit lamp or biomicroscope in a dimmed room. Topical anesthetic drops, dilating drops or a contact lens may be placed in the eye.

The surgeon administers from 50 to several hundred rapid bursts of energy to the affected areas of the eye. The patient may see flashing lights and may experience slight discomfort or brief, painful moments. The procedure may last from five to 30 minutes, and the patient is usually able to walk or drive home afterward. Follow-up treatments may be necessary.

Although photocoagulation may improve vision in some cases, it is not always a cure. It frequently cannot restore lost vision and may only serve to stop or impede the progression of a disease or disorder.

Berland, Theodore, and Richard A. Perritt. *Living With Your Eye Operation.* New York: St. Martin's Press, 1974.
Eden, John. *The Eye Book.* New York: Penguin Books, 1978.
Krames Communications. *The Retina Book.* Daly City, California: KC, 1987.
Medem Medical Library. How is Diabetic Retinopathy Treated? www.medem.com/search, 1997.
Reynolds, James D. "Lasers in Ophthalmology." HealthNet Library, CompuServe, 1989.
Schweitzer, N. M. J., ed. *Ophthalmology.* Amsterdam: Exerpta Medica, 1982.
Shulman, Jules. *Cataracts.* New York: Simon and Schuster, 1984.

photophobia Photophobia, or fear of light, is a condition in which the eyes have little tolerance for light. The eyes may experience pain as a result of exposure to light or may involuntarily squint or blink in response to light.

Photophobia is not a disease but, rather, a symptom or result of an ocular disease or disorder. Photophobia is a first sign of congenital glaucoma in infants. It may be caused by or seen in a multitude of disorders including IRITIS, corneal lesions, ALBINISM, cataracts, BLEPHARITIS, MIGRAINE, TRACHOMA, UVEITIS, some types of drugs, and SYMPATHETIC OPHTHALMIA. Since photophobia is a result or symptom of disorder, its occurrence should prompt an ocular examination.

pinguecula   See CONJUNCTIVA.

Plaquinil   See LUPUS.

pleoptics   Pleoptics or pleoptic methods are part of orthoptic training, the use of exercises to correct or improve vision disorders. Pleoptic methods use flashing devices to improve macular and foveal orientation and fixation in cases of amblyopia, a condition of blindness in one eye due to disuse.

The treatment consists of producing an afterimage on which the patient is taught to focus. The macular region of the retina is stimulated with a bright or dazzling light. When the light is turned off, the patient fixates on the macula's after-image, encouraging the individual to use the macula.

Pleoptic treatment may last several weeks to several years. Results of pleoptic treatment have been disappointing in light of early expectations, and the methods are now more widely used in Europe than in the United States.

pneumatic retinopexy   A fairly new procedure used to repair a retinal detachment. A retinal detachment occurs when the retina becomes separated from the back of the eye. Some detachments are caused by retinal holes or tears, which must be surgically repaired.

With pneumatic retinopexy, freezing treatment is placed around the retinal tear, after which an expanding gas bubble is injected into the eye. The gas pushes against the area of the retinal tear and closes it, eliminating the need for a scleral buckle.

The procedure requires only local anesthetic and often can be done in a doctor's office. It does not, however, work for all types of retinal detachments. Pneumatic retinopexy was first introduced in the United States in 1985.

posterior chamber   The posterior chamber of the eye is the area between the iris and the lens. It is the counterpart to the ANTERIOR CHAMBER located between the cornea and the iris. Both chambers are filled with AQUEOUS FLUID, the clear liquid that nourishes the cornea and lens and carries away waste.

The aqueous is produced by the CILIARY BODY epithelium. The ciliary body also has a muscle group that bends the lens of the eye to focus properly. The aqueous flows from the ciliary body into the posterior chamber to bring nutrients to the lens. It then flows through the pupil of the eye into the anterior chamber to reach the back of the cornea. After the fluid has circulated, it leaves the eye through the Schlemm's canal, a drainage point at the junction of the cornea and the iris.

The posterior chamber is the site of surgery for posterior intraocular lens implantations. As a part of cataract surgery, a plastic lens is often placed either in front of, or behind, the iris to replace the portion of natural lens lost to surgery. Posterior lens implantation places the artificial lens behind the iris.

Posterior is also a term used to describe the back portion of the eye behind the lens. This area is filled with the vitreous, a clear gel-like material that makes up 80 percent of the volume of the eye. The vitreous gives volume to the eye and supports the other organs within the globe.

The expanded definition or boundaries of the posterior area may include the retina, optic nerve, and portions of the CHOROID and SCLERA, which are positioned in the back of the eye. This area may be injected with antibiotics or other medications in the treatment of disease or infection. It may be the site of surgery as in retinal detachment operations, or vitrectomies. In retinal detachment surgery, the retina is reattached to the epithelial layer next to the choroid. During vitrectomy, the chamber behind the lens is drained of diseased vitreous gel and filled with a sterile saline solution.

The posterior section behind the lens may be subject to floaters, bits of debris or blood in the vitreous. Light passing through the vitreous casts shadows of the debris onto the retina, causing images of the debris to float through the field of vision. Floaters appear in normal vision and are not considered as a symptom of disease unless they appear suddenly or in large numbers.

potential acuity meter   (PAM)   A slit-lamp attachment used to assess the potential, usable vision of those with cataractous lenses or corneal opacities.

The PAM uses a prism system and self-illumination to project a small SNELLEN CHART through a clear section of the cornea or lens and onto the retina of the person being examined. In by-passing the opacities, the examiner can efficiently use the Snellen chart to measure visual acuity.

prisms   Prisms are inexpensive optical additions to prescriptive lenses that maximize use of remaining vision. They are used to improve ocular conditions such as NYSTAGMUS, DIPLOPIA, macular disease, or peripheral-field defects.

Prisms are horizontally incorporated into frames for prescriptive lenses or noncorrective spectacles to treat nystagmus, an uncontrollable jerking of the eyes that impairs focusing on an object. The prisms may relieve symptomatic headache and improve acuity and stabilization of vision.

Vertically applied prisms are used to treat diplopia, or double vision, due to retinal surgery. The prisms compensate for the impaired abilities of the extraocular muscles.

Those with macular disease may be helped by prisms. If the macula, or central section of sight, is impaired or destroyed, prisms can be placed to move the image from the FOVEA (central macular region) to an area outside the fovea that is usable.

Prisms such as the Fresnel prism are used for peripheral-field (side vision) defects. They are incorporated into prescription lenses or pressed onto noncorrective spectacles in sections above and below or to the sides of the usable central visual field. By moving the eyes or the head slightly, the user can see through the prisms into the restricted field.

progressive addition lenses   Seamless, multifocal lenses that allow the wearer a smooth transition from the distance portion of the lens into the reading portion. No line is visible, either to the wearer or anyone else. The power of a progressive addition lens gradually increases as the wearer looks from the distance portion to the reading portion, creating an appropriate lens power for every distance. A disadvantage of these lenses is that the sides tend to become distorted, making side vision appear to be wavy. Technology for creating these lenses, which first appeared in the late 1970s, continues to improve, however, and wearers find the distortion to be less troublesome as they get accustomed to the lenses.

proptosis   See EXOPHTHALMOS.

prosthesis   A prosthetic or artificial eye is used to replace an eye that has been enucleated, or surgically removed. Prosthetic eyes have been in existence for centuries. Ancient Egyptian cultures fashioned wax, plaster- or precious-stone eyes to adorn their dead.

Roman surgeon priests made artificial eyes for the living out of wood, shells, bone, ivory, stone, and precious metals. In the 16th century, Venetians developed the first glass eyes, but the precursor of the modern type of prosthetic was developed in the 17th century by French surgeons.

Before World War II, most prosthetic eyes were manufactured of glass in Germany and exported to other countries. After the war, plastic prosthetics were invented and manufactured throughout the world. Modern prosthetic eyes are made from glass or plastic by ocularists. They are custom shaped to match the eye socket of the individual and the coloring of the natural eye. Prosthetic eyes are generally nondistinguishable from natural eyes.

Two or more days after enucleation the eye socket is fitted with a plastic shell that will cradle the prosthesis. Three or four weeks later, the prosthetic eye is fitted. The eye is attached to the remaining extrinsic muscles in the orbit to ensure natural movement.

The prosthetic eye is worn constantly to prevent contraction of the eye socket. It is cleansed daily and may be lubricated with drops for this purpose. A slight mucous discharge is a normal characteristic of prosthesis wearers, but profuse discharge could indicate an infection.

Infection often stems from roughening of the prosthesis. The prosthesis should be polished once or twice a year to buff out scratches and reduce irritation, and should be checked for wear by a specialist at regular intervals. Most plastic prosthetic eyes last five years on average.

pterygium   See CONJUNCTIVA.

ptosis   A sagging of the upper eyelid. It may be congenital or acquired and can affect one or both eyes. The disorder may appear congenitally in children or in adults due to aging, nerve palsy, inflammation, styes, tumors, cysts, MYASTHENIA GRAVIS, oculomotor palsy, Horner's syndrome, or use of guanethidine eyedrops.

Mild ptosis that does not affect vision may require no treatment. Severe forms of the condition may affect vision by obstructing the pupil or may be cosmetically unattractive. After careful diagnosis as to the cause, ptosis may be corrected surgically in some congenital, nerve palsy, or age-related cases.

Surgery may be performed on children of three or four years of age or younger if the ptosis is unilateral and causing amblyopia. The surgery may be performed under local anesthetic for adults and general anesthetic for children. The type of surgical procedure used depends on the severity and underlying cause of each case.

Three surgical procedures are most commonly used. The *Fansanella-Servat* involves the removal of a portion of the lid from the inside. The outer skin is not incised. The shortened lid is lifted off the eye. This procedure is used to treat mild cases of ptosis. The *levator resection* is used to treat moderate cases. During this procedure several incisions are made in the lid. A sling is placed inside the lid to permanently lift it. The *frontalis suspension* is reserved for severe cases of ptosis. A section of the muscle that raises the eyelid is removed. The surface skin of the eyelid is usually involved in the incision. The shortened muscle keeps the lid elevated. Complications from eyelid surgery may include infection, bleeding, scarring, and corneal drying. Over- and under-corrections may occur.

Treatment of other forms of ptosis involves treating the underlying cause. Neostigmine may be prescribed in cases of myasthenia gravis. When surgery is contraindicated, special spectacles with an attached crutch to raise the eyelid may be prescribed.

R

radial keratotomy (RK)   A type of cornea surgery developed in the
Soviet Union by Dr. Syvatoslav Fyodorov. The surgery is designed to
improve myopia (nearsightedness). The ultimate goal of the surgery is to
restore the patient's vision to 20/20 without the use of contact lenses or
eyeglasses. The words *radial keratotomy* refer to the radial cuts or incisions
made on the cornea during surgery.

Those with mild myopia can expect the best results from radial keratotomy. Possible candidates must require glasses or contact lenses to correct
their vision. The best results are for those with a refraction between -2.00
to -4.00 diopters and a visual acuity level of 20/80 to 20/200. Those with
high myopia (-5.00 or greater) will not achieve the same results.

Although prospective RK patients must be mildly myopic, people with
very slight myopia are discouraged from undergoing surgery for such minimal correction. Those with corneal disorders, glaucoma or pre-glaucoma-
tous conditions, lenticular astigmatism, or other eye disorders are also
often not considered good candidates for this surgery.

The presurgical examination involves an external examination of the
eye, a vision acuity test, and a refraction test. Additional tests may include
corneascope photographs, a slit-lamp examination, intraocular-pressure
testing, motility studies, and cornea measurement and depth testing.

Approximately one hour before surgery, the patient is treated with two
or more sets of eye drops to dilate and anesthetize the eye. Many surgeons
also administer an antibiotic such as gentamicin sulfate.

In the operating room, the surgeon takes a number of exact readings
and measurements of the eye to determine the surgical plan. The cornea
is stamped with a trephine, a cookie-cutter-like instrument that marks an
incision pattern that the surgeon uses as a guide. The pattern includes a
center circular clear zone and a variable number of incision lines radiating
out from the clear zone. The surgeon uses a diamond blade to cut from the
clear zone circle outward. The procedure flattens or shortens the cornea,
to produce better refraction and improved vision.

The surgery is done on an outpatient basis (without overnight hospitalization) and generally requires 30 minutes per eye. The eye is covered
with a patch for 24 hours, and eye drops such as pilocarpine hydrochloride are used for a week.

After surgery the patient may experience pain, sensitivity to light, tearing, decrease or fluctuation of visual acuity, over- or undercorrection, and
astigmatism. Patients may achieve from 20/20 vision to 20/200 vision, or
experience no improvement at all.

Studies indicate that radial keratotomy improves vision in the majority of cases. However, the procedure remains a controversial one and the

prospective candidate for RK is encouraged to research the procedure, its risks and benefits and the surgeon involved to develop a reasonable expectation.

Waring, A. O., et al. "Results of the Prospective Evaluation of Radial Keratotomy (PERK) Study on Year After Surgery." *Ophthalmology,* vol. 92, no. 2 (February 1985): 177.

radiation burns   Burns caused by light. Ocular radiation burns can be caused by ultraviolet rays, infrared rays, X rays, microwaves, laser beams, and gamma rays.

Burns due to ultraviolet rays include SNOW BLINDNESS, welders' flash, and sun-lamp injuries. Ultraviolet waves do not penetrate the globe and therefore deliver a burn to the cornea, or clear, outermost covering of the eye. Symptoms of these burns are usually delayed two to nine hours and include extreme pain, a sensation of sand in the eyes, and severe light sensitivity. The burns heal themselves within two to three days but antibiotics or steroid drops may be prescribed. Ultraviolet burns can be prevented by wearing protective eyeglasses or goggles.

Eclipse blindness is an ultraviolet burn caused by watching the sun during an eclipse. Although the ultraviolet rays of the sun do not enter the globe, the heat generated within the eye during prolonged exposure to these rays produces a burn to the macula. The macula is the area of clearest sight within the retina, the light-sensitive layer at the back of the eye. The damage to the macula from an eclipse burn is irreversible and causes loss of central vision. An eclipse cannot be safely viewed directly. Sunglasses, photographic film, or film negatives afford no protection to the eyes. An eclipse may be safely viewed indirectly by observing the image of the sun projected onto a flat surface through a small hole in a piece of paper.

Infrared rays can penetrate the eye and may cause cataracts. In the past, ocular infrared burns were found among steel workers and glass blowers. The adoption of safety goggles and eyeshields has virtually eliminated the problem.

X rays may produce cataracts in threshold doses of approximately 1,000 rad but may vary with exposure times. Simple dental or diagnostic X rays will not endanger the eyes. X rays that are used therapeutically to treat lesions near the eyes should be given only when the eyes are appropriately shielded.

Microwaves may cause cataracts but only when the eye is in the direct line of the beam. According to current knowledge, microwave ovens constitute no threat to vision.

Lasers are intense beams of light that can enter the globe of the eye. They are used therapeutically in ophthalmology to heal hemorrhages in the retina. The beam is focused directly onto the point of therapy that is exposed to the light for a specific amount of time. Industrial lasers can produce retinal burns when viewed directly or by reflection off other objects.

Gamma rays can produce cataracts and loss of vision. The rays released by atomic bomb explosions resulted in mass amounts of cataract cases following the bombings of Hiroshima and Nagasaki during World War II.

radio information services   Radio channels and programs that provide news and information on community events. Many services read sections or complete issues of local newspapers and offer information of interest to visually impaired listeners.

Radio services may be broadcast on open, freely accessible channels or on closed channels that require a reception box available to the user through the broadcasting station. State radio information services are often titled Radio Reading Service, Radio Talking Book, or Radio Information Service. (See Appendix for listing by state.) Local cable television stations may provide similar services.

Television descriptive services such as Descriptive Video Service (DVS) and Washington Ear provide narration describing various visual features of dramatic television programs. During the program, the narrator supplies details of the costuming, lighting and physical actions taking place. The service uses a separate channel accessible through an adapter that is compatible with standard television and video cassette recorders with stereo capabilities.

Contact:

Descriptive Video Service, WGBH-TV
125 Western Avenue
Boston, MA 02134
617-300-5400 (ph)
617-300-1026 (fax)
http:\\main.wgbh.org

The Metropolitan Washington Ear, Inc.
35 University Boulevard East
Silver Spring, MD 20901
301-681-6636 (ph)
301-681-5227 (fax)
www.washear.org

Randolph-Sheppard Act   The Randolph-Sheppard Act of 1938 established an employment-opportunities program in which blind individuals could operate vending facilities on federal property. Amendments to the act, legislated in 1974, extended its scope to include federal property operated by all federal agencies or departments and added operational guidelines to be authorized by state licensing agencies.

The act amendments outlined procedures and regulations to ensure fair treatment between blind vendors, the licensing agencies, and the federal government, and established greater control and participation by the Rehabilitation Services Administration. In cases in which vending machines directly compete with blind vendors, the amendments allowed the income from the machines to accrue to the vendor or to be used by the state licensing agency as a sick fund or vacation/ retirement fund. (See BUSINESS ENTERPRISE PROGRAM.)

U.S. Department of Education. *Summary of Existing Legislation Affecting Persons with Disabilities.* Washington, D.C.: USDE, 1988.

reading machines   Machines that "read" printed material aloud via a voice synthesizer. They are used by visually impaired and blind persons who are unable to read with magnification.

Most reading machines, such as the Kurzweil Reading Machine, employ a computer-controlled camera that scans the lines of print and recognizes words from its programmed computer memory. These machines can read textbooks, articles, and tests, as well as a user's own written work. The voice synthesizer says each word aloud. The user puts the text on the glass plate of the scanner and pushes buttons on a control panel to activate the voice synthesizer. On several models, the user can control the speed, volume, and pitch of voice and can direct the machine to repeat material or to read punctuation marks.

The Optacon is an optical-to-tactual converting reading machine. It translates print into letter configurations that are read with the fingertips. The user slides a camera across a line of print with the right hand. Simultaneously, the left hand feels the letter configuration formed on an array of vibrating pins. The user must be extensively trained to use the machine.

reduced rates   Reduced rates for telephone and transportation fares are frequently available to legally blind individuals. Legal blindness is a term describing visual conditions of either visual acuity of 20/200 or less in the better eye, after correction, or a visual field of 20 degrees or less in the better eye, regardless of visual acuity.

Verification of legal blindness by a doctor or ophthalmologist may in some cases be used to obtain reduced monthly service rates for touch-tone dialing and speed calling. Telebraille devices may be offered to those who are deaf/blind and can read braille. Those with low vision may be eligible to receive free 411 information or large-number overlays for the telephone dial.

Interstate bus lines and Amtrak offer reduced fares to legally blind individuals as do many city public transportation systems. Identification cards may be necessary to obtain the reduced fare and are often issued by the individual transportation agency. An identification card verifying legal blindness can also be obtained from the American Foundation for the Blind.

refractive error   Refractive error, or ametropia, is an inability of the eye to focus properly. The cornea and the lens of the eye focus light on the retina, which transforms the light into electrical impulses. The impulses are sent to the brain, where they are interpreted and presented as an image. If the cornea and the lens are unable to effectively focus the light onto the retina, a refractive error is present and blurred vision results.

The four most common refractive errors are MYOPIA (nearsightedness), hyperopia (farsightedness), astigmatism (distorted image), and presbyopia (aging eyes). Refractive error is often caused by the length of the eye. An average eye is approximately 24 millimeters long. The lens and cornea are designed to work best with an eye this length. An eye that is longer or shorter than this length creates focusing problems. A longer-than-average eye is myopic, or nearsighted. A shorter-than-average eye is hyperopic, or farsighted.

An eye that is too curved or flat presents a distorted image and is termed *astigmatic.* The irregular shape causes the light to focus onto two different points, rather than the one focusing point of normal vision. Astigmatism may be present in myopic, hyperopic, or presbyopic eyes. A presbyopic eye is one in which the lens has lost its natural elasticity due to aging. The lens is unable to change shape to focus on near objects.

Refractive errors are easily detected in the routine eye examination. Contact lenses or eyeglasses may be prescribed to correct the error and allow the eyes to see clearly, or refractive surgery may be recommended. Although early diagnosis and treatment are encouraged because they produce clear vision, refraction errors are not worsened or improved by the use of corrective lenses or glasses.

refractive keratology   The first type of refractive surgery to reshape the cornea, refractive keratology has been widely replaced by photorefractive keratectomy (PRK) and laser in situ keratomileusis (LASIK) surgeries.

Refractive keratology was developed mainly in Russia. During the procedure, doctors use a special scalpel to score the surface of the cornea in order to reshape it. This type of surgery is most successful for mild cases of astigmatism and nearsightedness. Treating more severe cases sometimes resulted in fluctuating vision, a persistent glare and starbursts.

rehabilitation   Rehabilitation services are programs that provide training or support to disabled individuals from federal, state, or private agencies. Rehabilitation may be offered through a public or private residential school, within a program of special education in a public school (through an organization for the blind), by a private rehabilitation facility (through correspondence courses) or by state rehabilitation agencies.

All 50 states administer programs of VOCATIONAL REHABILITATION and daily living skills for the purpose of enabling disabled individuals to become independent, employed, integrated members of society. These agencies are listed under various names, such as Department of Rehabilitation, Commission for the Visually Handicapped, State Services for the Blind and Visually Impaired, and the Bureau of the Blind.

Each state program varies according to the range of services and training available and the amount of financial assistance provided. Services may include medical and vocational diagnostic services, physical restoration, home-management skills training, orientation and mobility instruction, braille instruction, communication-skills training, personal-management skills instruction, books and training supplies, transportation allowance, reader services for the blind, vocational rehabilitation, job-placement services, postemployment services, procurement of job-related equipment and occupational licenses, adaptive aids evaluation and selection, counseling, and family-member services.

Legally blind individuals may qualify for state rehabilitation services if they can provide certification of disability and if the state has a reasonable expectation that such individuals will benefit from receiving the services. Vocational rehabilitation services are provided if the disability results in a substantial handicap to employment and if the state has a reasonable expectation that the recipient will get or hold a job as a result of vocational training.

Rehabilitation services are available at little or no cost to the individual. Some aspects of the rehabilitation program may require financial contribution by the individual. In some states, services such as psychological counseling, equipment purchase, and transportation to school or school tuition may be financed by the state or a combination of the state, the individual, and grants or loans.

In all state programs, each individual's case is carefully evaluated by a rehabilitation counselor for the blind and/or a vocational rehabilitation counselor for the blind with input from the disabled person. Everyone eligible is given an individualized written plan that outlines the rehabilitation goals, the individual's skills and needs, and the process by which those needs will be met.

The plan may provide for a medical examination to ascertain the extent and limitations of the disability in order to assess suitable employment possibilities. Medical treatment or equipment, including surgery, psychiatric counseling, hospital services, prostheses, and eyeglasses, may be provided to reduce or alleviate the disability and improve productivity on the job.

Guidance counseling may be suggested to assess the individual's potential for rehabilitation, independent living, and appropriate employment.

Job training may be provided at home, rehabilitation centers, trade schools, or on-the-job settings. Educational tuition and expenses may be supplied if college is necessary to the vocational rehabilitation. The plan may furnish financial assistance during the rehabilitation process.

Rehabilitation services may be provided by social workers, occupational therapists, therapeutic recreation workers, vocational rehabilitation counselors, rehabilitation counselors, or orientation and mobility teachers.

Rehabilitation counselors or teachers are college-trained specialists who provide daily living skills training as well as communication-skills, recreational-skills, and low-vision aids training.

Daily living skills, also known as independent-living skills, concern personal and home management and are frequently taught in the home or in a rehabilitation facility. They include methods for grooming and self-care, dressing, eating, precane mobility, handling and identifying money, personal recordkeeping, labeling food and clothing, cooking, laundering, safety skills, household cleaning, sewing, and home repair.

Communication skills may include listening skills, handwriting, typing, telephoning, braille, procurement of large-print or recorded materials, and personal communication or nonverbal-communication skills instruction.

Recreational-skills training includes instruction in leisure activities and exposure to adaptive games, crafts, and hobbies. The availability of support groups, sports groups, and other social activities may be explored.

Low-vision evaluation is provided by an ophthalmologist or optometrist who recommends specific aids and often provides training. Rehabilitation teachers can provide training in the use of other nonprescriptive adaptive low-vision aids and appliances such as bold-line writing paper, talking clocks, or glare-free lighting.

Orientation and mobility teachers are college-trained specialists who provide instruction that allows the visually impaired individual to move safely and efficiently in the environment. Skills provided in the instruction include auditory skills, tactual skills, olfactory skills, kinesthetic awareness, perpendicular and parallel alignment, search patterns, recovery skills, use of reference points, soliciting assistance, time and distance estimation, sighted-guide technique, protective techniques, trailing, and use of the long cane and electronic travel aids.

Vocational rehabilitation enables the visually impaired individual to continue employment or train for new work. Vocational training may be offered by the state rehabilitation agency, a rehabilitation facility, a residential or public school, an organization for the blind, or a sheltered workshop.

College-trained vocational rehabilitation specialists work with individual to evaluate existing skills and aptitudes, evaluate and recommend occupations, outline needed skills, provide vocational skills training and education, and recommend and provide training of vocational aids or devices.

Vocational-rehabilitation training may result in employment in the mainstream of industry, employment in a business enterprise program (BEP), a vending, short order, or cafeteria-style stand business program supported by the federal funds, or employment in a sheltered workshop. The individual may also be employed at home as a homemaker and family-care provider.

The success of rehabilitation training varies by individual. The extent of the visual loss, the time in life when the loss occurred and the abilities and aptitude of the individual all affect the outcome. The length of time for rehabilitation services also differs and may continue six months or longer.

American Foundation for the Blind. *Rehabilitation Services.* New York: AFB, 1988.
California Department of Rehabilitation. *Client Information Booklet.* Sacramento, California: CDR, 1987.
California Department of Rehabilitation. *Rehabilitation is Here to Help.* Sacramento, California: CDR, 1986.
Lions Clubs International. *Rehabilitation of the Blind.* Oak Brook, Illinois: LCI, 1984.
National Association for Visually Handicapped. *The Adult Partially Seeing.* New York: NAVH, 1984.

rehabilitation center   A facility that provides rehabilitation services to persons with disabilities. Rehabilitation services may include medical, psychological, social, and vocational services. The program is designed to offer reeducation and restoration of the disabled individual to the greatest physical, social and economic level possible. Rehabilitation centers may be supported through federal, state, local, or private funding.

Programs offered may include testing, fitting, or training in the use of prosthetic and orthotic devices; prevocational or recreational therapy; physical and occupational therapy; speech and hearing therapy; psychological and social services; personal and work-adjustment counseling; vocational training; evaluation for control of a specific disability; orientation and mobility services for the blind; additional adjustment services for the blind; and employment for those with disabilities who cannot be readily absorbed into the competitive labor market.

rehabilitation engineering center   Rehabilitation engineering centers were first established in 1972 as facilities to develop ways to apply advanced technology in medical, scientific, psychological, and social areas for solving rehabilitation and environmental problems of disabled persons.

There are 15 rehabilitation engineering centers in the United States. Each works within a core area of research specialty.

The Smith-Kettlewell Institute of Visual Sciences, located in San Francisco, is the center devoted to the visual sciences. The center designs and modifies sensory aids for the blind and offers rehabilitation engineering services through collaboration with the Pacific Presbyterian Medical Center's low-vision services.

retinal edema   A condition in which the capillaries of the retina bleed, filling the spaces between retinal cells with fluid. Retinal edema may be present throughout the retina or it may be contained in a general area.

If the macula, the central indentation of the retina and section of sharpest sight, is spared, vision may be relatively unaffected at first. However, the macula tends to accumulate the fluid. In this case, MACULAR EDEMA occurs. The condition is characterized by inflammation of the macula and blurred or impaired vision. If untreated, macular edema may develop into cystoid degeneration, and central vision may be permanently lost.

Retinal edema is caused by DIABETES, hypertension, retinal vein obstruction, traction of the vitreous, inflammations such as UVEITIS and retinitis and cataract surgery.

Retinal edema is diagnosed with FLUORESCEIN ANGIOGRAPHY, a procedure in which fluorescein dye is injected into a vein in the arm and monitored as it passes through the veins of the retina.

Retinal edema may resolve spontaneously or persist. Persistent cases may cause permanent vision loss. Treatment of the condition varies according to the cause. Cases due to inflammation are treated with corticosteroids. Those conditions of edema caused by vascular problems and diabetes may be treated with photocoagulation, a treatment that uses a laser to seal leaking blood vessels. There is no treatment for edema due to traction or cataract surgery.

retinitis pigmentosa   (RP)   A group of inherited diseases that causes degeneration of the eye's retina. The disease affects 100,000 Americans, and approximately one in 80 persons carries the recessive gene for RP. There are approximately 1,560 new cases of RP diagnosed each year, or an average incidence of 6/1,000,000. RP and related retinal degenerative diseases, including USHER'S SYNDROME and other rare syndromes, affect 400,000 Americans and 4 million people worldwide.

Although the disease name includes "itis," no infection or inflammation is associated with these diseases. Retinitis pigmentosa is characterized by a degeneration of the rods and cones of the retina.

The retina of the eye receives the reflected light from an object. The light-sensitive rods and cones translate the light into electrical impulses that the retina sends to the brain through the optic nerve. The brain changes the impulses into an image. The rods of the retina function in dim light. They are responsible for detecting movement and shape. Scattered throughout the retina, they are accountable for peripheral vision. The cones, which discern detail and color, require brighter light to work effectively. They are packed into the central part of the retina, the macula, and are responsible for central vision.

Retinitis pigmentosa first affects the rods. As the rods are destroyed, vision in low light is decreased, and peripheral vision constricts. As the disease progresses, the cones are affected, and central vision is lost.

Retinitis pigmentosa is hereditary but rarely may accompany other diseases. When accompanied by a serious hearing loss, the disorder is termed Usher's syndrome. There are several types of RP. They include:

- Congenital RP, or Leber's congenital amaurosis, is apparent at birth or in infancy. This rare disease causes a steady, progressive loss of sight.
- Recessive RP is passed to the child of two individuals who carry the gene for RP but who may not have RP. There is a 25 percent chance that a child (male or female) of two carriers will have RP.
- Dominant RP is passed to the child of one affected parent and one unaffected parent. With each pregnancy, there is a 50 percent chance that each child (both male and female) will inherit the disease. Unaffected children usually will not pass on the disease to their children. Three genes thought to cause dominant RP have been discovered.
- Sex-linked RP is passed to a child by the mother, who is the carrier. Sons of a female carrier of sex-linked RP and an unaffected male have a 50 percent chance of having RP. Daughters of such a pairing have a 50 percent chance of being carriers but will not inherit the disease.

The genetic cause and inheritance pattern for sporadic RP is unknown. Research is being conducted to investigate new mutations as they appear with each new generation.

The most common symptom of RP is night blindness or difficulty seeing in dim light. There may be a progressive loss of peripheral or side vision, which results in tunnel vision. As the disease progresses, the individual may experience a loss of central vision. Many individuals may develop cataracts, or opaque sections on the lens of the eye. Some individuals may experience complete blindness as a result of RP, although most will retain some limited vision.

In most types of RP, the onset is during childhood or early adolescence. Congenital, recessive and disease-related types of the disease tend to be more severe than dominant RP. Sporadic RP varies in severity with the individual.

Retinitis pigmentosa is not easily diagnosed. Often during the ophthalmologic exam, a change in the appearance of the retina may indicate RP. However, other tests, such as an electroretinogram, may be necessary to confirm the diagnosis.

An electroretinogram, or ERG, measures the electrical activity of the retina when exposed to light stimulus. Drops are first placed in the eyes to dilate the pupils. Anesthetic drops are administered to the eye just before a contact lens attached to electrodes is placed on the cornea of the eye. The electrodes record the responses of the retina as lights are flashed in both dark and light environmental conditions.

There is no cure or treatment for retinitis pigmentosa. Vitamin-A therapy, topical treatment with DMSO, and light deprivation have been investigated as cures with disappointing results. Research is continuing in the areas of retinal cell transplantation, gene therapy, pharmaceutical therapy, and nutritional therapy. These areas of research are thought to be very promising for victims of RP.

Low-vision aids such as the night vision aid, prescriptive glasses, telescopes, large print, or closed circuit television may be helpful. Genetic counseling may alert families to some types of hereditary RP.

Finkelstein, Daniel. "Blindness and Disorders of the Eye." *The Braille Monitor* (December 1988): 578–579.

The Foundation for Fighting Blindness. "Frequently Asked Questions Regarding Retinitis Pigmentosa." www.blindness.org, 2000.

Pagon, Roberta A. "Retinitis Pigmentosa." *Survey of Ophthalmology,* 33, no. 3 (November–December 1988): 137–168.

Reynolds, James D. "Retinitis Pigmentosa," HealthNet Library. Columbus: CompuServe, 1989.

retinoblastoma   A malignant eye tumor that originates in the retina. It is the most common childhood ocular tumor and may be the most common congenital tumor of any kind.

Retinoblastoma may be either hereditary or sporadic. According to the U.S. Department of Health and Human Services, up to 40 percent of cases are hereditary. The hereditary type is usually present at birth and most frequently appears at approximately one year of age. It often affects both eyes. Children of families with a history of retinoblastoma should be examined regularly for tumors. Even without prior family history of retinoblastoma, all bilateral retinoblastoma tumors should be considered hereditary and capable of being passed to future generations.

The more common sporadic type of retinoblastoma is not hereditary. It usually affects one eye only and appears at approximately two years of age. All forms of the disease are evident by age five in almost all cases.

Symptoms of retinoblastoma may include redness, pain, and inflammation in the early stages. Once the tumor has grown larger, the eyes may cross or the pupil may change from black to white or gray. This change in pupil color, called leukokoria, is the actual appearance of the tumor itself, visible through the hole of the pupil.

Once the tumor has been diagnosed, treatment must be given immediately. Both types of retinoblastoma are life threatening and can grow and spread rapidly up the optic nerve to the brain.

Sometimes, the affected eye is enucleated, or removed. In the case of bilateral retinoblastoma, the more seriously affected eye may be enucleated and the less affected eye given radiation or chemotherapy treatments.

Retinoblastoma is caused by the absence of paired retinoblastoma genes on the 13th chromosome. This can occur from heredity and/or environmental causes. Although retinoblastoma has one of the highest rates of spontaneous regression among all tumors, the cause of regression is unknown.

retinopathy of prematurity   (ROP)   A condition that appears soon after birth, generally in premature infants, in which abnormal blood vessels develop in the retina. This condition may progress to a retinal detachment that may cause blindness.

Although the precise cause of ROP is unknown, it is a result of prematurity, with very low birth weight (less than 1,000 grams) as the major factor. These premature infants may develop an overabundance of blood vessels in the retina. This may resolve spontaneously or may result in hemorrhages and the development of fibrous tissue or scar tissue. High MYOPIA, UVEITIS, glaucoma, amblyopia, strabismus, and retinal detachment may follow as secondary conditions. Total blindness may result.

In approximately 80 percent of retinopathy of prematurity, the retinal vessels heal themselves within the first year of the child's life. Approximately 15 percent of the remainder of cases progress to mild or modest ROP. The remaining 5 percent of cases develop severe ROP with retinal detachment and other secondary conditions.

Treatment of ROP has recently included CRYOSURGERY, or freezing therapy. In cryosurgery, proliferative retinal vessels are sealed with a cryoprobe, an instrument with a tip cooled to between 30 and 70 degrees below freezing. This therapy has shown good results and, if the ROP is severe, has proven to be the most effective treatment. If retinal detachment occurs, it is difficult to treat, resulting in only 30 percent to 50 percent success rates.

Historically, ROP was called RETROLENTAL FIBROPLASIA and thought to be caused by an overabundance of oxygen used in the incubators of premature infants. Modern, well-managed neonatal intensive care units for premature infants monitor oxygen, electrolytes, vitamins, and nutrition, carefully maintaining each at the best level for normal growth and development. Despite these efforts, ROP may be unavoidable for very low birth weight premature infants.

retinoscope   An instrument used during the eye examination for determining the refractive power of the eye. The examiner shines the light of the retinoscope onto the eye from an arm's distance away.

As the light moves across the pupil, the speed and direction of the lights and shadows are evaluated and recorded. This data indicates to the examiner the refractive power of the eye and is used to determine nearsightedness, farsightedness, or astigmatism.

retrobulbar neuritis   A form of optic neuritis, or swelling of the optic nerve associated with MULTIPLE SCLEROSIS. Retrobulbar neuritis is commonly seen among younger patients with multiple sclerosis and is often a first symptom of the disease.

Symptoms of retrobulbar neuritis include sudden loss of vision in one eye accompanied by pain associated with eye movement. Blind spots, or scotomas, may appear within the field of vision as well as color blindness and difficulty seeing in bright light. Vision may be affected in the entire field or may begin in the center of the field and progress to peripheral fields. Retrobulbar neuritis also can be caused by a neurological lesion, and is not necessarily a symptom of multiple sclerosis.

The condition may be treated with the drug ACTH and oral steroids. Although recurrence is possible, the prognosis for remission is good. Patients usually recover partial or full vision within three months.

retrolental fibroplasia   (RLF)   The historical term for a disorder responsible for an epidemic of blindness during the 1940s and 1950s. During this period, it was the most common cause of visual impairment in children.

The condition appeared in conjunction with the widespread use of infant incubators. Premature infants or those in respiratory distress were placed into incubators supplied with 100 percent oxygen. The high levels of oxygen caused the retinal arteries and veins of the eyes to constrict. Once the infants were removed from the incubator and breathed normal air, the arteries and veins expanded and proliferated causing hemorrhages and the development of fibrous tissue or scar tissue.

The scar tissue blocked light from reaching the photosensitive rods and cones of the retina and resulted in partial or total blindness. Secondary disorders, including retinal detachment, glaucoma, UVEITIS, cataract, MYOPIA, and strabismus sometimes followed within months or years.

The epidemic of retrolental fibroplasia reached its peak in 1952, and by 1954 the link between high concentrations of oxygen and retrolental fibroplasia was accepted and medical practices were altered. The blood level of infants is now monitored carefully, and oxygen is used only in amounts sufficient to prevent brain damage or death.

RLF is sometimes confused with RETINOPATHY OF PREMATURITY (ROP), an eye disorder that occurs in premature infants of very low birth weight. Using the terms synonymously is not correct because it implies that ROP is caused by an overabundance of oxygen. In the current epidemic of ROP, oxygen use is not considered to be the cause.

Most of those who developed RLF are now adult and blind. Their condition affected the education system, since the majority of these children entered school during a short span of time. Demands for mainstreaming in education by the parents of RLF children forced public school systems to develop programs that exist today for all disabled children.

river blindness   See ONCHOCERCIASIS.

rubella   Rubella, or German measles, is known to cause blindness when contracted in utero during the first three months of pregnancy. Although the mother may feel little discomfort, the disease may cause vision impairment, mental retardation, hearing impairment, heart defects, and respiratory problems.

Ocular disturbances may include congenital cataract, glaucoma, iris, or retinal disorders or defects and undersized eyes. Cataracts may be bilateral or unilateral and may develop slowly or appear severe at birth. Severe cataracts may be removed, but the patient often requires removal of the posterior capsule at a later date. Those with congenital cataracts often develop amblyopia, dysfunction of one eye due to disuse.

Runyan, Marla   The first legally blind person ever to qualify for the U.S. Olympic team and a finalist in the 1,500 meters event at the 2000 games in Sydney. Runyan also broke the U.S. indoor record in the 5,000 meters category in February 2001.

Legally blind since the age of nine due to STARGARDT'S DISEASE, Runyan played soccer as a child but switched to track and field at age 14. She competed in the high jump by placing reflective tape on the bar, and learned to jump hurdles by counting the number of steps between jumps.

Born in Santa Maria, California, in 1969, Runyan graduated with honors from San Diego State University in 1991 with a degree in education of the deaf. She earned a master's degree in education of deaf-blind children from the same school, and works teaching handicapped children in Eugene, Oregon.

She was quoted as saying, "I think what I represent is achieving what you want in life. It's a matter of attitude. Some people have a negative attitude, and that's their disability." Runyan has been featured on numerous television sports and news shows, as well as in various publications.

S

sarcoidosis A systemic disease whose symptoms resemble those of tuberculosis. The disease is characterized by nodules in the skin and lymph nodes and fibrosis of the lungs. The disease most often affects young adults and produces ocular disorders in roughly half the cases.

Sarcoidosis causes posterior and anterior UVEITIS, an inflammation of the uveal tract, the pigmented portions of the eye including the CHOROID, the iris, and the CILIARY BODY. Prolonged uveitis may lead to secondary glaucoma, cataract, MACULAR EDEMA or scarring, and loss of vision. Uveitis is treated with local and systemic STEROIDS.

Sarcoidosis, which often produces no symptoms, is diagnosed with a Mantoux test, biopsy of the nodules, X rays, and blood tests. There is no cure for sarcoidosis.

Schirmer's test An ocular test used to determine the amount of moisture or tear production in the eye. The test is often conducted as a part of a routine eye examination or in response to patient complaint of dry eye.

The Schirmer's test is painless and involves the placement of one folded end of a thin strip of filter paper into the lower eyelid. The uninserted end of the strip projects forward, out of the eye. The strip is left in place for one to five minutes during which time the tears of the eye wet the strip.

A measurement is taken of the amount of moisture accumulated in the strip. Normal readings may be 12 millimeters or more, and dry readings may be from 1 to 5 millimeters.

sclera The tough, outer protective layer of the eye. It is seen as the white portion of the eye surrounding the colored iris but it lines the entire globe of the eye. The sclera joins the transparent cornea at the front of the eye and circles around to join the optic nerve at the back of the eye. The sclera lies atop the CHOROID, the vascular layer that supplies blood to the eye.

The sclera may appear red as a result of an infection or disorder of the CONJUNCTIVA, the mucous membrane lining the sclera and the inside of the lids. The sclera is also subject to SCLERITIS, or inflammation of the sclera. Scleritis is closely linked to rheumatoid arthritis, gout, and collagen disease. Symptoms include redness, pain, and erosion of the sclera. The condition is treated with systemic antiinflammatory agents but seldom with steroids, which destroy collagen and exacerbate scleral thinning.

scleritis An inflammation of the SCLERA, the outer protective layer of the eye. Scleritis produces a red, painful eye and sensitivity to light. Scleritis may be linked to rheumatoid arthritis, collagen disease, disorders of menstruation, and gout, but may develop for unknown reasons as well. It is particularly found among young women.

Scleritis leads to thinning of the sclera and may expose the underlying uveal pigment. If untreated, scleritis may lead to necrosis (death of tissue) or perforation of the globe. Scleritis is treated with systemic nonsteroidal antiinflammatory agents. Corticosteroids are usually contraindicated, because they encourage scleral thinning. Treatment generally is directed at the underlying condition.

scotoma   A blind spot or area of blocked vision in the visual field. It may be caused by eye injury, disease, or disorder or migraine headaches.

Each eye contains one scotoma. This is the blind spot in the normal field of vision caused by the OPTIC DISC. The optic disc is the part of the retina where the optic nerve meets the eye. It is here that the blood supply enters the eye. The optic disc contains no photosensitive rods and cones and is therefore unable to "see."

Scotomas may be present in either the central or peripheral field of vision. Macular diseases attack the macula, the point of clearest vision in the central field. A scotoma, or blind spot, develops that permanently blocks central vision but that usually leaves peripheral vision intact.

Scotomas caused by RETINITIS PIGMENTOSA and glaucoma block vision in the peripheral or side visual fields. These diseases continue to destroy peripheral vision until tunnel vision results.

Scotomas caused by migraines are temporary. They occur during the preheadache or prodrome stage of migraines and may forewarn of the subsequent headache. Migraine scotomas may appear in any part of the visual field and may move during the course of the prodrome or headache stages. These scotomas may simply block out vision or may be scintillating and shimmer or blink with bright or colored lights. Migraine scotomas usually last from five minutes to an hour. They tend to retreat with the onset of the migraine headache.

screening   Screening examinations are eye examinations that are used to detect the possibility of a visual disorder in individuals. General screenings are routinely performed on the population during patient eye and medical exams, driver's license renewals, and entrance to the armed forces.

Specific screening exams look for particular visual field losses or ocular diseases. Screening exams performed in retirement communities would concentrate on those diseases and disorders associated with aging, such as age-related maculopathy, cataract, and glaucoma. An exam performed on a patient complaining of lost vision would screen for scotomas (blind spots) or specific field losses.

Often, a screening examination leads to a diagnosis. Evidence of diabetic retinopathy found in a routine screening examination detects both the result of the disease and its underlying cause. Diagnostic examinations follow the screening exams. The diagnostic exam is used on those who test positive or who show indications of disease or a disorder on a screening exam. This examination confirms the presence of a disorder and diagnoses the cause.

senses   The body obtains information from all five senses plus the equilibrium and kinesthesis. The tendency is to rely on the sense of sight or to use the other senses to validate sight information when the same information can often be provided by the other senses alone.

When vision is lost or impaired, the affected person must learn to use the other senses in more effective ways. Contrary to the myth, the other senses do not become heightened, nor does ESP develop as compensation for the lost sight. Rather, the visually impaired person integrates the other senses with any remaining vision and uses them more effectively.

Most visually impaired persons have some remaining vision. This vision may range from clear vision within a limited central or peripheral field to being able to determine light. Individual vision may vary from one day to the next due to general health, diet, stress, fatigue, medication side effects, or environmental factors such as glare or artificial light.

Use of the residual vision may require the visually impaired person to adopt new head or body movements, or to use a visual aid such as a magnifier when viewing an object. The remaining vision may allow for information about the size, shape, color, or contrast of the object in view.

The sense of hearing is used for subject identification, direction, distance, size, and structure. Visually impaired people must learn to recognize and discriminate between sounds and to determine the relative distance and direction between the source of the sound and themselves, a concept termed localization. Localization is dependent on adequate binaural hearing, or balanced, relatively equal hearing in both ears.

Hearing may also be used in echolocation, listening for the echo of a sound rising from an object. The person using echolocation makes a sound such as clapping hands, whistling, or snapping fingers and listens for the faint echo that rebounds from the object. The echo's sound changes as the user gets closer to, or farther away from, an object. With practice, echolocation can be useful in determining the distance, size, or existence of an object in the area.

Echolocation users must have adequate binaural hearing and must be able to hear high-frequency sounds. The use of echolocation is more effective in certain environmental conditions. Hard, large surfaces such as walls and cars reflect echoes better than smaller, softer surfaces such as drapes or people. Echolocation is also related to facial vision. Facial vision is the ability to locate nearby obstacles, without touch, by a feeling of pressure on the face. The close objects reflect background noise in a particular manner that can be interpreted to locate objects. Facial vision depends on adequate binaural hearing.

The sense of touch involves every part of the body from the top of the head to the soles of the feet. Touch provides information about the size, weight, density, texture, and temperature of an object or the environment. Touch may be used to compensate for lost vision in specific tasks such as reading braille.

The sense of smell is used to determine location or landmarks, such as the corner bakery, to detect danger such as leaking gas or the presence of smoke, or to confirm information provided by another sense. Smell is closely linked to taste, which is used to identify foods and provide information about the freshness and texture of ingested foods or medications.

Kinesthesis is the body's ability to remember a movement. It is a muscle sense or awareness that allows the body to perform a movement or physical task with little mental concentration. This sense provides information about the tilt in surface or grade, allows one to effectively estimate distances and positions and enables one to touch-type and sign a signature without looking.

The equilibrium is the body's sense of balance. It provides information as to the position of the body and allows for balance in turning or changing position.

sensory aids   Any aids, devices, or systems that enable an individual to overcome, compensate, or alleviate the performance losses caused by an impairment of any of the senses. Sensory aids may either enhance remaining vision or replace the visual information with information in a tactile or auditory form.

Because sensory aids increase independence and are related to job performance, they are often associated with VOCATIONAL AIDS, or aids that enable an individual to perform a job. Such sensory aids include talking computers, electronic devices to enlarge print, reading machines, electronic braille devices, and telephone communication devices. (See ADAPTIVE AIDS.)

shaken baby syndrome   A medical term used to describe a form of child abuse in which a baby or child is shaken violently enough to cause trauma from acceleration forces. Also called shaken infant syndrome, this form of abuse can cause brain damage and bleeding in and on the surface of the brain. It also can result in ocular injuries such as retinal hemorrhages.

The American Academy of Ophthalmology has encouraged parents and caregivers to learn the symptoms of shaken baby syndrome and to make sure a baby who may have been shaken receives an eye exam, which can reveal evidence of shaking. More than 75 percent of all severely shaken babies have retinal hemorrhages, a symptom rarely seen with an accidental head injury.

Babies and toddlers have weak neck muscles, which give them little control over their relatively heavy heads. When shaken, their heads vibrate rapidly back and forth, which can cause devastating damage. It is estimated that 85 percent of children who are violently shaken sustain serious injury, including blindness, hearing loss, learning disabilities, permanent brain damage, paralysis, or even death.

Shaken baby syndrome was first discussed in medical literature in 1972, and public awareness of the syndrome has increased dramatically in recent years. There often are no obvious outward signs of injury to a baby who has been shaken, although the child may appear to be stunned and glassy-eyed or sluggish. Vomiting, difficulty in breathing, inability to lift or turn the head, lack of appetite, and seizures are signs of possible abuse.

The Survivor's Foundation. "Eye M.D.s Urge Parents to Request Eye Exam in Shaken Baby Cases." www.survivors-foundation.org, 2000.
American Humane Association Children's Division. "Shaken Baby Syndrome Fact Sheet." www.csfpa.org/pages/shaken.html, 2001.

sheltered workshops   Any protected work settings for disabled individuals. These work locations may be nonvocational work-activity centers, transitional rehabilitation training and employment centers, or long-term competitive employment centers that provide opportunities for self-support.

The first sheltered workshop was established in the Perkins School in 1840 as a separate work department. The idea was duplicated in other schools for the blind and later became separate workshops administered by voluntary organizations for the adult blind and state agencies.

The Wagner-O'Day Act of 1938 established a program in which federal agencies could purchase selected commodities from qualified workshops for the blind. The act was amended in 1971 as the JAVITS-WAGNER-O'DAY ACT to extend the authority to workshops for all severely disabled persons and to services as well as products.

Early workshops produced handmade objects for household use, including brooms, chair caning, and hand weaving. Modern sheltered workshops are often more industrial in nature and produce such products as military equipment, including the Kevlar helmet, tracheotomy kits, and kitchen gadgets sold to military commissaries.

Many workshops for the blind are associated with the National Industries for the Blind (NIB), a private nonprofit organization that develops industrial employment for blind and multihandicapped Americans. The NIB offers technical and management services and allocates federal government orders among its workshops.

sickle-cell disease   A term used to describe any condition that involves inherited sickle-cell hemoglobin of the blood. The disease is most common among those of African descent and those with ancestors from Puerto Rico, Cuba, Haiti, Jamaica, Italy, Sicily, Greece, Cyprus, Turkey, Syria, and

South India. Sickle-cell disease affects about 72,000 people in the United States—about one in every 500 Americans of African descent—and the disease trait is present in one of every 10 Americans of African descent.

The disease affects the hemoglobin of the blood, the matter in red cells that enables the blood to carry oxygen to the body. Normal hemoglobin, called hemoglobin A or C, is characterized by round red blood cells which flow easily through the body's vessels. Sickle-cell hemoglobin, hemoglobin S, is contained in sickle-shaped, elongated cells that resist flow and cause obstructions in circulation (microinfarctions), a lack of oxygen to the tissues (hypoxia), and the proliferation of additional sickle cells.

Sickle cells have a shorter life span than normal cells. Their rapid breakdown rate results in a lowered hemoglobin level, or anemia. For this reason, sickle-cell disease is often referred to as sickle-cell anemia.

Sickle-cell disease occurs when hemoglobin A is changed to hemoglobin S by a genetic substitution of one amino acid in the hemoglobin chain. If both parents are carriers of sickle-cell hemoglobin, there is a one in four chance that the child will inherit normal hemoglobin and not carry the trait.

There is a two in four chance that the child will inherit one trait for sickle-cell hemoglobin and one for normal hemoglobin. This child is a carrier of the trait and may develop very mild symptoms of the disease or none at all.

The remaining one in four chance is that the child will inherit both sickle-cell hemoglobin traits. In this case the child will develop sickle-cell disease.

Early symptoms of sickle-cell disease are manifested in infancy and include listlessness, aches in the arms, legs, stomach and back, poor appetite, and pallor. Patients experience "crisis" periods that involve intense bouts of these symptoms. A crisis may last one day to two weeks and is often preceded by an infection, cold, or sore throat. Crises may recur several times a year, but the patient remains quite healthy between occurrences.

In patients with sickle-cell disease, the vision is affected when blood vessels become blocked in the CONJUNCTIVA, CHOROID, or retina. In turn, this may cause anterior segment ischemia, pupil irregularity, iris atrophy, retinal degeneration, and loss of visual field.

A serious condition called sickle-cell retinopathy is a common result of sickle-cell disease. As vessels within the peripheral sections of retina become blocked, the retina becomes starved for oxygen. It develops new vessels that tend to be weak and hemorrhage. The neovascularization may cause leakage into the vitreous or retinal detachment. A loss of vision results.

Photocoagulation therapy, laser treatments, are performed once neovascularization has begun. This may stop the hemorrhaging but can cause complications such as vitreal neovascularization. Cryotherapy, freezing treatments, may be performed on the smaller areas of neovascularization.

Scleral buckling may be used to reduce the traction that causes retinal detachment. This normally simple procedure is difficult in cases of sickle-cell disease because there may be overlying bleeding that interferes with localization of the hemorrhage source, and since the procedure may trigger necrosis, localized tissue death, in anterior areas.

It is thought that the sickle-cell trait may have developed as a natural response to malaria, a more serious disease commonly found in descendant countries of those affected by the disease. Those with sickle-cell disease carry a high resistance to malaria. There is no cure for sickle-cell disease, but medical treatment and monitoring may lessen its effects. Doctors recently began using hydroxyurea, a drug often used to treat leukemia, on patients with sickle-cell disease. The drug has been found to reduce the painful crisis periods.

Galloway, N. R. *Common Eye Diseases and Their Management.* Berlin: Springer-Verlag, 1895.

Mayfield, Eleanor. "New Hope for People with Sickle-Cell Anemia." *FDA Consumer,* May 1996, p. 16.

Rhode, Stephen J., and Stephen P. Ginsberg. *Ophthalmic Technology.* New York: Raven Press, 1987.

Schweitzer, N. M. J., ed. *Ophthalmology.* Amsterdam: Excerpta Medica, 1982.

Sickle Cell Anemia Research and Education Inc. *Facts About Sickle Cell Anemia.* Oakland, California: SCARE, 1977.

sighted-guide technique   A method of guiding a visually impaired person. The sighted person holds the disabled person's arm in a relaxed position close to the body. The arm may be straight or bent at a right angle. The visually impaired person grasps the guide's arm just above the elbow. This position allows the sighted guide to walk a step ahead. The visually impaired person can then follow the guide's movements and directions.

The guide may inform the visually impaired person about steps or cracks in the path or overhead obstacles. The guide may pause when reaching the bottom or top landing of a flight of stairs. This alerts the visually impaired person that one last stair remains. When traveling through a narrow passage, the guide moves the guide arm behind himself so that his wrist is behind the small of his back. This alerts the visually impaired person to drop back. The guide then proceeds through the passage, and the visually impaired person follows single-file.

Partially sighted persons may be asked whether they prefer to take a sighted guide's arm in a darkened room. The sighted guide should never force assistance or lend assistance without first asking permission. Rehabilitation classes teach visually impaired persons how to break the grasp of well-meaning but unwanted guides. (See ORIENTATION AND MOBILITY.)

signature guide   An aid that enables the user to sign a signature within a specific space on a page. The guides may be made of plastic or metal and often have a rubber component that holds the guide in place.

Designs vary, but most guides are a template with a rectangular window or opening that conforms to the standard signature area of a check, credit card receipt, etc. The signature guide is placed on the paper with the lower straight edge of the opening centered on the signature line of the document. The individual uses the edge as a guide and signs the signature within the opening.

slate and stylus   The braille slate and stylus are tools used to print braille. The slate is made from two rectangular metal plates hinged together at one end. The upper plate has rows of small, open windows punched out of the metal. Directly underneath each window on the bottom plate is an indentation of a complete braille cell.

The braille cell is made up of six dots, two across and three down. Each dot is numbered. Different configurations or combinations of dots are used to stand for each letter of the alphabet. For instance, dot 1 stands for the letter A, and dots 1 and 2 stand for the letter B.

In order to make a braille letter with the slate and stylus, a card or sheet of braille paper is placed between the two metal plates of the slate. The stylus, a short metal prong fastened to a handle, is held in the palm and used to make the letters. The writer presses the stylus downward onto the paper within an open window. The stylus pushes the paper against the corresponding indentation of the braille cell dot on the bottom plate. A raised dot is formed on the reverse side of the paper. The writer continues to press against the correct dots in the cell until the correct letter is formed. The writing is read when the paper is turned over and the dots are facing upward.

Therefore, in order to write braille, which must be read from left to right, the slate and stylus user must write from right to left and reverse the normal configuration of dots on the braille cell. Rather than learning to picture each letter in reverse, braille writers learn the number configuration of the dots.

Snellen chart   The eye chart routinely used in the eye examination to determine central visual acuity. VISUAL ACUITY is the measurement of the amount of detail an individual sees as compared with the amount of detail a person with normal vision sees. The visual-acuity test involves reading the Snellen chart when positioned 20 feet away. The chart contains nine lines of letters, written in progressively smaller print.

Each line corresponds to a degree of vision. Line one corresponds to 20/200 vision; line two, 20/100; line three, 20/70; line four, 20/50; line five, 20/40; line six, 20/30; line seven, 20/25; line eight, 20/20; and line nine, 20/15. If an individual can read all nine lines, the vision is measured as 20/15, or able to read at 20 feet what a normally sighted person can read at 15 feet. If the person can read only the top line, or big E, that vision is measured as 20/200, or able to read at 20 feet what a normally-sighted person can read at 200 feet. This is classified as legally blind.

The Snellen chart has been criticized for inaccuracy since each line on the chart must cover a wide range of visual ability. Those with borderline vision may fall between two lines of ability and be incorrectly classified.

snow blindness   An eye injury caused by intense light reflected off snow. The bright light in prolonged exposure produces an ultraviolet burn on the cornea of the eye. Symptoms of snow blindness appear in both eyes, and include extreme pain, a feeling of sand in the eyes, and severe sensitivity to light. The symptoms are usually delayed two to nine hours after exposure. The burn heals itself within two to three days. Antibiotic or steroid drops may be prescribed to ease discomfort and discourage infection. Snow blindness can be prevented by wearing protective goggles or glasses.

Although the rays that cause snow blindness are the same as those that cause sunburn at the beach, sunbathers rarely get snow blindness. This is because most of the rays at the beach are coming from above and the eyes are afforded some protection by the eyelids, eyelashes, and eyebrows. In cases of snow blindness, the rays are reflected from the snow and enter the eye from below, a relatively unprotected position. (See RADIATION BURNS.)

Social Services Block Grant   The Social Security Act was amended in 1974 to establish, under Title XX, the Social Services Block Grant program. The program allows each state to provide social services to its residents in ways it deems most appropriate and effective. States may use Title XX funds to provide services to disabled persons. Funds may be used to prevent or reduce dependency, attain and maintain self-sufficiency, prevent neglect or abuse of either adults or children, improve or prevent inappropriate institutional care, and obtain institutional care.

Funds may also be used to improve state programs concerning day-care services of either children or adults, protective services, foster-care services, home-care management and maintenance services, transportation and health services, employment services, information and counseling services, and meal-delivery programs. Services must relate to the special needs of children and the elderly, and those who are blind, mentally retarded, emotionally disturbed, physically disabled, or drug or alcohol dependent.

The eligibility of recipients is determined by each state. Allotments to the state are proportionally set according to population. In fiscal year 2001, Congress allocated $1.725 billion for this program.

U.S. Department of Education. *Summary of Existing Legislation Affecting Persons with Disabilities.* Washington, D.C.: USDE, 1988.

Sonicguide The Sonicguide is an electronic travel aid developed and designed by Humanware, Inc. for the visually impaired. The device has three components: a pair of spectacles, earphones, and a control box for the electronic components and power supply.

The spectacle-mounted transmitting device sends out ultrasonic waves that bounce off objects in the user's path. The reflected waves are converted into audible tones heard in stereophonic earpieces. The pitch of the tone provides information as to the distance, position, and surface characteristics of the detected object. The device has a range of five meters.

Other similar devices are known by the trade names Kay binaural sensor and Sensory 6. Versions of the device are available for children, wheelchair users, and orientation and mobility instructors. Correct use of all such devices requires training from a qualified instructor.

Sorsby's fundus dystrophy (SFD) A rare genetic disorder that causes macular degeneration to occur at an early age, usually between the ages of 30 and 40. Researchers are interested in SFD because of its clinical similarity to age-related macular degeneration. Symptoms include retinal edema, hemorrhages, and exudates in the macular area. As the disease progresses, considerable scarring may occur. Symptoms usually occur first in one eye, with the other eye developing symptoms months or even years later. As with age-related macular degeneration, central vision is affected first.

The disorder was first addressed in 1949 in a study of five British families who were afflicted by the disease. It has been identified in patients in Europe, North America, South Africa, Australia, and Japan.

special education See EDUCATION.

sports and recreation Sports and recreation activities benefit all persons, both disabled and able-bodied, by developing self-assurance and confidence, competitive spirit and athletic skills, and by providing stress reduction, comradeship, and fun. Local, state, regional, national, and international competitions exist for participation in sports by visually impaired persons as well as persons with other disabilities.

Although some sports or games require some adaptation to allow full participation by visually impaired individuals, many do not. Adaptation is dependent on the participant's eye condition, general health and interests and requirements of the sport.

A visually impaired jogger or runner may run alone on a track with high contrast or distinctive texture to differentiate the path or on a track specially equipped with guide ropes or poles for visually impaired athletes.

A visually impaired person may run with a sighted partner while holding onto the guide's elbow, a stick held between the two, or a rubberbandlike tether.

Competitive games in track and field exist for visually impaired athletes. Competitive events include the triple jump, shot put, long jump, javelin throw, discus, and meter races.

Bicycling is possible when the rider rides a tandem bike with a sighted partner in the front, or pilot, position. The visually impaired person sits behind in the stoker position and provides the power base for the pair. Tandem cycling may take the form of leisurely recreation or competitive riding.

Bowling programs and tournaments are offered through blind bowling or athletic associations. Bowling lanes can be adapted with a portable bowling rail that is assembled and placed next to the aisle as a banister guide.

Skiing clubs and programs are available to visually impaired skiers. Many ski areas have staff to teach or accompany blind individuals in either nordic (cross country) or alpine (downhill) skiing.

Nordic skiing is pursued in flat terrain at fairly slow, controllable speeds. Since nordic skiing generally follows tracks made from previous skiers, the sport is only minimally dependent on a sighted guide who calls directions to the visually impaired skier.

Alpine or downhill skiing is a faster sport that relies on excellent communication between the visually impaired skier and the sighted guide. The guide calls out directions to indicate turns and guide the partner around obstacles. Often, visually impaired skiers wear tunics or shirts printed with "Blind Skier" to advise sighted skiers of their presence.

Ice skating, speed skating, or roller skating may be pursued with a sighted guide. The guide may call out directions or may skate in tandem, allowing the partner to hold onto his elbow or a stick held between the two.

Swimming is a popular sport for recreation or competition. A pool with rope lane markers makes swimming laps possible without a sighted guide. Some visually impaired swimmers prefer to use an outside lane that borders the side of the pool and to count the number of strokes required to reach complete a lap.

Competitive blind swimmers are tapped on the head or hand at the end of each lap to indicate the approach of the pool wall. The tapper taps just as the swimmer should start the turn. This enables the visually impaired swimmer to duplicate the turning techniques of nondisabled swimmers in safety.

Boating or canoeing is usually pursued with a sighted guide partner who takes the lead position in the craft. The guide supplies continuous information on obstacles, rapids, or changes in direction. All boaters should wear personal flotation devices.

Horseshoes may be played by adapting the horseshoes by color or texture. The post can be accented with a bright color or by an auditory cue.

Horseback riding is widely available and pursued in the company of a sighted rider who provides information concerning directions and overhead obstacles. Riders may be required to wear a safety helmet.

Exercising and weight lifting programs are available in gyms and fitness centers that provide individualized instruction. Weight lifting or power lifting requires no adaptation for blind participants but may necessitate a "spotter" or guide to monitor the lift.

Judo and wrestling are two sports that need no adaptation for participation by visually impaired individuals. The referee makes verbal calls concerning scoring and penalties.

Gymnastics programs are available through athletic organizations and local gymnasiums. The visually impaired individual may participate in all activities including the uneven bars, balance beam, floor exercise, and vault. A "spotter" or guide may monitor the activity, and an additional layer of floor matting and padding covering all metal parts may be recommended.

Competitive or recreational darts are played on the Audio Dart Game. The dart board talks to control the game. It informs players when it is their turn, the score earned, and the status of the game as it progresses.

Balls of all types including basketballs and children's playground balls are adapted with inner bells or beeps that alert the visually impaired user to the location of the ball. Goal ball is a game played exclusively by the visually impaired. The object is to roll a ball containing bells past the opposing team and into the goal net. Each team consists of three players who alternately roll and defend. The floor is marked with tape to accent the goals and boundaries. See Appendix 11 for sports organizations. (See TOYS AND GAMES.)

Stargardt's disease   An inherited disease that causes people to lose central vision, usually in the first or second decade of life. It is sometimes referred to as juvenile macular degeneration. Doctors estimate that between 17,000 and 25,000 people in the United States have Stargardt's disease.

The disease typically starts between the ages of six and 15. Some children lost most of their central vision quickly, while others experience a slow and gradual loss of sight. Researchers in May 1998 identified a gene that causes Stargardt's disease. The gene causes cells to produce a protein that functions only in the retinas of the eyes. Discovery of this gene is significant for several reasons. It will allow doctors to develop a specific test for Stargardt's disease, which frequently is confused with other vision problems, and, it may move researchers closer to finding the cause of age-related macular degeneration.

steroids   Drugs used in the treatment of eye diseases and disorders. They are most often used to combat inflammation in the eye. Steroids may be prescribed in pill, ointment, or drop form. They are most often topically applied, because systemic (taken internally) steroids may have more serious side effects.

Steroids increase the eye's susceptibility to infection and may encourage the multiplication of viruses such as HERPES SIMPLEX. Topical steroids may immediately cause a rise in intraocular pressure, which may lead to glaucoma. Over time, systemic steroids may encourage cataract development. Thereafter, steroids should be prescribed for a specific disorder and only if other drugs have proven ineffective. They should be taken only as directed and should not be used for extended periods of time.

stroke   An interruption of blood flow to the brain. Stroke is the third most common cause of death in the United States after heart attack and cancer. According to the American Heart Association, about 600,000 Americans experience stroke each year.

More than 75 percent of those who suffer strokes each year are over 65. The incidence of stroke increases by more than 100 percent with each decade over 65. Men suffer 30 percent more strokes than women. Blacks suffer 60 percent more strokes than whites, and evidence suggests that people from poor socioeconomic backgrounds are more susceptible than those from affluent circumstances. Strokes tend to run in families, occur more commonly in the southeastern part of the United States, and occur most often during phases of extreme weather temperatures.

A stroke is a type of cardiovascular disease. Blood is brought to the brain via four large arteries. The brain cannot store nutrients, so it needs a constant supply of blood to furnish oxygen and nutrients and carry away carbon dioxide and other waste materials. When the flow of blood is interrupted, a stroke occurs. Any cessation of blood to the brain can cause damage, including paralysis, loss of consciousness, loss of speech, loss of mental functioning, loss of vision, and death.

Strokes are caused by a blockage or bursting of one of the arteries to the brain. These types of strokes, called cerebral thrombosis and cerebral embolism are the most common types of stroke. They account for up to 80 percent of all strokes suffered in the United States.

ARTERIOSCLEROSIS, hardening of the arteries, is the cause of more than half of all strokes. Arteriosclerosis causes fatty plaque to form inside the walls of the arteries, which slows or stops the flow of blood. This causes a stroke called a thrombotic stroke or cerebral thrombosis.

Platelets, blood-clotting cells in the blood, may cling to the arteriosclerotic plaque and form blood clots that can block an artery. Often, such a clot is jarred loose and floats through the blood stream until it becomes lodged in a smaller blood vessel. The blood flow is cut off and a stroke occurs. This type of stroke is called an embolic stroke.

Blood vessels weakened by injury or hypertension (high blood pressure) may break and allow blood to flow into or around the brain and destroy tissue. This causes a stroke known as a cerebral hemorrhage or a subarachnoid hemorrhage. A cerebral hemorrhage is when blood flows into the brain, and a subarachnoid hemorrhage is when a blood vessel on the surface of the brain ruptures and bleeds into the space between the brain and the skull.

Strokes can be categorized by severity into three types: transient ischemic attack, stroke in progress, and completed stroke. Transient ischemic attacks (TIA) precede more severe strokes in about 10 percent of cases. A transient ischemic attack is a blockage of one small blood vessel to the brain. Stroke symptoms such as loss of vision or tingling in the limbs may last from a few minutes to 24 hours, then disappear. TIAs are usually a warning sign of a more serious stroke to follow.

A stroke in progress is a stroke that begins suddenly and steadily worsens during the following few hours or days. The symptoms may include a tingling or numbness of a limb or one side of the body that develops into total paralysis.

A completed stroke is one in which the blood has been interrupted in its flow, and brain damage has occurred. This may result in paralysis to one side of the body, vision loss of one half of the field of vision or one eye, slurred speech, mental confusion, coma, and death.

All three types of stroke may impair vision. Total vision may be lost in one eye, or one-half of the visual field of both eyes may be lost. This condition is called HEMIANOPSIA and is also present, temporarily, in migraine headaches. Loss of vision may be a result of stroke, a symptom of a stroke in progress, or a TIA, a warning sign of a more serious stroke to follow.

Double vision may result from a stroke if the muscles of one eye become paralyzed or damaged. The weakened muscles may not be able to focus the eye properly on an object that the unimpaired eye views. The brain receives images of two different objects, and double vision occurs.

If the stroke damages the brain stem, NYSTAGMUS may occur. Nystagmus is a constant, involuntary movement of the eyes. The condition may impair vision, but the patient can often learn through rehabilitation to work with the condition to see adequately.

Patients suffering from any stroke symptoms require immediate medical attention. The symptoms may be temporary or sustained and include weakness or tingling of face or limbs, difficulty with speaking or understanding speech, hemianopsia, blurring of vision, double vision, total loss of vision in one eye, headache, dizziness, inability to swallow, mental confusion, and loss of memory.

Treatment of stroke may include the use of anticoagulants or blood thinning drugs to reduce the risk of arteriosclerosis. In the case of TIAs, a surgical procedure called carotid endarterectomy may be called for if the stroke was caused by a stenosis or narrowing of the carotid artery. The stenosis is caused by arteriosclerotic plaque that is removed during the procedure.

After a stroke, patients may enter rehabilitative therapy to regain lost abilities. Physical therapy may help restore coordination and use of impaired limbs. Occupational therapy may assist in the recuperation of hand movements and provide alternative methods for performing daily tasks. Speech therapy may improve the ability to communicate. Often, psychiatrists, psychologists, social workers, and vocational rehabilitation counselors may be called on to assist in the rehabilitation process.

Those who survive stroke usually maintain a plateau or a period of no change in condition after the stroke. The plateau may last for hours or days. The recovery period may be rapid or last months and range from complete restoration of abilities to maintenance of long-lasting or permanent impairments. The degree of recovery is dependent on the damage done to the brain, the type of stroke and the condition and age of the patient.

In the last 30 years, death due to stroke has been reduced 30 to 40 percent. In 1950, the death rate due to stroke was 88.8 per 100,000 people. In 1985 the rate was 32.8 per 100,000. The rate continues to fall, and since 1973, the average rate of decline has been 5.5 percent per year. From 1988 to 1998, the stroke death rate dropped 15.5 percent.

This may be because of increased awareness of stroke risk factors. Several conditions are recognized as risk factors for stroke. They are hypertension, heart disease, diabetes, high red-blood-cell count, TIAs, cigarette smoking, and obesity. Treatment or control of these conditions may reduce the risk of stroke.

subluxation of the lens   Subluxation of the CRYSTALLINE LENS occurs when the lens becomes partially displaced due to a break in the fibers of the ZONULES that hold it in place. The condition may be congenital or acquired. It may be caused by a blow to the eye or other injury, MARFAN'S SYNDROME, homocystinuria (a metabolic congenital disorder associated with mental retardation), and aging.

Symptoms of subluxation of the lens include rapid changes in vision and increased myopia (nearsightedness) due to the increased mobility of the lens. On examination, the iris may appear wobbly or tremulous, and the lens may be visible in the pupil. The lens may subluxate up and out, as in Marfan's syndrome, down and in, as in homocystinuria, backwards into the vitreous, a condition called posterior subluxation, or forward into the ANTERIOR CHAMBER, a condition called anterior subluxation.

Subluxated lenses may develop cataracts or may become trapped in the pupil. Aqueous fluid production forces the trapped lens into the anterior chamber, where it may cause a rise in intraocular pressure, or secondary glaucoma.

When the lens has drifted to the anterior chamber, the pupils are dilated and the patient is set in a supine position to encourage the lens to fall back into place behind the iris. If the lens falls into place, the pupils are immediately constricted with miotic drops, although recurrences are common. If the lens fails to move into position, it is surgically removed, or a peripheral iridectomy is performed to allow aqueous flow.

When the lens moves into the POSTERIOR CHAMBER, it may be left untouched if it does not cause UVEITIS or cataract. In such cases, the lens may be removed. If the lens moves from the central pupil area, becomes completely dislocated or detached or is removed, the eye becomes aphakic, or without a lens. Aphakic characteristics such as lack of accommodation, enlarged image, and color distortion can be corrected with prescription contact lenses or spectacles.

Sullivan, Anne   Anne Mansfield Sullivan Macy was the teacher and companion to Helen Keller. Born in 1866 in Feeding Hills, Massachusetts, she developed TRACHOMA at age five. The eye disease arose from the poverty and unsanitary conditions of her environment and slowly destroyed her sight.

In 1874, she was sent to a state poorhouse in Tewksbury where she remained off and on for six years. Five unsuccessful operations were performed on her eyes that alleviated the pain but did not improve her sight.

In 1880, Sullivan entered the Perkins Institution for the Blind in Boston. During her time at the Institution, she received two eye operations that improved her vision. Sullivan graduated from Perkins in 1886, as valedictorian of her class.

In 1887, Sullivan was recommended by the Perkins Institution as a teacher for a deaf-blind child named Helen Keller. Sullivan went to live with the Keller family and battled with the unruly child, attempt-ing to teach her the fingerspelling for various objects in the environment. Keller was unable to link the importance of the spelling to the meaning of the object until one day at the well when Sullivan poured water on Keller's hand while fingerspelling W-A-T-E-R into the other hand.

Keller went on to master the manual and braille alphabet under the tutelage of Sullivan on whom Keller bestowed the lifelong title of "Teacher." Keller attended and graduated from Radcliffe in 1904, with the assistance of Sullivan, who attended classes with Keller and translated class lectures and texts.

When Keller began writing articles and her book *The Story of My Life*, John Macy, an editor and Harvard instructor, was recommended to the two women as an editor and writing assistant. Macy and Sullivan married in 1905, and Keller lived with the couple. Sullivan continued to assist Keller in her writing and lecturing career. The marriage grew troubled and Macy sailed alone to Europe in 1913. In 1914, Polly Thomson joined Sullivan and Keller as a companion and assistant.

In 1929, Sullivan's right eye was removed to relieve constant pain. Her vision in the remaining eye and her general health deteriorated rapidly.

Sullivan died in 1936. Her ashes reside next to those of Helen Keller and Polly Thomson.

surgical procedures   Surgery may be required in the treatment of an eye disorder or disease. According to the type of disorder, surgery may be indicated immediately or reserved as a later alternative in cases that do not respond to medication.

Cataract removal is the most common surgery performed in the United States. There are two main types of cataract surgery: phacoemulsification and extracapsular.

During phacoemulsification, which is the most common method of cataract removal, a small incision is made on the side of the cornea, and a tiny probe is inserted into the eye. The probe produces ultrasound waves that break up the cloudy center of the lens. The lens can then be removed, using suction.

In extracapsular surgery, a slightly longer incision is made on the side of the cornea, and the surgeon removes the hard center of the lens. The remainder of the lens is then removed using suction.

Once the cloudy lens has been removed, it is usually replaced with a clear artificial lens called an intraocular lens (IOL). The IOL becomes a permanent part of the eye and does not require any additional care or attention. The person wearing the IOL does not feel or see it. In some cases, patients cannot have an IOL, due to problems that occur during surgery or another eye problem. In these cases, a soft contact lens or glasses may be used instead.

Certain types and conditions of glaucoma necessitate surgery. Two major forms of surgery are IRIDECTOMY and filtering surgery, called TRABECULECTOMY. An iridectomy is a surgical procedure in which a portion of the iris is removed to eliminate the blockage of angle-closure glaucoma and prevent further attacks. A trabeculectomy bypasses damaged meshwork and creates a new drainage tract to allow the aqueous to flow from the eye.

CORNEAL TRANSPLANT, or keratoplasty, uses a donor cornea to replace all or part of a diseased cornea and restore vision. A section of donor cornea is measured to the precise needs of the host and removed from the donor cornea with scissors. A corresponding section of host cornea is measured and removed. The donor cornea is placed into the remaining cavity and sewn into position with small stitches or sutures.

Tear duct surgery is often indicated in cases of WET EYE. Obstructions are cleared surgically by simple probe and irrigation or silicone intubation procedures, or the more serious surgical procedure, a dacryocystorhinostomy.

A TARSORRHAPHY is a surgical procedure in which a section of the eyelids is stitched together at the corner of the eye. The surgery is performed in the treatment of dendritic ulcers, Bell's palsy, thyroid disease, or any disorder in which the eye is in danger of overexposure or drying.

ENUCLEATION is the surgical removal of the eyeball. Enucleation is performed when the eye contains a malignant tumor, when the eye is blind and causes pain, and when the eye is nearly blind and sympathetic ophthalmia (an inflammation that occurs in both eyes as a result of injury to one eye) is a risk.

RADIAL KERATOTOMY (RK) surgery is elective surgery designed to improve MYOPIA (nearsightedness). The surgery uses radial cuts or incisions to reshape the cornea.

sympathetic ophthalmia   A rare condition in which one eye becomes inflamed as a result of an injury or trauma to the other eye. The condition is most common among children and occurs following a perforation injury or surgery. It also can occur if a foreign body remains in the eye, causing great irritation.

Sympathetic ophthalmia occurs when the injured eye remains inflamed and infected due to insufficient or delayed cleansing. Over a period of two weeks to several months, an inflammatory response occurs in the UVEA. Examination of the choroid reveals the presence of eosinophils, giant cells and lymphocytes, serious signals that threaten sight in the eye.

After a period of two weeks to several years, the inflammation spreads to the unaffected eye. Symptoms of blurred vision or PHOTOPHOBIA develop. An eye examination with the slit lamp reveals the presence of granulomatous keratic precipitates on the posterior surface of the cornea, a condition that endangers vision.

Sympathetic ophthalmia can be prevented by earnest attention to cleansing and care of the affected eye or by enucleating (surgically removing) the initially injured eye within a two-week period following the injury. Any severely injured eye that remains inflamed or infected up to a two-week period may need to be removed to prevent sympathetic ophthalmia.

If sympathetic ophthalmia occurs after the two-week time period, the condition may be treated with local and systemic steroids. The treatment is often successful, but the condition is inclined to recur.

synechiae   A condition in which the iris adheres to either the cornea or the lens. The iris/cornea adhesion is termed anterior synechiae and the iris/lens adhesion is termed posterior synechiae. Synechiae of either type may be caused by anterior UVEITIS, an inflammation of the iris and/or ciliary body. Anterior synechiae may be caused by perforation of the cornea or injuries.

Posterior synechiae may cause a blockage of aqueous flow and an iris bombe, in which the iris bows forward unnaturally. This interferes with the flow of AQUEOUS FLUID and causes secondary glaucoma, a disease in which the accumulation of aqueous fluid causes a rise in intraocular pressure.

Symptoms of synechiae include redness, pain, oversensitivity to light, pus in the anterior chamber on examination, constricted pupil, and inability of the pupil to dilate. Synechiae is treated according to its cause. Since the condition generally includes inflammation of the iris, or IRITIS, the treatment usually involves local steroids and mydriatic drops to dilate the pupil. Some injury-induced synechiae may be self-limiting.

synthetic speech   Artificial speech created by speech synthesizers. Speech synthesizers convert printed speech into spoken words to put information into, or remove information from, a computer. The first speech synthesizer was invented in 1936 by H. W. Dudley, a scientist at Bell Labs. The machine required an operator with a keyboard and foot pedals to provide the pitch, timing, and intensity of speech. Dudley's machine was called a voice coder, but soon became known as "The Voder."

Many commercially available personal-computer software programs may be used with synthesizers that read material that appears on the computer screen or information sent to it from the computer.

Speech synthesis may be used to access personal electronic mail and general print information as well. Electronic mail or E-mail is a system of receiving and sending personal communications through the personal computer. It is an instant, and with the use of Braille printers or speech synthesis, private form of communication accessible to individuals with visual impairments.

General print information is accessible via speech synthesis through reading machines such as the Kurzweil Reader. Printed material placed on the scanning screen is scanned and read aloud. The voices of synthetic speech read English words and numerals and are available in various forms of male, female, or robotic voice, adult or child voice, voice pitch, speed, and volume. Some synthesizers offer foreign languages, talking calculators, singing, music with several octaves of pitch, musical keyboards, and sound effects.

The voice is projected over an internal speaker, external speaker, earphones, or telephone, depending on the type of hardware. Often, a section of the standard keyboard, a hand or foot switch or a keyboard on a control box is used to control that section of the screen that will be read and how it will be read. Most programs offer options of reading the text letter by letter or word by word and verbalization of the punctuation.

Synthetic speech is a breakthrough in independence for those with visual impairments. The individual can privately transmit and receive personal documents and produce work-related material independently. It allows free access to information at times and in situations convenient to the individual, and not dependent on the assistance of others. Many advances are being made in this area as technology continues to develop.

ABLEDATA. *Speech Synthesizers.* Newington, Connecticut: ABLEDATA, 1989.
Chong, Curtis. "Speech Output for the IBM Personal Computer." *The Braille Monitor* (January 1986): 37–47.
Hagen, Dolores. *Microcomputer Resource Book for Special Education.* Reston, Virginia: Reston Publishing Company Inc., 1984.
Lauer, Harvey, and Leonard Mowinski. *Recommending Computers for the Visually Impaired: A Moving Target or a Losing War?* HealthNet Library. Columbus, Ohio: CompuServe, 1989.

syphilis   A venereal disease caused by the spirochete *Treponema pallidum.* The disease may cause ocular disorders both congenitally and after birth.

Approximately 800 cases of congenital syphilis were reported in 1998. Syphilis is transmitted congenitally from the infected mother to the fetus through the womb after the fourth month of pregnancy when the spirochete can pass through the placenta. Congenital syphilis may result in vision loss and ocular impairment, deafness, dental defects, mental retardation, organ damage, and death.

Ocular damage may involve severe KERATITIS, or corneal inflammation, and chorioretinal scarring. Although the infection is present at birth, the keratitis may develop later in life between ages 5 and 25. Severe keratitis may be treated with medication but may result in corneal opacification and PHOTOPHOBIA.

Syphilis contracted after birth can cause chorioretinal scarring, IRITIS (an inflammation of the iris), and optic nerve atrophy or degeneration. Syphilis can be diagnosed with a Wasserman test, a blood test to determine the presence of the spirochete in the blood. An eye examination may also determine the presence of the disease and is often used to confirm the diagnosis.

Syphilis is treated with ANTIBIOTICS, and ocular disorders are treated with medication. If treated in the early stages, the damage resulting syphilis may be mild. Congenital syphilis can be prevented if the disease of the mother is treated and controlled before the fifth month of pregnancy. Toward this purpose, most states have developed laws that require testing for syphilis at the beginning of each pregnancy.

Centers for Disease Control. "Congenital Syphilis—United States," 1998. www.cdc.gov., 1999.

T

tactile aids   Tactile aids provide information that visually impaired individuals access through the sense of touch. These may include braille materials, braille-marked tools, or adaptive aids.

Braille materials, printed materials that are read with the fingertips, are reproduced by transcribers, publishers, and printing houses such as the American Printing House for the Blind. Braille markings are found on adaptive aids such as rulers, measuring cups, and clocks in place of printed letters or numbers. A Braillewriter is a six-key typewriter for typing braille. It produces raised dots onto specially designed, heavy braille paper.

The SLATE AND STYLUS are writing tools used to write braille. The user places a sheet of braille paper between the two metal plates of the slate. The stylus, a short metal prong fastened to a handle, is held in the palm and pressed downward onto the paper within an open window. The stylus pushes the paper against the corresponding indentation of the braille cell dot on the bottom plate. A raised dot is formed on the reverse side of the paper. The writing is read when the paper is turned over and the dots are facing upward.

Templates and writing guides are frames used in writing on lines or in specified spaces. Window openings in the templates serve as a guide for signing checks or writing letters. Raised line paper is writing paper with embossed lines to enable the user to follow a straight writing path.

PAPERLESS BRAILLE or cassette braille is an information system that is stored on audio cassette tapes and accessed in braille. The user runs his fingers over display cells to read the text and pushes a button to access the next segment of recorded material. The user can produce, edit, and record braille with the system. It can be adapted for use with computer terminals, calculators, and typewriters.

A raised-line drawing kit is a board covered with a soft underlay of rubber. The user places a sheet of acetate over the board and draws on it, creating raised lines and an embossed picture.

Tactile color is a standardized system of 12 distinctive colors, each assigned a specific texture. This allows visually impaired persons to better participate in creating or enjoying visual artwork. It is also useful in mapmaking, for labeling, and as an educational resource.

A thermoform machine is a device that heats a sheet of plastic paper so that it may be molded to whatever shape is placed beneath it. Thermoform machines produce copies of braille and can be used to create raised line maps or graphs.

Tactile maps and globes are three-dimensional maps that are used as an orientation aid. They contain raised surfaces, textures, and braille markings and are designed to be read with the fingertips, in a manner similar to braille.

The Cranmer abacus is an abacus that has been adapted to prevent the beads from accidentally sliding. It is used to perform mathematical computations.

The Optacon is a reading machine that converts print into tactual letter configurations. The user scans a small camera over a line of print with the right hand, while resting the left hand on an electronic array. The machine electronically converts each letter into a print letter configuration formed on the array by vibrating pins and read by the left index finger.

See ADAPTIVE AIDS.

targeted jobs tax credit   See WORK OPPORTUNITY TAX CREDIT.

tarsorrhaphy   A surgical procedure in which a section of the eyelids is stitched together at the corner of the eye. The surgery may be performed in the treatment of dendritic ulcers, Bell's palsy, thyroid disease, or any disorder in which the eye is in danger of overexposure or drying. Tarsorrhaphy is reversible and may be used temporarily.

tax benefits   Additional income tax deductions are available to legally blind individuals. The amount that may be deducted varies depending on marital status and age. A married blind individual, for instance, may deduct an additional $850. Single blind individuals may deduct an additional $1,100. To qualify for the deduction, an individual must be legally blind, which means he or she must have a visual acuity of 20/200 in the better eye, after correction, or a visual field of 20 degrees or less in the better eye after correction. The individual must attach to the tax return a statement from an ophthalmologist confirming legal blindness.

Some medical expenses, such as eyeglasses, necessary home improvements, dog guides, tuition for special education, prosthetic eyes, and, in some cases, attendant care, also may be deducted from income if itemized.

Taylor slate   One of the earliest manipulative/ tactile aids for visually impaired students studying mathematics. The slate measures about 11 by 17 inches, with holes running across and up and down in columns. Each hole looks like a plus sign (+) overlying an "X." The one-inch pegs have the same shape as the holes and are stored in a tray on the slate when not in use. At one end of each peg there is a bar, and at the other end there are two conical projections. The angle at which each peg is inserted into the hole determines the numerical value represented. Very popular through the 1930s and into the 1940s, the Taylor slate is no longer used.

tear system   The tear or nasolacrimal system is the system that the eye uses to produce, maintain and eliminate tears from the eye. Tears protect, nourish, and moisturize the eye. Without proper tear function, as in dry eye, the cornea and CONJUNCTIVA may become dry and develop disorders.

In the normal eye, the tear film is made up of three layers, which are produced by the lacrimal gland and accessory lacrimal glands and cells. The lacrimal glands are located in the ORBIT and inner eyelid. The accessory glands and cells are located in the conjunctiva.

The top layer of tears is formed by the secretion of the meibomian glands and is oily in nature. The second layer is composed of watery tears from the lacrimal glands, and the third layer, which lies next to the cornea, is of mucouslike consistency and is produced by accessory glands. The layers are maintained by constant blinking and are all necessary for proper health of the eye.

Tears are constantly being produced and drained from the eye. They drain through lacrimal puncta, holes in each inner corner of the upper and lower lids. The tears are gathered in the lacrimal sac, an organ at the junction of the nose and lower lid. The tears then pass under the tissue to drainage ducts in the nasal cavity.

The nasolacrimal system is subject to functional disorders, obstructions and infections that may result in WET EYE, DRY EYE, or DACRYOCYSTITIS. Inadequate drainage of tears leads to wet eye. Wet eye may be a congenital or acquired condition. Congenital wet eye occurs as a result of obstructions to the nasolacrimal ducts. Symptoms include tearing, crusting of the lids or eyelashes, mucous discharge, and inflammation of the lacrimal sac.

Obstructions often clear spontaneously within the first 12 months of life. After this time, obstructions are cleared surgically by simple probe and irrigation or silicone intubation procedures or the more serious surgical procedure, dacryocystorhinostomy, which connects the lacrimal sac to the nasal cavity.

Acquired obstructions usually occur in middle age, and most commonly among women. Tearing becomes severe and annoying. The simple procedures of probe and irrigation or silicone intubation are often ineffective, and a dacryocystorhinostomy is indicated.

The condition of dry eye may occur as a result of poor tear production (called keratoconjunctivitis sicca), poor tear quality, or inadequate blinking, which leaves the eye open to the drying elements or which does not properly wet the entire surface of the eye.

Symptoms of dry eye include burning, irritation, redness, and loss of corneal luster. Conditions that can cause dry eye include SARCOIDOSIS, rheuma-toid arthritis, vitamin-A deficiency, pemphigoid, TRACHOMA, Stevens-Johnson syndrome, chemical burns, neuroparalytic and exposure KERATITIS, and AGING.

Dry eye may lead to corneal damage, permanent corneal scarring, and opacification. Once the cornea has opacified, vision is lost.

Treatment of dry eye includes treating the underlying cause or disease and the administration of artificial tears. In some cases, ANTIBIOTICS may be prescribed, and the use of home vaporizers or humidifiers may be advised. Surgery may be performed to close the tear drainage ducts to ensure better utilization of reduced tear production. If the cornea is severely scarred and vision is lost, a CORNEAL TRANSPLANT, or keratoplasty, may be indicated. However, those with dry eye conditions are generally poor candidates for a successful corneal transplantation.

Dacryocystitis is an inflammation of the tear drainage sac caused by an infection. It usually affects one eye only and may become a chronic disorder. It is most commonly found in adult females, and may be caused congenitally, from a blockage or obstruction of the tear duct or from a trauma or injury. The resulting infection is caused most often by bacteria such as *Staphylococcus aureus* and beta-hemolytic streptococcus, and by fungi such as *Candida albicans*. Symptoms may include constant tearing, swelling, discharge, and tenderness of the eye. A culture of the discharge may identify the infecting agent.

Dacryocystitis is usually treated with warm compresses and topical or systemic antibiotics. Blocked nasolacrimal ducts of infants may be massaged to encourage dilation. If the duct fails to open, it may require probe and irrigation therapy. If the condition produces an abscess, it may be drained.

telebraille   A braille telephone device for deaf-blind persons. Manufactured by Telesensory Systems, Inc., the device is a modified TDD (telecommunications device for the deaf) system, which provides braille input and output. The system contains a standard TDD, including a standard alphabet keyboard and visual character display, plus a braille keyboard and refreshable braille display.

The telebraille can be used to communicate with other standard TDDs over telephone lines or as an aid in communication for deaf-blind persons. In a conversation, the sighted person types words onto the standard TDD unit. The text is translated into braille and is read by the deaf-blind person on the refreshable display. To reply, the deaf-blind person types words on the braille keyboard, they are translated to text and read by the sighted person on the visual display. There have been several versions of the telebraille. The latest is TeleBraille III.

terminology   There is no complete consensus on terms concerning the topic of blindness and vision impairment. Rehabilitation experts, doctors, educators, legislators, and other leaders in the field determine and define terminology according to their own preferences and viewpoints.

Over the past 150 years, visual impairments have been described by numerous terms, including medically blind, economically blind, braille blind, educationally blind, functionally blind, partially seeing, partially blind, vocationally blind, legally blind, low vision, visually defective, visually handicapped, visually impaired, visually disabled, and visually limited. In recent years, those involved in the field of blindness and vision impairment have made strides to standardize terms to eliminate confusion or misinterpretation. The following definitions combine common aspects of terms drawn from a variety of sources.

An *impairment* refers to a recognizable defect or malfunctioning of an organ or any part of the body, such as an eye. The defect or malfunction can be diagnosed and defined by a medical doctor. A visually impaired person may range from an individual with no sight to someone with low vision.

A *disability* is the effect the impairment has on the individual to function. It is the limitation, restriction, or disadvantage due to the malfunction.

The word *handicap* stems from "cap in hand," a reference to beggars. Because of this negative connotation, the word *disability* is often the preferred term. A handicap may be defined as a disadvantage in the performance of tasks as a result of expectations or attitudes about the impairment. Disabilities are not necessarily handicaps. When the term visually handicapped is applied to a child it usually refers to the requirement for special educational provisions due to the sight loss.

Visually limited refers to an individual's difficulty in using vision under average circumstances. A visually limited person may be able to see with corrective lenses or optical aids.

Blind is a term many reserve for those with no vision or light perception only. Legally blind is a term defined by the federal government to determine eligibility for benefits. Legal blindness involves central visual acuity of 20/200 or less in the better eye with correction or a field of vision of 20 degrees or less in the better eye with correction.

Partially sighted or *partially seeing* is defined as a central visual acuity between 20/70 and 20/200 in the better eye with correction. *Low vision* is defined as a central visual acuity of between 20/50 and 20/200 in the better eye with correction or a visual field of 20 to 40 degrees or less in the better eye with correction. Low vision, partially sighted, and visually impaired are often used interchangeably to describe individuals with some usable vision, regardless of how little.

Fully sighted individuals are those who have correctable vision to 20/20. The terminology does not include a term for those individuals with correctable vision between 20/20 and 20/50. These people fall between the definitions for the terms fully sighted or low vision.

American Foundation for the Blind. *Low Vision Questions and Answers.* New York: AFB, 1987.

Barraga, Natalie C. *Visual Handicaps and Learning.* Belmont, California: Wadsworth Publishing Company Inc., 1976.

ERIC Clearinghouse on Handicapped and Gifted Children. *ERIC Digest: Visual Impairments.* Reston, Virginia: ERIC, 1982.

Foundation for the Junior Blind. *California Services for Persons with Visual Impairments.* Los Angeles: FJB, 1987.

Kelley, Jerry D., ed. *Recreational Programming for Visually Impaired Children and Youth.* New York: American Foundation for the Blind, 1981.

National Association for Visually Handicapped. *Problems of the Partially Sighted.* New York: NAVH, 1980.

National Information Center for Handicapped Children and Youth. *General Information about Handicaps and People with Handicaps.* Washington, D.C.: NICHC, 1982.

Scholl, Geraldine T. *Foundations of Education for Blind and Visually Handicapped Children and Youth.* New York: American Foundation for the Blind, 1986.

Timolol   A drug, in the form of timoptic eye drops or Blocadren tablets, prescribed for open-angle glaucoma and high blood pressure. The drug is a beta-adrenergic blocking agent that also decreases the amount of fluid produced within the eye and increases the fluid elimination rate. The drug has been found to lower intraocular pressure by 26 to 38 percent.

Timolol should not be used by pregnant or nursing women or those who cannot tolerate oral beta-blocking drugs. Care should be exercised by those with upper respiratory disorders such as asthma, hay fever, or allergies. Some patients may suffer side effects that include decreased heart rate, increased possibility of congestive heart failure, lowered blood pressure, insomnia, tingling in the arms or legs, dizziness, depression, and fatigue. Patients may also experience visual problems, including hallucinations, disorientation, personality change, memory loss, and abdominal disorders including diarrhea, constipation, cramps, nausea or vomiting. Reactions such as sore throat, fever, blood system disorders, or upper respiratory difficulties indicate an allergy to the drug.

Psychotropic or psychiatric drugs may interact with Timolol to cause serious problems. Timolol raises the effectiveness of antidiabetic medications. Physicians of diabetics taking Timolol may need to reduce present dosages of insulin or oral medication while the patient is taking Timolol. Timolol also lowers the effectiveness of digitalis, so physicians of heart-disease patients may need to increase the dosage of digitalis while the patient takes Timolol. Timolol may also interact with certain prescription blood pressure medications and over-the-counter cold remedies. These should not be taken with Timolol without a physician's advice.

Symptoms of Timolol overdose include heart failure, decreased heart rate and blood pressure, and upper respiratory problems. Overdose patients require proper treatment at a hospital emergency room. Timolol should be decreased slowly, over a period of time. Abrupt discontinuance can cause serious problems.

tobacco amblyopia   A condition in which the vision is lost due to the use of tobacco. The toxic effects of tobacco constrict the vessels of the body and interfere with circulation. As a result, the optic nerve swells, a condition known as optic neuritis.

Early symptoms of tobacco amblyopia include painless blurring or loss of central vision that may be accompanied by numbness or tingling in the fingers. If allowed to progress, the blurring may spread to the peripheral visual fields, and optic nerve damage may result. Reduction or elimination of tobacco usage in conjunction with proper nutrition usually restores vision. Patients may be instructed to supplement the diet with additional vitamins, such as B_{12}.

tomography   Also known as computerized axial tomography, tomography is a test that records the way tissues react when exposed to X rays. The computerized process measures the resistance of the soft tissues to the passage of the rays and translates the measurements to pictures on film or video screen. The process intensifies and contrasts sections of the eye, eye orbit and brain, which are indistinguishable with X rays alone.

The process is a computer scan that can isolate segments of the eye as slight as three millimeters thick. It can outline the CRYSTALLINE LENS apart from the surrounding AQUEOUS FLUID and point out tumors to the back of the eye, such as in the CHOROID, which would be invisible to standard X rays. Computerized axial tomography can often be used as a safer alternative to more expensive and risky procedures that require hospitalization, such as injection of air or radiopaque dyes.

tonography   A test to determine the fluid pressure within the eye, called intraocular pressure. The test is conducted as part of the routine annual eye examination.

A *tonometer* is used to conduct the test. This is a small instrument probe that is attached to a biomicroscope or slit lamp. The biomicroscope is an instrument that illuminates and magnifies the front part of the eye. The examiner looks through the biomicroscope as the test is conducted.

The test is painless. The eyes are prepared by first inserting anesthetic drops. Next, the examiner gently touches a strip of paper laced with fluorescein dye to the inside of each lower lid. The released orange dye mixes with the eye's tears and covers the cornea.

The examiner shines a blue light on each eye and then gently touches the cornea with the tonometer. When the probe touches the cornea, a pattern is created in the dye. The intraocular pressure is measured by the amount of force needed to create the pattern. A normal reading varies from 14 to 21. A higher reading may indicate the presence of glaucoma. The procedure is regularly performed as a glaucoma screening test and often is a step in presurgical evaluations to determine whether surgery is immediately prudent.

tonometer   See TONOGRAPHY.

toxic amblyopia   A condition in which vision is lost as a result of the absorption of toxic agents or the deficiency of nutrients. The condition, also known as nutritional amblyopia, is usually bilateral, and although in the case of wood alcohol and arsenic poisoning the vision loss is irreparable, it generally tends not to be permanent.

Some poisons induce a central vision blurring or scotoma, a blind spot. These include tobacco, ethyl alcohol, methyl alcohol, carbon disulphide, halogenated hydrocarbons, aromatic amino and nitro-compounds, sedatives such as barbiturates, opium, and morphine, anti-infective compounds and other drugs, and the metals lead and thallium.

Other compounds produce a reduction of the peripheral field, or tunnel vision. These include organic arsenic, quinine, carbon tetrachloride, methyl iodide, and the drugs salicylic acid, hydrocupreine derivatives, ergot, and aspidium.

Alcohol and tobacco amblyopia are common conditions. Overuse of either compound affects the optic nerve and OPTIC DISK, causing optic atrophy. A slow, progressive loss of central vision and, often, color vision follows. Both conditions are associated with poor nutrition or diet, which also affects ocular function. Treatment with VITAMINS and minerals as well as reduction of alcohol and tobacco use often restores vision.

Vitamin and mineral deficiencies are linked to nutritional amblyopia. Lack of vitamin A in the diet causes blindness. A lack of zinc prevents the body from using adequate vitamin A stored in the body. Thiamine and B_{12} deficiencies may cause optic neuropathy and vision loss. Generally, intensive vitamin therapy and proper nutrition can restore lost vision.

toxocariasis   An infection caused by dog tapeworm eggs called *Toxocara canis*. Human infection occurs with ingestion of infected fecal material. An estimated 10,000 cases of toxocariasis occur annually in humans in the United States.

The larvae causes acute CHORIORETINITIS, an inflammation of the CHOROID and retina. The infection spreads rapidly, involving the vitreous and clouding it with inflammatory cells. As the center portion of the globe becomes involved, the condition is termed endophthalmitis. Complete loss of sight in the affected eye may result. The condition may be treated with steroids, and vitrectomy (removal and replacement of the vitreous) may be performed in advanced cases.

toxoplasmosis   An infection caused by the parasite *Toxoplasma gondii*, a protozoan carried by wild or domesticated animals such as cats. Toxoplasmosis causes CHOROIDITIS (or posterior uveitis), an inflammation of the CHOROID. More than 60 million people in the United States are probably infected with the toxoplasma parasite, according to the Division of Parasitic Diseases of the Centers for Disease Control and Prevention. Very few people develop symptoms, however, because the immune system keeps the parasite from causing illness.

Toxoplasmosis occurs when the parasite infects the body and enters the blood stream through ingestion of infected material. Adult infection is usually moderate, but the parasite may be transmitted through the placenta and can cause serious infections in children. Congenital toxoplasmosis affects the brain and eyes and may cause epilepsy or mental developmental problems. Both eyes may develop choroiditis or CHORIORE-TINITIS of the macular region, a vision-threatening disorder.

The *Toxoplasma* parasite lives in fundus lesions of the eye, which can be dye tested to confirm a diagnosis. However, the diagnosis must be carefully made since a large portion of the population has been infected with the parasite at some time even though they may be unaware of any symptoms of the infection.

Symptoms of toxoplasmosis chorioretinitis or choroiditis include blurred vision and the appearance of floaters, possibly preceded by a fever. Treatment of the condition is unsatisfactory but may include systemic steroids or a combination of steroids and antibiotics if the infection threatens the macular region of the retina.

Most cases resolve themselves over time, leaving chorioretinal scarring near the macula. Recurrences are common and tend to originate on the borders of scarred areas.

See UVEITIS.

toys and games   Although many familiar toys and games played by sighted individuals are appropriate for use by those with little or no vision, others, which have been specially adapted, are available through adaptive-aids catalogs and organizations that serve the visually impaired.

Many games differ little from the original versions and merely require tactile markings for numbers, letters, or space delineation to be adaptable. Others are original games specially designed for the needs and goals of the visually impaired.

Board and card games are adapted with raised dots, braille, large print, a change in playing pieces or some other type of tactile marking. Playing cards are printed in large print, braille, or a combination of the two for use by both sighted and visually impaired players.

Checkers is played on an adapted board with raised and recessed squares using square and round playing pieces. Chess is played on a similar board which may be drilled to hold pegs projecting from under the chess pieces. Since each piece is distinguishable by shape, the only adaptation may be a point on top to distinguish the white from the black.

Many popular games such as Monopoly, Scrabble, bingo, backgammon, cribbage, dice, dominoes, Chinese checkers, and tic tac toe have been modified with large print, braille, or shape changes for use by the blind and visually impaired. Board games can be adapted at home by adding glue dots or lines that harden when dry or large-print or braille labels.

Puzzles are available in a variety of forms ranging from children's puzzles, which chime or play a tune when the pieces are in place, to large-print crossword puzzles, to the tactually marked Rubik's Cube.

Balls of all types, including basketballs and outdoor game balls, are available with bells or electronic beepers placed inside to alert the visually impaired user as to the location of the ball. Other adaptations for sports exist, including a bowling rail, which is placed next to the aisle as a bannister guide for visually impaired bowlers.

Educational toys and games for children are available in a myriad of designs. They range from simple tactual clocks to more sophisticated toys, such as the Flexi-Formboard (developed at Smith-Kettlewell Eye Research Institute, available from Adaptive Communication Systems), which contains plastic shapes that fit into a corresponding puzzle board. Placing a shape in its correct location on the board activates a battery-operated toy.

Other such games include modules to teach fine motor skills, braille and large-print spelling machines, math and reading games, bright or fluorescent materials to stimulate visual interest in children with low vision, sensory-stimulation games, biology and science models. (See SPORTS AND RECREATION.)

trabeculectomy   A surgical procedure performed to treat open-angle glaucoma, a condition in which the intraocular pressure builds within the eye to cause damage and vision loss.

Intraocular pressure is controlled by the flow of AQUEOUS FLUID, a watery liquid that flows through the ANTERIOR CHAMBER, nourishing the avascular lens and cornea and carrying away waste. The intraocular pressure rises when the aqueous fluid of the anterior chamber is unable to properly drain from the eye through the trabecular meshwork.

A trabeculectomy bypasses the damaged meshwork drainage systems and creates a new drainage duct from the eye. During the procedure, the SCLERA, or white part of the eye, is dissected to make a "trapdoor" opening or flap. A block of tissue as thick as the sclera and corneal tissue and containing trabeculum is removed.

Often, an IRIDECTOMY is then performed. A peripheral iridectomy is the removal of a peripheral section of iris blocking the anterior angle and deterring aqueous fluid drainage.

After the iridectomy, the opening is sutured shut in a loose stitch that will serve as a trapdoor drainage canal for the aqueous and relieve the intraocular buildup. The conjunctival covering of the sclera is then stitched closed.

A trabeculectomy is performed with local or general anesthesia in a hospital operating room. The procedure usually takes less than an hour.

The patient remains hospitalized for up to three days, and eye drops are prescribed for up to one month. Heavy lifting, bending or strenuous activity is not permitted for one month. The results of trabeculectomy surgery vary greatly, depending on factors such as inflammation, scarring, and healing of the drain.

Complications associated with trabeculectomy include flattened anterior chambers, scarring of the drainage site (which results in continued glaucoma), infection, inflammation, and hemorrhage. Approximately one-third of all trabeculectomy patients develop cataracts. (See SURGICAL PROCEDURES.)

trachoma   A contagious disease of the eyelids, CONJUNCTIVA and cornea. It is a leading cause of blindness in the world and may affect over 500 million people. It has caused blindness in about 6 million people according to the World Health Organization. While practically unknown in the United States, the infection is widespread in underdeveloped countries with poor sanitation and medical care.

Trachoma is caused by the bacteria *Chlamydia trachomatis* and may be linked to bacterial infections caused by agents Koch-Weeks bacillus, Morax Axenfeld diplobacillus, and the gonococcus bacillus. It thrives in overcrowded conditions in which a lack of clean water and poor sewage disposal, sanitation, and hygiene exist. In such conditions, the highly communicable disease may infect an entire community.

The infection attacks both eyes, scarring the conjunctiva inside the eyelid and eventually spreading to the cornea. Initial symptoms include pain, oversensitivity to light, and impaired vision. The eye produces a surplus of tears and a discharge. Muscle spasms develop in the eyelids, and the eyelashes turn inward, which further inflames the cornea. As the cornea becomes more scarred, it becomes more opaque, and blindness may result.

Trachoma can be successfully treated in the early stages with sulpha drugs, ANTIBIOTICS, or surgery. Advanced stages of the disease resist treatment and often result in blindness. A drug called azithromycin is being used in some countries, with good results. Trachoma can be prevented by improving sanitary conditions, such as the water supply, personal hygiene, and medical care. (See WORLD BLINDNESS.)

transpupillary thermotherapy   (TTT)   A new experimental laser treatment for patients who have the wet form of age-related macular degeneration, especially those who have a condition known as occult choroidal neovascularization.

Occult choroidal neovascularization is a condition in which the abnormal blood vessels that grow beneath the macula in the wet form of age-related macular degeneration are hidden beneath layers of tissue. Because a doctor must be able to see the abnormal vessels in order to treat them with traditional laser therapy or photodynamic therapy, patients with occult choroidal neovascularization were considered unsuitable for those treatments.

TTT involves using a low-intensity laser to apply heat to the area in which the abnormal blood vessels are growing. The heat raises the temperature of the retina, causing the blood in the abnormal vessels to clot. This stops the blood vessels from leaking, and reduces the size of lesions in the area of the blood vessels. This is beneficial because the fluid and blood that leak from the vessels damage the light-sensitive photoreceptor cells in the macula.

Trials showed that about 20 percent of the 15 patients who participated in a pilot study experienced a slight improvement in vision. All but a few patients showed a notable decline in the thickness of the retina, which doctors say indicates that the growth and leakage of new blood vessels had been stopped—at least temporarily. Researchers are continuing to move forward with TTT and say that the procedure appears to be promising in the area of treatments for macular degeneration.

trauma   Ocular trauma is any injury to the eye. Ocular trauma, even seemingly minor injuries, should be examined promptly and thoroughly by a physician. A trauma may be blunt (concussive) or perforating (invading the inner eye). An estimated half million serious eye injuries occur each year, with 25,000 of them resulting in blindness.

The eyelids are often the first line of defense in an injury, and if closed in time can minimize the severity of the injury. However, in protecting the eye, the eyelids are often damaged. A contusion, or blunt blow from a ball or fist, will result in hemorrhaging and swelling under the skin. This will appear as a "black eye" and will heal itself.

Minor cuts to the eyelids that are located away from the lid margin often do not require stitching. However, cuts that involve the eyelid margin are considered serious and may require surgical repair performed in an hospital operating room.

Care must be taken during examination and treatment to ensure that the eyelid properly closes. If left uncovered, the cornea could become damaged, and loss of vision may result.

Nasolacrimal (tear duct) injuries may result in constant tearing and must be surgically repaired. Often the area must be allowed to partially heal before final surgery can be performed. In this case, and in minor injuries of the nasolacrimal area, a tiny silicone tube is inserted into the tear duct to ensure correct healing.

The CONJUNCTIVA and the cornea are subject to injury by foreign bodies, lacerations and burns. The conjunctiva is the membrane that covers the white part of the eye (SCLERA) and the inside of the eyelids. The cornea is the clear protective covering of the eye.

Foreign bodies may become lodged in the conjunctiva or cornea. Conjunctival foreign bodies usually wash out of the eye by the flushing action of the tears. However, foreign bodies that imbed in the cornea are painful and require removal by a physician.

Minor lacerations to the conjunctiva are usually not treated. Lacerations that produce significant bleeding in the sclera should be examined for a more serious injury. Nonperforating lacerations such as scratches and abrasions, including those caused by overwear of contact lenses, cause pain to the cornea but are usually self-healing. In the case of corneal abrasion, the cornea can be comfortably examined with anesthetic drops, but the continued use of the drops is discouraged since they delay healing. Treatment may include antibiotic drops and temporary eye patching.

Chemical burns to the cornea are serious and vision threatening. The burns cause permanent, severe corneal scarring, which precludes vision. Burns caused by acid or lye should be flushed immediately and profusely with water. The eyes must receive emergency care by an ophthalmologist.

Thermal burns such as those caused by sunlight are generally not serious to the cornea and are self-healing or treated with antibiotic drops. There may be substantial pain, however, and the lids may be burned and require treatment.

Blunt injuries can also cause damage to portions of the inner eye. Hyphema, hemorrhaging into the anterior chamber of the eye can be caused by injury. The patient is usually instructed to rest prone for up to three days to prevent secondary bleeding, which may cause glaucoma. Blood staining of the cornea may be permanent and cause an opacity that interferes with vision.

Contusion may cause radial tears or splits in the iris and CILIARY BODY from the sclera. This may reduce the angle of the ANTERIOR CHAMBER and contribute to or cause glaucoma.

Severe contusion involving the lens may cause cataract, although the process of opacification set in motion by the injury may take years to mature and be noticeable. A blow may also cause the lens to become completely dislocated or subluxated (partially displaced). A displaced lens is associated with secondary glaucoma.

The vitreous may hemorrhage or become detached after a blunt injury. Vitreal hemorrhages generally are self-limiting, but a detached vitreous can result in a retinal tear or detached retina.

The retina may hemorrhage and develop macular edema as a result of a contusion. Blows to the eye may result in retinal tears which could lead to a retinal detachment.

Blunt injuries may cause tears in the choroid, optic atrophy, and hemorrhaging into the optic nerve sheath, conditions that can result in permanent vision loss.

Severe contusion injuries such as automobile accidents may involve the side of the cheek and one eye. This often results in a blow-out fracture of the orbit. The orbit is forced backwards, the orbital floor is fractured, and the bone is displaced downward. A plastic implant is placed in the floor of the orbit to correct the situation.

Perforating wounds pass the cornea and enter the inner eye. Perforating injuries are caused by pointed instruments such as scissors, darts, sharp tools, or glass. Any perforating wound is considered an emergency and may be subject to infection. The prognosis for the health of the eye and the preservation of the vision depends on the depth of the wound and the care taken to clean and repair the wound. If the wound penetrates the cornea alone, it may be cleaned and sutured with excellent prognosis.

If the lens has been breached, cataract or aphakia (an eye without a lens) may eventually become the result. If the eye is further invaded, retinal damage and detachment are possible.

Perforating injuries are treated immediately with a preventative tetanus injection and systemic and local antibiotics. X rays are often ordered to locate the presence of foreign bodies in the wound. Foreign bodies that breach the inner eye can cause infection and blindness.

Metal particles associated with some occupations can cause iron salt deposits to gather in the eye and result in blindness. The particles can be removed with a surgical procedure that employs a magnet.

Pellets from pellet guns cause massive damage to the eye upon entry. The entire eye is usually enucleated, or removed. Some glass or plastic particles that enter the eye may be of materials that are well tolerated by the eye and do not require removal.

Sympathetic ophthalmia must be considered after any perforation injury. This condition involves the spread of inflammation from a steadily inflamed eye to the uninjured eye over a period of two weeks.

The infected eye may be removed during the two-week period, to prevent sympathetic ophthalmia. If the condition develops after the two week period it may be treated with steroids but may continue to recur.

Galloway, N. R. *Common Eye Diseases and Their Management.* Berlin: Springer-Verlag, 1985.

Reynolds, James D. *Ocular Trauma.* HealthNet Library. Columbus: CompuServe, 1989.

Rhode, Stephen J., and Stephen P. Ginsberg. *Ophthalmic Technology.* New York: Raven Press, 1987.

trephine   A surgical instrument used in ophthalmologic procedures. The metal instrument looks much like a small, round cookie cutter attached to a handle. The round section comes in various diameter sizes, ranging from three to five millimeters. The size of the trephine is etched onto the handle for identification.

The trephine is generally used as a marker. When pressed gently onto the cornea, it makes a distinct, temporary indentation for the surgeon to follow. The trephine is used in corneal transplant surgery to mark duplicate sections of cornea from host and donor, and in RADIAL KERATOTOMY (RK) surgery, to mark the optical zone for radial cuts.

trichiasis   A condition in which the eyelashes grow inward into the eye. The lashes rub against the cornea, causing pain and infection. This may occur spontaneously or be caused by an injury, infection, or disease such as trachoma. The lashes can be removed with epilating forceps to immediately remedy the disorder. If regrowth is a problem, the lash roots can be destroyed by electrolysis.

trifluridine   An antimetabolite drug used in the treatment of ocular herpes. It is also known by the names TFT, F3T, and Viroptic. Trifluridine, along with idoxuridine, was one of the first drugs developed to treat herpes keratitis, an inflammation of the cornea caused by the herpes virus.

Trifluridine is a toxic drug since it is activated by the enzymes contained in healthy human cells. Since it cannot differentiate between healthy and viral cells, it may attack and destroy normal cells along with the unwanted viral cells. Because of its toxicity, trifluridine is not to be taken intravenously. It is available in ointment or drop form only.

Trifluridine drops are used nine times per day for a period of two to three weeks.

Trifluridine is not a cure for herpes keratitis. It is effective only when the virus is active in the body. It is ineffective during periods when the virus is latent or inactive.

trifocal lenses   Three lens prescriptions put into one pair of contact lenses or eyeglasses. Trifocal lenses are prescribed when bifocals are not sufficient for clear vision at all distances. Those who need trifocals are usually over 40 and suffering from presbyopia, aging of the eyes. As the eye ages, it loses the ability to bring close objects into focus.

The three sections of the trifocal include a reading section for close work, a distance section for seeing objects five feet away or farther, and a section for the midrange between the two.

The placement and size of the segments within the lens frame is determined by the wearer's needs. The largest section is generally the one most often used.

Trifocal wearers must develop head and eye movements in conjunction with their new lenses. It may be necessary to move the head up or down in order to match the section of lens to the object viewed.

tumors   Tissue growths that can form in any part of the body and eye. Tumors may be malignant (cancerous) or benign (noncancerous).

Malignant tumors carry specific characteristics. The cells of these tumors differ from the cells of the encompassing tissue, tend to grow quickly and uncontrollably, do not stop growing once they have reached a particular size, and tend to spread or metastasize to other parts of the body. Malignant tumors may be life threatening.

Three common malignant tumors found in the eye are MALIGNANT MELANOMA, RETINOBLASTOMA, and metastatic tumors. All are serious disorders that benefit from early diagnosis and treatment.

Malignant melanoma is a tumor that develops from the melanin-laden cells in the CHOROID, iris or CILIARY BODY. The tumor may develop spontaneously or from a mole. This type of tumor usually grows and metastasizes at a slow rate and generally affects one eye only.

Symptoms of melanoma include redness, inflammation, vision loss, glaucoma, and distortion of the pupil. Melanoma is usually treated by enucleation, or removal of the eye, but may be subjected to chemotherapy or radiation treatments during a period of observation. The cause of melanoma is unknown.

Retinoblastoma is a malignant tumor of the retina found in young children. The tumor spreads rapidly and may metastasize up the optic nerve to the brain.

The tumor is hereditary or may develop sporadically. The more common sporadic type usually is limited to one eye and appears at approximately two years of age. The hereditary type often affects both eyes, appears near one year of age, and can be passed to future generations.

Symptoms of retinoblastoma include redness, pain, inflammation, crossed eyes, and change in pupil color. Immediate treatment includes enucleation. In cases in which both eyes are involved, the more affected eye may be removed and the less affected treated with radiation, chemotherapy, or cryotherapy (freezing treatments).

Retinoblastoma has one of the highest rates of spontaneous regression, but little is known about the causes for regression. The development of the tumor is caused by the absence of paired retinoblastoma genes on the 13th chromosome, a condition that may occur through heredity or environmental conditions.

Metastatic tumors are malignant tumors that originate in another organ of the body and metastasize to the eye. Metastatic tumors affect both eyes approximately 25 percent of the time.

Symptoms of the secondary ocular tumor may be apparent before those of the primary tumor. Symptoms may involve pain, redness, glaucoma, and vision loss or interference. Once a diagnosis has been made, the primary tumor is appropriately treated. Treatment of the ocular tumor may involve surgery, chemotherapy or radiation treatment.

Basal-cell carcinoma and squamous-cell carcinoma are two similar-looking malignant tumors found on the eyelids. They each first appear as a small bump and then develop into a saucer-shape with a raised rim.

The tumor is removed and sent for biopsy to determine the identity of type. If left untreated, the basal-cell carcinoma may spread to the underlying bone but rarely metastasizes further. Advanced basal-cell carcinoma is treated with radiation therapy.

Squamous cell carcinoma is a more serious tumor. It may metastasize to the lymph nodes of the upper or lower lids. This type of carcinoma may be treated with chemotherapy or radiation treatment.

Rhabdomyosarcoma is a rare malignant tumor of the ORBIT. It affects children and is characterized by rapid growth. Early treatment with radiation gives the best hope for a cure.

Benign tumors differ little from encompassing tissue, grow more slowly than malignant tumors and often stop growing at a certain point. Benign tumors do not spread to other parts of the body. In the case of benign ocular tumor, the growth may be left intact if it does not interfere with sight.

Benign tumors may develop in any part of the eye. The strawberry nevus and the cavernous hemangioma are two commonly found in the eyelids. The nevus, or strawberry nevus, is a tumor that appears as a pinkish or red raised mark on the skin. It is present at birth but is often undetectable until later in life when it starts to grow. It rarely becomes malignant and may spontaneously regress. The nevus may be left untreated.

The cavernous hemangioma is a deeper tumor that may appear as a blue raised area on the lid. The tumor tends to expand during periods of crying. This tumor may spontaneously regress or may be treated by freezing methods.

Benign tumors of the orbit include the pseudotumor, or a mass of inflamed tissue found in the orbit. Symptoms of pseudotumor are EXOPHTHALMOS, or bulging forward of the eyes, and double vision. If a biopsy reveals nonmalignant tissue, the tumor may be treated with steroids.

See CANCER.

ultrasonography   The use of sonic waves in ophthalmologic tests. High-frequency sound waves are used to probe and view the inner eye when other instruments prove ineffective. The sonic waves are directed to the eye, and the echoing sounds are translated into a picture of it.

Ultrasonography is used to examine the tissues of the eye for the presence of tumors, retinal detachments or fractures. Ultrasonography may be performed after glaucoma surgery to review results. It is used to take measurements of the eye or to determine the health of the underlying retina in presurgical tests for cataract surgery.

The A-SCAN applies ultrasonography to measure the length of the eye to determine the correct strength of intraocular lens needed for cataract surgery. The B-SCAN uses the sound waves to view a retina obscured by a dense cataract.

unemployment   See EMPLOYMENT, EMPLOYMENT DISINCENTIVES.

Uniform Anatomical Gift Act   (UAGA)   Legislation that allows for the donation of the body or body parts, including eyes and corneas, for transplantation or research. It was approved by the National Conference of Commissioners on Uniform State Laws in 1968. Since that time, all 50 states and the District of Columbia have adopted some form of this act.

The act permits any individual over 18 years of age and of sound mind to donate his entire body or parts of his body to any organ bank, hospital, medical school, surgeon, or physician. It further allows a donor to specify an individual as the recipient of the organs for therapy or transplantation.

The gift or donation can be specified in a written will or document. The document may be as simple as a card carried by the donor or, as is offered in 43 states, a signed section of the driver's license. However, family members must confirm the donation at the time of death, so it is important that they be notified in advance of intent to donate.

universities   There are no universities or colleges exclusiveiy for blind or visually impaired students. It is generally considered desirable for them to attend the same institutions of higher learning as nondisabled students. Section 504 of the Rehabilitation Act of 1973 mandates that no qualified disabled individual can be excluded solely on the basis of disability from participation in any program, including educational programs, that receive federal financial support.

Although programs vary on campuses across the country, most offer a number of "core" services: interpreters, readers, notetakers, counselors, and tutors. These services are usually available from a university or college Office of Disabled Student Services. Many university programs rely on federal, state, and private grants to expand services for disabled students. There is a trend for higher education institutions to offer specialized technology to meet the educational and employment needs of the disabled students they serve.

The Center on Disabilities at California State University, Northridge (CSUN), near Los Angeles, is widely regarded as a model for other university programs. CSUN serves a disabled student body of approximately 3 percent of the entire student population, a figure twice that of the national average.

In addition to offering core services, CSUN's Office of Disabled Student Services has taken a leadership role in delivering technological services to the disabled student body and the professionals who serve them. This office has established a Technology Group, a critical mass of programs and professional personnel, that:

• Conducts one of the largest conferences in the world on the subject of Technology and Persons with Disabilities. Some scholarships are available for parents and persons with disabilities, making it one of the most accessible conferences in the country for these groups.

• Established a Computer Access Lab offering the latest in peripherals (braille printers, speech synthesizers) and software such as the VISTA large-print program for blind and visually impaired users.

• Conducts training in technology for rehabilitation counselors and employers throughout California, Arizona, Nevada, Guam, Saipan, and American Samoa.

• Conducts engineering research through projects such as the Universal Access System, which provides access to any computer through a laptop computer.

• Hosts a monthly radio show on KIEV (Los Angeles) on the subject of Technology and Persons with Disabilities.

Other CSUN-sponsored conferences include those concerning learning disabilities, art for disabled persons, and employment-related topics.

Students entering universities or colleges may receive funding for personal readers or educational materials from the state agency for the blind. Federal transition services offered through state commissions for the blind or vocational-rehabilitation agencies are a federal priority but are not mandated.

Contact:

CSUN Center on Disabilities
1811 Nordhoff Street
Northridge, CA 91330-8340

818-677-2578 (voice and TTY)
818-677-4929 (fax)
www.csun.edu/cod

Usher's syndrome   An inherited condition combining a serious hearing loss and a progressive loss of vision caused by RETINITIS PIGMENTOSA (RP). According to the RP Foundation Fighting Blindness, there are between 10,000 and 15,000 people with Usher's syndrome in the United States. It is the major cause of deaf-blindness.

There are three known types of Usher's syndrome. Type I individuals are born with a profound hearing loss and retinitis pigmentosa. Individuals with Type II are born with a mild to moderate hearing loss and generally have a less severe form of RP. Type III Usher's syndrome is characterized by hearing loss and vision loss due to RP that are both progressive.

Retinitis pigmentosa is characterized by a degeneration of the rods and cones (light-sensitive cells) of the retina. The retina of the eye receives the reflected light from an object, and the rods and cones translate the light into electrical impulses that the retina sends to the brain through the optic nerve. The brain changes the impulses into an image.

The rods function in low light or darkness and are responsible for detecting movement and shape. They are scattered throughout the retina and are accountable for peripheral or side vision. The cones discern detail and color and require light to work effectively. They are concentrated into the central section of the retina, the macula, and are responsible for central vision.

Retinitis pigmentosa attacks the rods first, then the cones. As the disease progresses, night vision diminishes and peripheral or side vision is lost. Over long periods of time, central vision is affected. The vision loss may not be apparent for several years. Tunnel vision and night blindness may become noticeable during adolescence, and progressively worsen.

Roughly 30 percent of those with retinitis pigmentosa report a hearing loss, some of whom may be considered to have Usher's syndrome. Usher's syndrome accounts for up to 3 percent of all cases of profound deafness. The hearing loss is caused by a malfunction in the sensory cells of the inner ear by an unknown cause. The loss is generally present at birth or follows shortly after birth.

Usher's syndrome can be diagnosed. The hearing loss is easily detected with audiometric testing. RP can be diagnosed by the characteristic changes that take place in the retina. Tests such as an electroretinogram and a visual-field test may be performed to confirm the diagnosis.

Usher's syndrome affects individuals of all races, ethnic and cultural backgrounds and is equally prevalent among males and females. It is a recessively inherited disorder that requires the necessary gene from both the mother and father. A pairing of two carriers of the gene results in a one in four chance of producing Usher's syndrome. A pairing of a carrier and a noncarrier of the gene seldom results in Usher's syndrome, but the gene is passed on to future generations. At present, there is no method for determining a gene carrier other than tracing family history of the disease. Genetic counseling may be beneficial in prevention of the disease.

Scientists made significant progress in the late 1990s to learn more about the defects that cause Usher's syndrome. Researchers think there are nine different genes that contain mutations that cause various types of Usher's syndrome. They are currently working to develop rodent models of Usher's syndrome that will help them understand how the genes function and how mutations in the gene lead to the hearing and vision loss that is typical of the disease.

There is no cure for Usher's syndrome or retinitis pigmentosa although a specified amount of vitamin A has been found to slow the progression of RP in some people. The hearing loss tends to remain stable, but since it is an inner ear loss, surgery is not possible to restore hearing. Some individuals without any residual hearing have been candidates for cochlear implants. Many of those with residual hearing have benefited from hearing aids.

The progressive sight loss is untreatable. Each case is unique and unpredictable. The retina may degenerate rapidly or over a period of decades. Usually, some central vision is maintained through middle age. Most Usher's syndrome patients who become legally blind retain some central vision.

Cataracts, a clouding of the eye's lens, may develop in patients with RP and Usher's syndrome. If the cataract is removable, the surgery does not improve retinal degeneration but can restore the visual acuity lost to the opacity of the cataract.

In the research for a cure or treatment for Usher's syndrome and retinitis pigmentosa, experiments and studies involving DMSO applications and light deprivation have had less than satisfactory results. Usher's syndrome patients may maximize their residual vision with low-vision aids. Optical aids such as Corning or NOIR glasses, telescopes, microscopes, and night-vision aids may be useful. Nonoptical and electronic aids such as the Wide Angle Mobility Light, large print, talking computers, and closed-circuit television may further independence. However, these low-vision aids cannot restore vision that has been lost to RP or Usher's syndrome.

Annala, L. "Facing the Future with Usher's Syndrome." Workshop on Usher's syndrome (December 2–3, 1976). Helen Keller National Center, Sands Point, NY.

Boardman, L. "My Son has Usher's Syndrome." *The Deaf-Blind American.* (June 1985): pp. 50–60.

The Foundation Fighting Blindness. *Usher Syndrome Gene Identified.* Hunt Valley, Md.: The Foundation for Fighting Blindness, 2001.

Pimentel, A. "Handling the Upper, Secondary and College Usher's Syndrome Student." Workshop on Usher's syndrome (December 2–3, 1976). Helen Keller National Center, Sands Point, NY.

Roehrig, A. "Living with Usher's Syndrome." Workshop on Usher's syndrome (December 2–3, 1976). Helen Keller National Center, Sands Point, NY.

RP Foundation Fighting Blindness. *Answers to Your Questions about Usher's Syndrome.* Baltimore, Maryland: RPFFB, 1988.

Vernon, McCay, Joann A. Boughman and Linda Annala. "Considerations in Diagnosing Usher's Syndrome: RP and Hearing Loss." *Journal of Visual Impairment and Blindness,* 76 (1982): 258–261.

uvea   The uvea, or uveal tract, is a heavily vascularized layer that supplies blood to the eye. It includes the melanin-pigmented portions of the eye: the iris and CILIARY BODY in the front of the eye and the CHOROID to the back of the eye.

The iris is the colored portion of the eye. It controls the size of the pupil, which regulates the amount of light that enters the eye. The ciliary body lies just behind the iris and is attached to the lens of the eye. The ciliary body produces AQUEOUS FLUID and moves the lens to focus properly. The choroid is a layer of blood vessels between the retina and the SCLERA, or white part of the eye. It nourishes and supports the eye.

Disorders of the uvea may include inflammations, injuries or infections. A common disorder, UVEITIS, is an inflammation of the uveal tract. It can be caused by an injury or other illness present in the body or can appear spontaneously from an unknown cause. In addition, each section of the uvea is subject to inflammation, including IRITIS, CYCLITIS, and CHOROIDITIS.

uveitis   An inflammation of the uveal tract of the eye. The uveal tract includes the iris, the CILIARY BODY, and the CHOROID. The entire tract is highly vascularized and contains the pigment melanin, which is also found in the skin. Uveitis may occur because of an injury, in connection with another disease of the eye or body, or spontaneously. The disorder is usually categorized as either anterior or posterior uveitis.

Anterior uveitis (or IRIDOCYCLITIS) occurs when the inflammation involves the iris and the ciliary body. The iris is the colored part of the eye. It controls the pupil, which opens and shuts to regulate the light that enters the eye. The ciliary body lies behind the iris and is connected to the lens of the eye. The ciliary body produces AQUEOUS FLUID and moves the lens to focus the eye properly. Symptoms of anterior uveitis include redness, light sensitivity, blurred vision, and extreme pain, especially when focusing on near objects. A thorough ophthalmologic examination may be needed to determine the cause of uveitis. Additional tests such as X rays of the chest, skull or sinuses, blood tests, and examinations for arthritis or other diseases may be necessary.

Usually, a specific cause for anterior uveitis is not found, and the condition is determined to have occurred spontaneously. Other diseases and disorders may cause uveitis and include arthritis, tuberculosis, SARCOIDOSIS, sinus disorders, venereal disease, ulcerative colitis, and injuries.

The prognosis for anterior uveitis is generally good, unless the eye develops complications due to recurrences. Recurrent uveitis may result in cataracts or secondary glaucoma due to increased intraocular pressure. Mild anterior uveitis is treated with the application of steroid eye drops to reduce the inflammation. Acute uveitis may be treated with steroid pills or injections. In both cases, cycloplegics, drops that widen the pupil, such as atropine sulfate, may be prescribed to restrict the focusing power of the inflamed eye and allow for a rest period.

Posterior uveitis involves the choroid and is also called CHOROIDITIS. The choroid is a layer of blood vessels between the retina and the SCLERA, or white part of the eye. The choroid nourishes and supports the eye.

Posterior uveitis is not usually as painful as anterior uveitis. There may be redness of the eye, blurred or lost vision, light sensitivity, and the appearance of floaters (small dark spots that seem to float through the field of vision). If the uveitis remains in the area of peripheral vision, the symptoms may not be noticed.

Posterior uveitis, like anterior uveitis, may occur spontaneously. It has been associated with toxoplasmosis, tuberculosis, sarcoidosis, venereal disease, viruses, and injuries. If untreated, posterior uveitis can spread from the choroid to the retina and the vitreous. If the inflammation involves the macula, permanent central vision loss may occur. When the inflammation spreads into the vitreous and entails the center of the globe, the condition is called endophthalmitis, which may be treated with ANTIBIOTICS and possibly reversed. Treatment for posterior uveitis includes steroid eye drops or pills. In more serious cases, immunosuppressive medications may be used. (See IRITIS.)

In 1990 researchers at the University of Iowa identified a gene defect that they believe is the cause of a new clinical syndrome they call hereditary uveitis. The proper name of the syndrome is autosomal dominant neovascular inflammatory vitreoretinopathy (ADNIV). Many of the features of the syndrome are common to those found in uveitis.

In 1992, researchers established that the gene that causes ADNIV is located on the long arm of chromosome 11. They are still working, however, to isolate the particular gene that they believe causes ADNIV.

V

venous occlusion   A condition that results from a blockage to a retinal vein. The disease usually involves the central retinal vein, or CRV. The damage to the retina occurs when blood flows into the eye from the undamaged arteries but cannot flow from the eye due to the blockage. Hemorrhaging and swelling occur, and vision is damaged.

The condition may occur suddenly or over a period of days. The vision may regress to 20/400 or worse, but there is rarely accompanying pain. The cause of the disease is unknown, but it is suspected that it occurs as a result of an intraluminal thrombosis, or a blood clot in the lamina cribrosa of the optic nerve.

Because of the high occurrence of CRV obstruction and ARTERIOSCLERO-SIS of the central retinal artery, it is believed that arteriosclerosis may lead to the obstruction. Open-angle glaucoma, orbital or global trauma, and optic-nerve or orbital tumors may also lead to occlusion.

Treatment for venous occlusion includes therapy for the underlying cause, if apparent, and may include anticoagulation medications and photocoagulation therapy. Laser surgery may be advised to help reduce macular swelling, prevent abnormal growth of new vessels, or prevent bleeding. It is not, however, always successful. Once a venous occlusion has occurred, vision loss can be permanent. Complications of venous occlusion include neovascular glaucoma (20 percent chance), neovascularization, and retinal detachment.

Branch-vein occlusion occurs because the vein crosses over a hard arteriosclerotic arteriole (small part of an artery that ends in capillaries). It can cause central vision loss, neovascularization and glaucoma.

VersaBraille   See PAPERLESS BRAILLE.

veterans   According to the Blinded Veterans Association, there are approximately 120,000 visually impaired veterans in the United States. Many more veterans become blind or visually impaired each year due to common eye diseases such as age-related maculopathy, glaucoma, and RETINITIS PIGMENTOSA.

The U.S. Department of Veterans Affairs (VA) provides a wide range of benefits to American veterans, including those with vision impairments, and their families. The vision loss does not need to occur during military service in order for a veteran to qualify for benefits.

Veterans who receive an honorable discharge are eligible for all benefits, including educational benefits. Those receiving general discharges qualify for all benefits except educational. Those who receive dishonorable and bad-conduct discharges are not eligible for veterans benefits. Those who receive other than honorable discharges may or may not qualify for some benefits. These cases are reviewed individually by the VA. Veterans rated nonservice-connected are required to complete an income questionnaire (means test) when applying for medical care and may be denied medical care depending on the results.

Those who originally enlisted after September 7, 1980, and those who entered military service after October 16, 1981, must complete the shorter of two possible terms in order to qualify for benefits: either 24 months of continuous active duty or the full period for which the individual was called to active duty. This does not apply to veterans with a service-connected disability or who were discharged near the end of an enlistment term because of a disability incurred or aggravated in the line of duty or due to hardship.

The U.S. Department of Veterans Affairs provides the benefits through three major offices:

1. The Veterans Benefits Administration administers compensation, pensions, GI loans, insurance, education, and job-training programs, including vocational-rehabilitation and disability benefits. The Veterans Administration operates the Blind Rehabilitation Service, which administers programs for blinded veterans at VA Blind Rehabilitation Centers and Clinics.
2. The National Cemetery System administers death benefits. These include burial expenses and compensation to surviving spouses and children.
3. The Veterans Health Services and Research Administration administers health-care benefits, such as hospitalization, nursing-home care, domiciliary care, outpatient medical and dental treatment, beneficiary travel, alcohol- and drug-dependency treatment, Agent Orange or nuclear radiation exposure treatment, prosthetic appliances, readjustment counseling centers, medical care for dependents, overseas benefits, appeals, and blind aids and services.

Aids and services are available to blind veterans who are eligible for medical services. Veterans are considered blind if they meet the specifications of legal blindness. Most blind veterans qualify for an annual review by the Visual Impairment Services Team (VIST), adjustment to blindness training, home improvements and structural alterations to homes, low-vision aids and training, approved electronic and mechanical aids for the blind (as well as their repair and replacement), and dog guides and the cost of the dog's medical care.

In order to inform blind veterans of the benefits available to them, Congress chartered the Blinded Veterans Association (BVA) to serve veterans with severe vision loss. The organization works through a field service program and an outreach employment program to help veterans obtain services, benefits, rehabilitation training, and employment. (See REHABILITATION.)

Another group, the Blinded American Veterans Foundation (BAVF), was formed in 1985 by three American veterans who had lost their sight while serving in Korea and Vietnam. The BAVF has three primary goals: research, rehabilitation, and reemployment. It does not maintain a membership, but serves as a clearinghouse for research and educational efforts and advancements.

The BAVF supports medical research concerning blindness and other sensory disabilities, participates in outreach programs to learn the needs and concerns of veterans with sensory disabilities, and conducts informational programs directed at government, business, and the general public. It also has developed a national volunteer corps to help veterans with sensory disabilities.

The BAVF funded the research and development of the Americane, a sensory aid that has been certified by the Department of Veterans Affairs and distributed to more than 2,500 blind veterans.

Contact:

The Blinded American Veterans Foundation
P.O. Box 65900
Washington, DC 20035-5900
www.bavf.org

The Blinded Veterans Association
477 H Street
Northwest Washington, DC 20001-2694
202-371-8880
www.bva.org

vidarabine   See ARA-A.

visual acuity   The measurement of the amount of detail an individual sees in relation to the amount of detail someone with normal vision sees. Visual acuity is stated as an equation with 20 as the first number, a slash mark and a second number of either 15, 20, 25, 30, 40, 50, 70, 100 or 200, such as 20/20. The first number of the equation, 20, indicates the distance at which the measurement is taken. The second number indicates the distance at which a normally sighted person can see specific detail or print.

Normal or "perfect" vision is written as 20/20. Someone with 20/20 vision sees detail at 20 feet that a normally sighted person sees at 20 feet. Someone with 20/100 vision sees detail at 20 feet that someone with normal vision could see at 100 feet.

The eye chart usually used for the visual acuity test is called the SNELLEN CHART. Using this chart as a measurement, the individual can be given a visual acuity range from 20/15 to 20/200. A measurement of 20/200 means that the individual was only able to see the largest letter on the chart, the big E.

The term *count fingers* refers to an individual who cannot see the big E, but who can count the number of fingers the examiner holds up. *Hand motion* is the term used to describe someone who cannot see the separate fingers, but who can discern some movement when the hand is waved.

Light perception, or LP, describes the person who can perceive only light or its absence. NLP, or no light perception, refers to one who is unable to discern any light.

Visual-acuity measurements help describe legal definitions for blindness. These classifications determine eligibility for federal benefits. Someone with corrected vision of 20/50 in the better eye is classified as having low vision. An individual with corrected vision of 20/200 in the better eye is classified as legally blind.

visual aids   See ADAPTIVE AIDS.

visual field   The area in which a person can see. This area or field is measured in degrees. A person with normal vision can see objects within a field of about 150 degrees with one eye and 180 degrees with both eyes when looking straight ahead. The central 60 degrees seen by both eyes is called CENTRAL VISION. It is also known as "seeing" vision, because it is the vision you use to look directly at something.

The vision on either side of these 60 degrees is called PERIPHERAL VISION. This is the vision surrounding what you are looking at. It describes side vision, or the things you see out of the "corner of your eye." Peripheral vision is also called "traveling" vision.

A loss of visual field can occur in the central vision, the peripheral vision or both. An individual with a visual field of 40 to 20 degrees of a possible 180 in the better eye is classified as having low vision. Someone with a field of 20 degrees or less of the possible 180 in the better eye is classified legally blind.

vitamins   Vitamins are essential to the health of the eyes and maintenance of vision. Vitamin A, or retinol, is an element most closely tied to vision. The retina contains light sensitive rods and cones, which receive light and provide information about the seen object. This information is converted by the retina to electrical impulses sent to the brain. The brain translates the impulses into an image.

The cones are responsible for central vision, detail, and color, and require light to function. The rods are responsible for peripheral vision and function in low light.

The rods contain the pigment rhodopsin, or visual purple, which is chemically very similar to vitamin A. When light strikes a rod, the rhodopsin is broken down and used up. In order to make new rhodopsin and continue to function, the rod must draw on vitamin A within the body. Without replenishment of vitamin A, the rod will eventually be destroyed.

The first sign of vitamin-A deficiency is night blindness. In dim light the eye depends on the rods to maintain vision. When the rods are not functioning, night blindness occurs.

Vitamin-A deficiency causes XEROPHTHALMIA, a leading cause of blindness in developing countries of the world. According to Helen Keller International, xerophthalmia impairs the vision of 5 million to 10 million children annually, and causes irreparable blindness to 500,000 of these.

Vitamin A is found in yellow vegetables such as carrots and is stored in the body for long periods of time in the liver. A normal diet that includes vegetables and vitamin A-rich foods will prevent vitamin-A deficiency.

Vitamin-B deficiency may cause vision loss. A deficiency of thiamine, vitamin B_1, affects the optic nerve, which carries the electrical impulses to the brain, thus interrupting or interfering with the message. This condition, referred to as nutritional amblyopia, produces scotomas, or blind spots, in the field of vision. Thiamine supplements can often correct and restore vision lost to B_1 deficiency.

Vitamin-B_2 (riboflavin) deficiency may cause cornea disease or KERATITIS, and vitamin-B_6 (pyridoxine) deficiency may cause vascular congestion and corneal neovascularization. Vitamin-B_{12} deficiency, or pernicious anemia, is associated with RETROBULBAR NEURITIS (swelling of the optic nerve). Treatment with adequate dosages of these vitamins usually reverses or improves the conditions caused by their lack.

Vitamin C, in large doses, has been shown to be effective in drawing fluid away from the eye and reducing elevated intraocular pressure associated with glaucoma. It is not used as a treatment for glaucoma but rather as a diet supplement.

Vitamin C may be effective in the prevention of cataracts and retinal disorders such as diabetic retinopathy and age-related maculopathy. Cataracts and retinal damage may be caused by an excess of free radicals, chemicals that are generated by a normal body process called oxidation. Since vitamin C is an antioxidant, a diet containing vitamin C may decelerate the process of developing cataracts or retinal disorders. Because subsequent research and studies in this area differ in their conclusions, this theory remains controversial.

Vitamin-C deficiency, or scurvy, may lead to ocular hemorrhage. For any hemorrhage of the eye not related to DIABETES, hypertension or another cause may be investigated as a symptom of scurvy. Vitamin-C treatment may produce results in a week.

An excess of vitamin D may cause opacities in the cornea or CONJUNCTIVA and scleral calcification. Overdosage in infancy may produce optic atrophy, optic neuritis, or convergent strabismus.

Researchers at the Department of Newborn Medicine at the Royal Alexandra Hospital in Edmonton, Alberta, have found that a dose of vitamin E given within 12 hours of birth may reduce the incidence of severe forms of RETINOPATHY OF PREMATURITY. This has not been confirmed in other studies and remains an unproven controversial form of treatment.

Supplements of vitamins A, C, and E may be prescribed in combination to retard the progression of diabetic retinopathy, age-related maculopathy, and cataracts, help maintain the health of blood cells and vessels of the retina, and assist in the healing process after surgery.

Zinc is necessary to healthy vision and is contained in the highest concentration in the body in the retina. Zinc allows vitamin A to be released from the liver and is used in the process of metabolism in the retina. Since a zinc deficiency prevents the body from using the available vitamin A, it may cause the same effects as a vitamin-A deficiency.

Vitamin products that claim to help guard against age-related macular degeneration and other diseases are available. Most doctors, however, warn that vitamins, while important in maintaining eye health, are not miracle cures for eye diseases.

Carden, Robert G. "Vitamins for Healthier Eyes." *Let's Live,* September 1984, pp. 10–11.

Editors of Prevention Magazine. *Prevention's New Encyclopedia of Common Diseases.* Emmaus, Pennsylvania: Rodale Press, 1984.

Havener, William H. *Ocular Pharmacology.* St. Louis: C.V. Mosby Company, 1970.

Helen Keller International. *Facts About Helen Keller International.* New York: HKI, 1987.

Vaughn, Lewis, ed. *The Complete Book of Vitamins and Minerals for Health.* Emmaus, Pennsylvania: Rodale Press, 1988.

Yukin, John. *The Penguin Encyclopedia of Nutrition.* New York: Viking Press, 1985.

vocational aids Any devices that allow an individual to perform any facet of a job. Vocational aids are often called sensory aids, because frequently they are devices that compensate for a loss of one of the senses.

Vocational aids for visually impaired individuals compensate for a lack of vision or a reduced field of vision. The aid may be an adapted form of an old device that has been marked with raised dots, braille, or large print. It may have an auditory signal or voice output component, or may be designed in a new form to compensate for the user's lack of sight.

Vocational aids may be categorized by type, including:

- BRAILLE devices, such as a brailler or braille typewriter, a braille shorthand machine, braillex (which records braille information in digitized form), digicassette (which records and stores braille on magnetic tape from a braille keyboard), or paperless braille (which records and stores braille information to discs).

- Calculators, such as those that provide a braille paper tape or printout of the display, electronic tone calculators that sound out a series of beeps to indicate a number, and talking calculators.

- Computers and computer-related items, such as punched-card readers (which enable users to determine characters on punched computer cards), voice-prompting automatic data-entry terminals, braille printers and embossers (which interface with computers), talking computer terminals or software with speech output or synthesis, or talking telephone directories (which respond vocally to typed requests).

- Magnifying aids, such as simple hand-held magnifiers or mounted magnifiers, loupes, bioptics, telescopic devices, and closed-circuit television (CCTV) systems.

- Illumination aids, which may be as simple as replacing low-wattage bulbs with higher-wattage light bulbs, may also include devices to reduce glare and flicker, special lamps, or hand-held flashlight magnifiers.

- Measuring aids, such as circuit testers (which emit a tone when a circuit or test cable attachment is complete), talking frequency measurers, auditory meter readers, brailled calipers, auditory or tactile dial indicators, electronic levels, tactually marked protractors, saw guides and tape measure, and auditory thermometers or pressure gages.

- Reading aids, such as the Kurzweil Personal Reader, the Optacon, and speech output for the Optacon.

- Recorders, such as cassette recorders and playback machines with variable-speed playback or time-compression systems.

- Tactile aids, such as the Sensory Quill, raised-line drawing kits, tactile maps, phone adaptors for determining tactually which lines on a multi-line phone are activated, or Lamp Activated Signal Terminal for telephone system workers.

- Organizational aids, such as large-print or braille label makers, talking label makers, and file folders differentiated by color.

- Time-keeping aids, such as raised-dot marked watches, talking clocks, metronomes, and raised-dot or talking stop watches.

- Tools, including adaptive chiseling guides, dovetailing guides, drill positioners, tactually marked framing squares, light probes for determining indicator lights, and copy holders.

vocational rehabilitation   Vocational rehabilitation services are programs that provide vocational training or support to disabled individuals from federal, state, or private agencies. Vocational rehabilitation enables visually impaired individuals to continue employment or train for new work. Vocational rehabilitation may be offered through a public or private residential school, within a program of special education in a public school, through an organization for the blind, by a private rehabilitation facility, by a sheltered workshop, through correspondence courses or by state rehabilitation agencies.

All 50 states administer programs of vocational rehabilitation and daily living skills for the purpose of enabling disabled individuals to become independent, employed, integrated members of society. These agencies are listed under various names, such as Department of Rehabilitation; Commission for the Visually Handicapped: State Services for the Blind and Visually Impaired; and the Bureau of the Blind.

Each state program varies according to the range of services and training available and the amount of financial assistance provided. Services may include medical and vocational diagnostic services, rehabilitation training, physical restoration, braille instruction, communication-skills training, books and training supplies, transportation allowance, reader services for the blind, vocational rehabilitation, job-placement services, postemployment services, procurement of job-related equipment and occupational licenses, ADAPTIVE AIDS evaluation, and selection, counseling, and family-member services.

Legally blind individuals may qualify for state rehabilitation services if they can provide certification of disability, if the disability results in a substantial handicap to employment, and if the state has a reasonable expectation that the recipient will get or hold a job as a result of vocational training.

Rehabilitation services are available at little or no cost to the individual. Some aspects of the rehabilitation program may require financial contribution by the individual. In some states, services such as psychological counseling, equipment purchase, transportation to school, or school tuition may be financed by the state or a combination of the state, the individual, and grants or loans.

In all state programs, each individual's case is carefully evaluated by a vocational-rehabilitation counselor for the blind with input from the disabled individual. College-trained vocational-rehabilitation specialists evaluate existing skills and aptitudes, evaluate and recommend occupations, outline needed skills, provide vocational-skills training and education, and recommend and provide training in the use of vocational aids or devices.

Every eligible individual is given an Individualized Written Plan that outlines the rehabilitation goals, the individual's skills and needs, and the process that will be taken to meet those needs.

The plan may provide for a medical examination to ascertain the extent and limitations of the disability, in order to assess suitable employment possibilities. Medical treatment or equipment, including surgery, psychiatric counseling, hospital services, prostheses, and eyeglasses, may be provided to reduce or alleviate the disability and improve productivity on the job.

Guidance counseling may be suggested to assess the individual's potential for rehabilitation, independent living, and appropriate employment. Job training may be provided at home, rehabilitation centers, trade schools, or on-the-job settings.

Educational tuition and expenses may be supplied if college is necessary to the vocational rehabilitation. The plan may furnish financial assistance during the rehabilitation process, as well as transportation costs, job referral and placement services, and job modification or reevaluation services.

Vocational-rehabilitation training may result in disabled individuals being employed in the mainstream of industry. These individuals earn and work at the same level of productivity as their sighted peers. Others may be employed in a Business Enterprise Program (BEP). These are usually vending, short order or cafeteria-style stands, or small businesses that are given priority for operation within federal facilities such as post offices, federal offices, or military institutions. The BEP is administered through the state vocational-rehabilitation agency and is supported by federal funds.

An individual may work in a sheltered workshop. A sheltered workshop is any place of employment that protects employment of the disabled. The individual may also be employed at home as a homemaker and family care provider.

The success of vocational-rehabilitation training varies by individual. The extent of the visual loss, the time in life when the loss occurred, and the abilities and aptitude of the individual all affect the outcome. The length of time for rehabilitation services also differs and may continue six months or longer.

American Foundation for the Blind. *An Introduction to Blindness Services in the United States.* www.afb.org/into_document_view.asp?documentid=930, 2001.

American Foundation for the Blind. *Rehabilitation Services.* New York: AFB, 1988.

California Department of Rehabilitation. *Client Information Booklet.* Sacramento: CDR, 1987.

California Department of Rehabilitation. *Rehabilitation is Here to Help.* Sacramento: CDR, 1986.

Lions Club International. *Rehabilitation of the Blind.* Oak Brook, Illinois: LCIRB, 1984.

National Association for Visually Handicapped. *The Adult Partially Seeing.* New York: NAVH, 1984.

W

Weihenmayer, Eric   Eric Weihenmayer is a blind speaker, writer, and adventurer who in 2001 became the first blind person to climb Mount Everest, the highest peak on Earth. Weihenmayer, who was born in 1969, began the climb in March and reached the summit shortly after midnight on May 25. He relied on his sense of touch and followed other climbers who wore bells during the ascent.

Born with retinoscheses, a degenerative eye disorder, Weihenmayer knew as a child that he would become blind by the time he was 13. He credits his family with helping him to develop and keep a positive outlook and to overcome the disadvantages that resulted from his blindness.

In addition to mountain climbing, Weihenmayer enjoys acrobatic sky-diving, scuba-diving, long-distance biking, running marathons, skiing, ice climbing, and rock climbing. He is determined that his blindness will not stop him from attaining his goals and has become an inspiration for blind people all around the world. The National Federal of the Blind sponsored Weihenmayer's Everest climb.

Weihenmayer has become well known to corporations and schools as an inspirational speaker. He has been featured in *Life, People, Sports Illustrated, Inside Edition, The Today Show, Good Morning America,* the Learning Channel, and many other newspapers, magazines, radio, and television shows. He recently completed his first book, *Touch the Top of the World: A Blind Man's Journey to Climb Further than the Eye Can See.* He lives in Englewood, Colorado, with his wife, Ellie, and daughter, Emma.

wet eye   a condition in which the eye contains an overabundance of tears due to inadequate tear drainage. It may be an annoying condition but rarely affects visual acuity.

Tears are constantly being produced and drained from the eye. They drain through lacrimal puncta, holes in each inner corner of the upper and lower lids. The tears are gathered in the lacrimal sac, an organ at the junction of the nose and lower lid. The tears then pass under the tissue to drainage ducts in the nasal cavity.

When the tears fail to drain adequately, wet eye occurs. This may be a congenital or acquired condition. Congenital wet eye occurs as a result of obstructions to the nasolacrimal ducts. Symptoms include tearing, crusting of the lids or eyelashes, mucous discharge, and inflammation of the lacrimal sac.

Obstructions often clear spontaneously within the first 12 months of life. After this time, obstructions are cleared surgically by simple probe and irrigation, silicone intubation procedures, or the more serious surgical procedure of dacryocystorhinostomy.

The probe and irrigation procedure is a five-minute operation that involves syringing the obstructed area under general anesthetic. The silicone intubation consists of inserting and looping a tiny silicone tube through the tear-duct system to link the upper and lower puncta. The tube is tied and left in the tear-duct system for several months. A dacryocystorhinostomy is a surgical operation that connects the lacrimal sac to the nasal cavity.

Acquired obstructions usually occur in middle age, and most commonly among women. Tearing becomes severe and annoying. The simple procedures of probe and irrigation or silicone intubation are often ineffective, and a dacryocystorhinostomy is indicated.

work opportunity tax credit (WOTC)   A federal tax incentive aimed at getting employers to hire individuals from seven groups that are seen as disadvantaged for employment purposes according to government guidelines. The WOTC replaces the targeted jobs tax credit, which had expired at the end of 1994. The new program went into effect September 30, 1996.

The groups targeted as disadvantaged for employment purposes are qualified veterans, qualified food-stamp recipients, qualified ex-felons, and qualified youth during the summer months. Also, it includes vocational rehabilitation referrals, which include workers with a physical or mental handicap; high-risk youth; and some workers who recently received some types of federal assistance.

Employers who choose to employ the WOTC may claim a credit of 35 percent of qualified first-year wages paid to an employee from one of the designated targeted groups. Tax credits generally range from a maximum of $2,100 for a full-time worker and $1,050 for a qualified summer employee.

world blindness   Blindness is an international problem that exists in both developed and developing countries. Because of differences in methods used to gather statistics and differences in definitions of blindness, statistics measuring the number of blind persons in the world vary. According to 2001 statistics from the World Health Organization (WHO), there are an estimated 40 million to 45 million blind people in the world. WHO projects the number will double by the year 2025, unless decisive public health action is taken.

Blindness is more prevalent in developing countries, where up to 85 percent of the population may have little or no access to hospitals in urban areas. Throughout Africa, South America, and Asia, blindness rates are increasing with the growth of the population. Four major causes of blindness in developing countries are cataract, TRACHOMA, XEROPHTHALMIA, and ONCHOCERCIASIS. Cataract is the leading cause of blindness in all parts of the world. In developed countries, sight is restored with cataract surgery and extraction. In developing countries, an estimated 16 million adults have cataract-induced vision loss due to lack of trained personnel and facilities to perform cataract surgery. In most countries of Africa and Asia, cataracts account for half of all blindness.

Cataract is any opacity in the eye's normally CRYSTALLINE LENS. The vision may be completely obstructed in specific areas of the visual field. Cataracts commonly worsen progressively over time.

The most common form, senile cataract, is a natural result of aging, although heredity, nutrition, general health and environment may influence the onset. There is no preventative treatment for senile cataracts, but they can be removed surgically. In developing countries, cataract extraction is often performed in mobile clinics or surgery units operated by mission or governmental agencies.

Trachoma, a contagious ocular disease caused by a chlamydial eye infection, may have a prevalence of as much as 500 million people worldwide and has caused blindness in about 6 million people. The infection causing the disease is due to the TRIC agent *Chlamydia trachomatis*. The infection is linked to bacterial infections caused by agents Koch-Weeks bacillus, Morax Axenfeld diplobacillus, and the gonococcus bacillus. Trachoma thrives in overcrowded conditions in which poor sewage disposal, sanitation, and personal hygiene, along with a lack of clean water supply, exist. In such conditions, this highly communicable disease may infect an entire community.

The disease first appears as a form of CONJUNCTIVITIS on the inside of the upper eyelids, later followed by symptoms of irritation, light sensitivity, and tearing. As the infection progresses to the cornea, it may cause ulceration leading to scarring, opacification, and vision loss.

Trachoma is treated with topical antibiotic eye ointment for several weeks. However, vision loss due to corneal scarring may be irreversible. Trachoma is prevented by improving environmental factors such as providing a clean water supply and employing simple methods of good personal hygiene.

XEROPHTHALMIA is the leading cause of blindness in children of developing countries. According to Helen Keller International, xerophthalmia annually affects 5 million to 10 million children in the world and completely destroys the vision in 350,000 of these per year. The disease occurs worldwide but is found most commonly in Asia and Africa. Children under six years of age are at greatest risk.

Xerophthalmia results from a lack of vitamin A in the diet. It occurs as a result of malnutrition and is closely associated with measles, diarrhea, and acute respiratory infection in vitamin-A-deficient children. Early symptoms include night blindness and Bitot's spots, a result of the drying of the CONJUNCTIVA leading to a sloughing of conjunctival epithelial cells.

The disease causes fundamental changes in the conjunctiva and cornea, which can lead to blindness. In severe cases, the cornea ulcerates and can perforate, causing AQUEOUS FLUID loss and collapse of the ANTERIOR CHAMBER. The cornea becomes opaque, and the eyeball is destroyed.

Xerophthalmia can be detected during an eye examination or by electroretinogram, a method impractical in field work. Treatment of the disease consists of three megadoses of 200,000 IU vitamin A by mouth, coupled with a protein- and calorie-rich diet, and treatment of any accompanying systemic infection.

One 200,000 IU vitamin-A dosage may be administered twice a year as a preventative measure. Other preventatives include enrichment with vitamin A of a commonly ingested staple such as tea or sugar, nutrition education and improvement in diet.

ONCHOCERCIASIS is a disease caused by the filarial worm, *Onchocerca volvulus*, transmitted by the Simulium blackfly. The disease occurs mainly in West Equatorial Africa, Central America, and South America. It is estimated to have infected over 18 million people and blinded an estimated 270,000 people. Visual impairment is projected for 20 percent of all those infected.

Onchocerciasis occurs when the worm infests the human body. The human becomes host to the worm, which may live up to 15 years within the body's skin, organs, and blood.

The disease causes corneal inflammation, or KERATITIS, corneal scarring, and vision loss. The inflammation can also cause chronic IRIDOCYCLITIS and glaucoma.

Prior to 1986, there was no effective medical treatment for onchocerciasis. Prevention of the disease consisted of vector control, using insecticides to rid the community of the worms, avoidance of breeding sites such as rivers and open waterways, wearing protective clothing, and excising of skin nodules that contain the worms.

Since 1986, human trials have shown that a drug, ivermectin, discovered by Merck, Sharp and Dohme Inc., is highly effective in killing the micro-filariae in humans and does so with few adverse reactions. The drug is available for worldwide distribution from Merck, Sharp and Dohme Inc., free of charge to onchocerciasis-control programs under the trade name Mectizan.

World blindness can be addressed by strengthening infrastructures and training health workers in the community being served. Indigenous people can be trained to become community health workers. The workers can maintain health-screening projects to diagnose and treat eye diseases in the earliest stages. Health education and awareness programs can improve personal hygiene, environmental conditions, sanitation, and nutrition. Mobile teams and surgical units can provide specialized treatment, surgery, and follow-up care.

Bath, Patricia E. "Blindness Prevention Through Programs of Community Ophthalmology in Developing Countries." In *Ophthalmology*. Vol. 2. Edited by K. Shimizu and J. Oosterhuis. Amsterdam: Excerpta Medica, 1979.

Cupak, K. "The Importance of Eye Camps in Underdeveloped Countries." In *Ophthalmology*. Vol. 2. Edited by K. Shimizu and J. Oosterhuis. Amsterdam: Excerpta Medica, 1979.

Helen Keller International. *Facts About Helen Keller International.* New York: HKI, 1987.

Helen Keller International. Diseases/causes.www.hki.org/diseases/index.html, 2000.

Phillips, Calbert I. *Basic Clinical Ophthalmology.* London: Pitman Publishers Limited, 1984.

World Health Organization. *Available Data On Blindness (Update 2000).* New York: WHO, 1987.

World Blind Sailing Championship   A competition started in 1992, when it was hosted by a blind group in New Zealand. The championship was held again in 1994 in Australia and in 1997 in England. Sailing is an activity in which blind people can participate and excel. In 1999, 29 four-person teams participated in the championships held that year in Miami.

A team includes two visually impaired crew and two sighted guides. One of the visually impaired persons is the helmsman, responsible for steering the boat around the course. The other controls the foredeck. The sighted guides, who are experienced sailboat racers, give verbal instructions to the visually impaired crew.

X, Y, Z

xanthelasma   Yellow plaques that form on the eyelid. The plaques consist of fat deposits and suggest that the body may be unable to process fats or cholesterol. Xanthelasma occasionally accompanies DIABETES, hypercholesterolemia, and histiocytosis. The blood should be tested for cholesterol and treated by diet or medication as indicated.

The condition is harmless and does not affect vision. Xanthelasma may be removed but may recur.

X-Chrom lens   See CONTACT LENSES.

xerophthalmia   A disease caused by a vitamin-A deficiency in the diet. It may occur as a result of malnutrition, protein malnutrition, or diarrhea. Early symptoms of the disorder include night blindness, conjunctivitis, and tearing.

Xerophthalmia is the second leading cause of blindness in the world and a leading cause of blindness in children in third world countries. Helen Keller International cites that xerophthalmia visually impairs 5 million to 10 million children worldwide each year and blinds 350,000 of these. Although the disease occurs worldwide, it is most concentrated in Southern Asia and Northern Saharan Africa. Children under six years of age are at greatest risk.

The disease causes fundamental changes in the cornea, CONJUNCTIVA, and anterior segments of the eye, which can lead to blindness. In severe cases, the cornea is perforated and AQUEOUS FLUID is lost. As a result, the ANTERIOR CHAMBER flattens, the iris adheres to the cornea, and the eyeball is destroyed. Xerophthalmia can be detected during a corneal examination or by electroretinogram, a method impractical in field work. Treatment of the disease consists of megadoses of 200,000 IU of vitamin A by mouth, coupled with a protein- and calorie-rich diet, and treatment of any accompanying systemic infection.

The vitamin-A dosage may be administered twice a year as a preventive measure. Other preventatives include enrichment of a commonly ingested staple such as tea or sugar with tasteless form of vitamin A, nutritional education, and improvement in diet.

Bath, Patricia E. "Blindness Prevention Through Programs of Community Ophthalmology in Developing Countries." In *Ophthalmology*. Vol. 2. Edited by K. Shimizu and J. Oosterhuis. Amsterdam: Excerpta Medica, 1979.

Cupak, K. "The Importance of Eye Camps in Underdeveloped Countries." In *Ophthalmology*. Vol. 2. Edited by K. Shimizu and J. Oosterhuis. Amsterdam: Excerpta Medica, 1979.

Helen Keller International. *Facts About Helen Keller International.* New York: HKI, 1988.

Phillips, Calbert I. *Basic Clinical Ophthalmology.* London: Pitman Publishers Limited, 1984.

World Health Organization. *Available Data On Blindness (Update 2000).* New York: WHO, 2000.

YAG laser   The YAG, or Neodymium: Yttrium-Aluminum-Garnet, laser is used in the postsurgical treatment of cataract-removal patients. After extracapsular cataract surgery, many patients experience opacification of the cataract capsule left behind in the eye. The YAG laser is used to create an opening in the capsule to restore vision.

The physician focuses the laser to a fine point on the capsule and releases a series of 500,000 watt explosions of energy that destroy the capsular matter. Because the laser can be so minutely focused, the physician can aim the beam accurately and avoid surrounding tissue or an intraocular lens resting on the opaque capsule.

The procedure is quick and painless and is most often performed without local anesthesia. The patient is able to walk or drive home after treatment.

The YAG laser is unique in its ability to perform this procedure because, unlike other lasers, it is not dependent on pigmented tissue to be effective. The argon and other lasers depend on pigment such as that found in the IRIS of the eye or in blood flowing through blood vessels in tissue. The pigmented tissue absorbs the energy from the argon laser and is destroyed. However, cataracts or their remaining capsules contain no pigmentation and are immune to the power of the argon laser.

In the past, when the postoperative vision declined due to this clouding of the capsule, a second surgery, a posterior capsulectomy, was necessary to restore good vision. The YAG approach is viewed as a safer, quicker procedure with fewer possible complications.

zonule   The zonules, or zonule of Zinn, is the group of thin, tightly drawn fibers that hold the lens in place in the eye. The thousands of threadlike fibers are attached to the ciliary muscle and work with the muscle to change the shape of the lens.

In order to focus on objects at different distances, the lens must adjust or accommodate. To focus on a near object, the lens must thicken and bulge forward. The ciliary muscle contracts, allowing the zonule to slacken and the lens to thicken and protrude forward. To focus on a distant object, the lens must flatten. The ciliary muscle expands, the zonule is pulled taut, and the lens flattens.

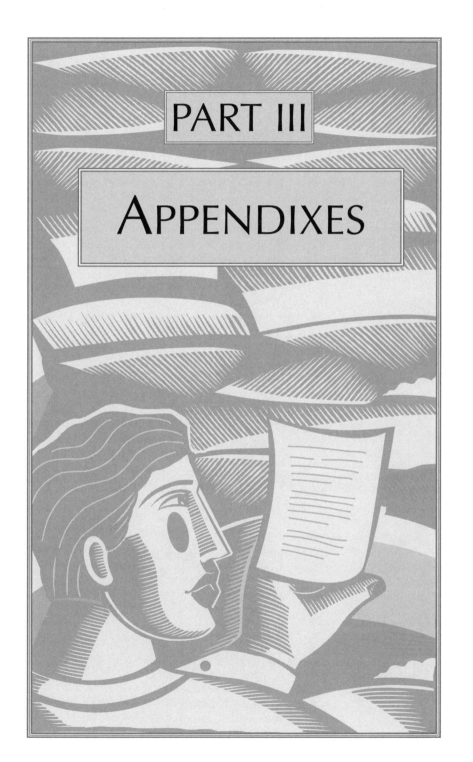

PART III

APPENDIXES

APPENDIX 1
COMPANIES

American Thermoform
  Corporation
1758 Brackett Street
La Verne, CA 91750
800-331-3676; fax 909-593-8001
http://www.atcbrleqp.com

Arkenstone, Inc.
555 Oakmead Parkway
Sunnyvale, CA 94086
800-444-4443; fax 408-328-8467
http://www.arkenstone.org

Artic Technologies
55 Park Street
Troy, MI 48083-2753
248-588-7370; fax 248-588-2650
http://www.artictech.com

Bavisoft
P.O. Box 8
Dewitt, NY 13214
http://www.bavisoft.com

Berkeley Systems, Inc.
1700 Shattuck Avenue
Berkeley, CA 94709
415-540-5535; fax 415-540-5115

BIT Corporation
52 Roland Street
Boston, MA 02129
617-666-2488; fax 617-666-4646

Blazie Engineering
105 East Jarrettsville Road
Forest Hill, MD 21050
410-893-9333; fax 410-836-5040
http://www.blazie.com

Duxbury Systems, Inc.
270 Littleton Road
Unit 6
Westford, MA 01886-3523
978-692-3000; fax 978-692-7912
http://www.duxburysystems.com

Enabling Technologies Company
1601 Northeast Braille Place
Jensen Beach, FL 34957
561-225-3687; fax 561-225-3299
http://www.brailer.com

Henter-Joyce, Inc.
11800 31st Court North Street
St. Petersburg, FL 33716
800-336-5658; fax 813-803-8001
http://www.hj.com

HumanWare, Inc.
6245 King Road
Loomis, CA 95650
800-722-3393
http://www.humanware.com

IBM Accessibility Center
11400 Burnett Road
Building 901, Room 5D-014
Austin, TX 78758
www.ibm.com/able

Independent Living Aids
200 Robbins Lane
Jericho, NY 11753
800-537-2118; fax 516-937-3906
http://www.independentliving.
  com

Lernout & Hauspie
52 Third Avenue
Burlington, MA 01803
781-203-5000; fax 781-238-0986
http://www.lhsl.com

LS&S Group, Inc.
P.O. Box 673
Northbrook, IL 60065
1-800-468-4789;
  fax 847-498-1482
http://www.lsgroup.com

NanoPac, Inc.
4823 South Sheridan Road

Suite 302
Tulsa, OK 74145-5717
918-665-0329; fax 918-665-0361
http://www.nanopac.com

Noir Medical Technologies
P.O. Box 159
South Lyon, MI 48178
1-800-521-9746; fax 734-769-1708

Talking Computers, Inc.
140 Little Falls Church Road
Suite 205
Falls Church, VA 22046
703-241-8224 or 1-800-458-6338

Telesensory Corporation
520 Almanor Avenue
Sunnyvale, CA 94086

408-616-8700; fax 408-616-8720
http://www.telesensory.com

Tojek & Associates
17355 Mierow Lane
Brookfield, WI 53005
414-784-4979

Transceptor Technologies, Inc.
2001 Commonwealth Boulevard
Suite 205
Ann Arbor, MI 48105
313-996-1899

Vision Technology, Inc.
8501 Delport Drive
St. Louis, MO 63114-5905
1-800-560-7226; fax 314-890-8383
http://www.visiontechinc.com

APPENDIX 2
DISABILITY DATABASES

ABLEDATA
8401 Colesville, Road
Suite 200
Silver Spring, MD 20910
800-227-0216
http://www.abledata.com/index.
  htm

Accent on Information
P.O. Box 700
Bloomington, IL 61701
309-378-2961; fax 309-378-4420

Ageline
American Association of Retired
  Persons
601 E Street NW
Washington, DC 20049
800-424-3410
http://www.aarp.org

Assistive Device Database System
Assistive Device Resource Center
California State University
6000 J Street
Sacramento, CA 95819
916-278-6916

BRS Information Technologies
1200 Route 7
Latham, NY 12110
518-783-7251

Combined Health Information Database (CHID)
National Institutes of Health
Box CHID
9000 Rockville Pike
Bethesda, MD 20892
301-468-6555
http://chid.nih.gov

CompuServe
232 N. Main Street
Marysville, Ohio
937-642-0002
http://www.compuserve.com

CTG (Closing the Gap) Solutions
P.O. Box 68
Henderson, MN 56044
507-248-3294; fax 507-248-3810
http://www.closingthegap.com

Dialog Information Services
3460 Hillview Avenue
Palo Alto, CA 94304
1-800-324-2564

Easter Seals Project ACTION
700 Thirteenth Street, NW
Suite 200
Washington, DC 20005
202-347-3066; fax 202-347-4157
http://www.projectaction.org

ERIC
Educational Resources Information
   Center
U.S. Department of Education
Office of Educational Research and
   Improvement
National Library of Education
555 New Jersey Avenue, NW
Washington, DC 20208-5721

202-219-2289
http://www.ed.gov

Job Accommodation Network (JAN)
West Virginia University
P.O. Box 6080
Morgantown, WV 26506
800-526-7234
http://janweb.idci.wvu.edu

MEDLINEplus
National Library of Medicine
8600 Rockville Pike
Bethesda, MD 20894
301-594-5983 or 1-888-346-3656
http://www.medlineplus.gov

The National Rehabilitation Information Center (NARIC)
1010 Wayne Avenue
Suite 800
Silver Spring, MD 20910
301-562-2400; fax 301-562-2401
http://www.naric/com

SPECIALNET
GTE Educational Network
   Services
5525 MacAuthur Boulevard
Suite 320
Irving, TX 75038
800-927-3000 or 214-751-0964
www.gte.net

APPENDIX 3
DOG-GUIDE SCHOOLS

Canine Companions for
   Independence
P.O. Box 446
Santa Rosa, CA 95402-0446
866-224-3647 or 1-800-572-2275
http://www.caninecompanions.
   org

Eye Dog Foundation for the
   Blind, Inc.
512 N. Larchmont Boulevard
Los Angeles, CA 90004
602-276-0051

Fidelco Guide Dog Foundation, Inc.
P.O. Box 142

Bloomfield, CT 06002
203-243-5200; fax 203-243-7215

Guide Dog Foundation for the
   Blind, Inc.
371 East Jericho Turnpike
Smithtown, NY 11787
516-265-2121; fax 516-361-5192
http://www.guidedogs.com

Guide Dogs of America
13445 Glenoaks Boulevard
Sylmar, CA 91342
818-362-5834; fax 818-362-6870

Guiding Eyes for the Blind, Inc.
611 Granite Springs Road
Yorktown Heights, NY 10598
914-245-4024; fax 914-245-1609
http://www.guiding-eyes.org

Leader Dogs for the Blind
1039 Rochester Road
Rochester, MI 48063

810-651-9011; fax 810-651-5812
http://www.leaderdog.org

Pilot Dogs, Inc.
625 West Town Street
Columbus, OH 43215
614-221-6367; fax 614-221-1577

Seeing Eye, Inc.
P.O. Box 375
Morristown, NJ 07960
1-800-539-4425
http://www.seeingeye.org

Southeast Guide Dogs, Inc.
4210 77th Street East
Palmetto, FL 33561
813-729-5665; fax 813-729-6646
http://www.guidedogs.org

Upstate Guide Dog Association
P.O. Box 165
Hamlin, NY 14464
716-964-8815

APPENDIX 4
FEDERAL AGENCIES

U.S. DEPARTMENT OF EDUCATION

Center for Libraries and
   Educational Improvement
400 Maryland Avenue, SW
Room 613
Washington, DC 20202
202-254-6572

Clearinghouse on Handicapped and
   Gifted Children
1920 Association Drive
Reston, VA 22091
703-620-3660

Division of Blind and Visually
   Impaired

330 C Street, SW
Washington, DC 20202
202-732-1316

National Council on the
   Handicapped
330 C Street, SW
Room 3118
Washington, DC 20202
202-453-3846

National Institute on Disability and
   Rehabilitation Research
400 Maryland Avenue, SW
Washington, DC 20202
202-205-5666; TDD 202-205-4756

Office of Special Education and
Rehabilitative Services
330 C Street, SW
Room 3132
Washington, DC 20202
202-732-1241

Office of Special Education
Programs
330 C Street, SW, Room 3086
Washington, DC 20202
202-732-1007

Office of the Secretary
400 Maryland Avenue, SW
Washington, DC 20202
202-732-3000

Rehabilitative Services
Administration
330 C Street, SW
Washington, DC 20202
202-732-1282

U.S. DEPARTMENT OF HEALTH AND HUMAN SERVICES

Administration for Children, Youth,
and Families
Donahoe Building
400 Sixth Street, SW
Washington, DC 20024
202-755-7762

Administration on Aging
North Building, Room 4760
200 Independence Avenue, SW
Washington, DC 20201
202-245-0724

Health Care Financing
Administration
200 Independence Avenue, SW
Washington, DC 20201
202-245-6726

Health Resources and Services
Administration
Bureau of Health Professions
5600 Fishers Lane

Rockville, MD 20857
301-443-5794

Health Services Administration/
Division for Maternal and
Child Health
Bureau of Health Care Delivery and
Assistance
5600 Fishers Lane
Room 605
Rockville, MD 20857
301-443-2170

National Center for Health Statistics
3700 East-West Highway
Hyattsville, MD 20782
301-436-8500

National Institutes of Health/
National Eye Institute
Building 31, Room Ao3
Bethesda, MD 20892
301-496-2234

Office of Human Development
Services
200 Independence Avenue, SW
Room 309F
Washington, DC 20201
202-245-7246

Office of Policy Planning and
Legislation
200 Independence Avenue, SW
Room 306E
Washington, DC 20201
202-245-7027

Office of the Secretary
200 Independence Avenue, SW
Room 615F
Washington, DC 20201
202-245-7000

Social Security Administration
6401 Security Boulevard
Baltimore, MD 21235
301-965-1234

U.S. DEPARTMENT OF LABOR

Employment Standards
Administration
Branch of Special Employment

200 Constitution Avenue, NW
Washington, DC 20210
202-523-8727

Office of Federal Contract Compliance Programs
200 Constitution Avenue, NW
Washington, DC 20210
202-523-9475

Office of the Secretary
200 Constitution Avenue, NW
Washington, DC 20210
202-523-8165

U.S. Employment Service
Patrick Henry Building
601 D Street, NW
Washington, DC 20213
202-376-6750

VETERANS ADMINISTRATION

Blind Rehabilitation Service
810 Vermont Avenue, NW
Washington, DC 20420
202-233-3232

Department of Medicine and Surgery
810 Vermont Avenue, NW
Washington, DC 20420
202-223-2596

Department of Veterans Benefits
810 Vermont Avenue, NW
Washington, DC 20420
202-233-2044

Office of the Administrator
810 Vermont Avenue, NW
Washington, DC 20420
202-223-3775

OTHER AGENCIES

Architectural and Transportation Barriers Compliance Board
1111 18th Street, NW
Suite 501
Washington, DC 20036
202-653-7834

Committee for Purchase from the Blind and Other Severely Handicapped
Crystal Square 5
Suite 1107
1755 Jefferson Davis Highway
Arlington, VA 22202-3509
703-557-1145

Equal Employment Opportunity Commission
Office of Legal Counsel
2401 E Street, NW
Room 222
Washington, DC 20507
202-634-6460

Library of Congress National Library Service for the Blind and Physically Handicapped
1291 Taylor Street, NW
Washington, DC 20542
202-287-5100 or 1-800-424-9100

President's Committee on Employment of People with Disabilities
1111 20th Street, NW
Washington, DC 20036
202-653-5044

Small Business Administration
1441 L Street, NW
Washington, DC 20416
202-653-6605

U.S. Department of Justice
Civil Rights Division/Coordination and Review Section
10th Street and Constitution Avenue, NW
Washington, DC 20530
202-633-2151 or 202-724-7678 (TDD)

U.S. Office of Personnel Management
Governmentwide Selective Placement Programs Division
1900 E Street, NW
Room 5A09
Washington, DC 20415
202-632-5491

APPENDIX 5
NATIONAL ORGANIZATIONS

Affiliated Leadership League
1030 15th Street, NW
Suite 468
Washington, DC 20005
202-775-8261

American Academy of
  Ophthalmology
P.O. Box 7424
San Francisco, CA 94120
415-561-8500
http://www.eyenet.org

American Association for Pediatric
  Ophthalmology and
  Strabismus
P.O. Box 193832
San Francisco, CA 94119
415-561-8505

American Association of Certified
  Orthoptists
St. Louis Children's Hospital
  Eye Center
One Children's Plaza
Room 2, South 89
St. Louis, MO 63110
314-454-2122
http://www.orthoptics.org

American Association of the
  Deaf-Blind
814 Thayer Avenue
Silver Spring, MD 20910

American Council of the Blind
1155 15th Street, NW
Washington, DC 20005
202-467-5081
http://www.acb.org

American Council on Rural
  Special Education
Kansas State University
2323 Anderson Avenue
Suite 226

Manhattan, KS 66502
785-532-2737
http://www.ksu.edu/acres

American Diabetes Association
National Service Center
P.O. Box 25757
1600 Duke Street
Alexandria, VA 22313
703-549-1500 or 1-800-232-3472

American Foundation for the Blind
11 Penn Plaza
Suite 300
New York, NY 10001
212-502-7660 or 800-232-5463;
  TDD 212-502-7662
http://www.afb.org

American Optometric Association
243 North Lindbergh Boulevard
St. Louis, MO 63141
314-991-4100 or 1-800-365-2219
http://www.aoanet.org

American Society of Cataract and
  Refractive Surgery
4000 Legato Road
Suite 850
Fairfax, VA 22030
703-591-2220; fax 703-591-0614
http://www.ascrs.org

American Society of Contemporary
  Medicine, Surgery and
  Ophthalmology
820 North Orleans Street
Suite 208
Chicago, IL 60610
312-440-0699

Associated Services for the Blind
911 Walnut Street
Philadelphia, PA 19107
215-627-0600

Association for Education and
Rehabilitation of the Blind and
Visually Impaired
206 North Washington Street
Suite 320
Alexandria, VA 22314
703-548-1884

Association for Macular Diseases
210 East 64th Street
New York, NY 10021
212-605-3719

The Association for Persons with
Severe Handicaps
29 W. Susquehanna Avenue
Suite 210
Baltimore, MD 21204
410-828-8274 or 800-482-8274;
TDD 410-828-1306
http://www.tash.org

Association of Radio Reading
Services
University of South Florida,
WRB 209
Tampa, FL 33620
813-974-4193

Association on Handicapped
Student Service Programs in
Postsecondary Education
P.O. Box 21192
Columbus, OH 43221
614-488-4872

Blind Children's Center
4120 Marathon Street
P.O. Box 29159
Los Angeles, CA 90029
213-664-2153

Blind Children's Fund
230 Central Street
Auburndale, MA 02166
617-332-4014

Blind Outdoor Leisure
Development
533 East Main Street
Aspen, CO 81611
303-925-8922

Blinded Veterans Association
477 H Street, NW
Washington, DC 20001
202-371-8880 or 800-669-7079

Braille Institute of America
741 North Vermont Avenue
Los Angeles, CA 90029
323-663-1111 or 800-272-4533
http://www.brailleinstitute.org

Corneal Dystrophy Foundation
1926 Hidden Creek Drive
Kingwood, TX 77339
713-358-4227

Council for Exceptional Children
1110 North Glebe Road
Suite 300
Arlington, VA 22201
703-620-3660 or 888-221-6830;
TDD 703-264-9446
http://www.cec.sped.org

Council of Citizens with
Low Vision
1400 North Drake Road
Kalamazoo, MI 49007
616-381-9566

Delta Gamma Foundation
3250 Riverside Drive
Columbus, OH 43221
614-481-8169
http://www.deltagamma.org

Eye Bank Association of America
Inc.
1725 Eye Street, NW
Suite 308
Washington, DC 20005
202-775-4999

Eye Bank for Sight Restoration
210 East 64th Street
New York, NY 10021
212-980-6700

Eye Research Institute of the Retina
Foundation
20 Stanford Road
Boston, MA 02114
617-742-3140

Fight for Sight
381 Park Avenue South
Suite 809
New York, NY 10016
212-679-6060

Foundation Fighting Blindness
11435 Cronhill Drive
Owings Mills, MD 21117-2220
410-568-0150 or 1-888-394-3937;
   TDD 1-800-683-5551
http://www.blindness.org

Friends of Eye Research
99 West Cedar Street
Boston, MA 02114
617-523-0303

Glaucoma Research Foundation
200 Pine Street
Suite 200
San Francisco, CA 94104
415-986-3162 or 800-826-6693
http://www.glaucoma.org

Guide Dog Users
14311 Astrodome Drive
Silver Springs, MD 20906
310-598-5771 or 888-858-1008
http://gdui.org

Helen Keller International
90 Washington Street
15th Floor
New York, NY 10006
212-943-0890
http://www.hki.org

Helen Keller National Center for
   Deaf-Blind Youth and Adults
111 Middle Neck Road
Sands Point, NY 11050
516-944-8900;
   TDD 516-944-8637
http://www.helenkeller.org

International Eye Foundation
7801 Norfolk Avenue
Bethesda, MD 20814
301-986-1830
http://www.iefusa.org

International Institute for Visually
   Impaired, 0-7
311 W. Broadway
Suite 1
Mount Pleasant, MI 48854
989-779-9966; fax 989-779-0015
http://www.blindchildrenfund.org

International Society on
   Metabolic Eye Disease
1125 Park Avenue
New York, NY 10128
212-427-1246

In Touch Networks
15 West 65th Street
New York, NY 10023
212-769-6270 or 800-456-3166

Joint Commission on Allied Health
   Personnel in Ophthalmology
2025 Woodlane Drive
St. Paul, MN 55125
651-731-2944 or 800-284-3937
http://www.jcahop.org

Joslin Diabetes Center
One Joslin Place
Boston, MA 02215
617-732-2400
http://www.joslin.org

Knights Templar Eye Foundation
5097 North Elston Avenue
Chicago, IL 60630
773-205-3838

Lions Club International
300 22nd Street
Oak Brook, IL 60570
630-571-5466
http://www.lionsclubs.org

March of Dimes Birth Defects
   Foundation
1275 Mamaroneck Avenue
White Plains, NY 10605
914-428-7100
http://www.modimes.org

Maynard Listener Library
171 Washington Street
Taunton, MA 02780
617-823-3783

Myasthenia Gravis Foundation
123 West Madison Street
Suite 800
Chicago, IL 60602
312-853-0522 or 800-541-5454
http://www.myasthenia.org

Myopia International Research
 Foundation
1265 Broadway
Room 608
New York, NY 10001
212-684-2777

National Accreditation Council for
 Agencies Serving the Blind and
 Legally Visually Handicapped
260 Northland Boulevard
Cincinnati, OH 45246
513-772-8449

National Association for Parents of
 Children with Visual Impairments
P.O. Box 317
Watertown, MA 02272
617-972-7444 or 800-562-6265

National Association for Visually
 Handicapped
22 W. 21st Street
New York, NY 10010
212-889-3141
http://www.navh.org

National Association of Blind
 Teachers
c/o American Council of the Blind
1155 15th Street, NW
Washington, DC 20005
202-467-5081

National Association of State
 Directors of Special Education
Suite 320
1800 Diagonal Road
Alexandria, VA 22314
703-519-3800; TDD 703-519-7008
http://www.nasdse.org

National Association of Vision
 Professionals Prevention of
 Blindness Society

1774 Church Street, NW
Washington, DC 20036
202-234-1010
http://www.members.tripod.com/
 charlie216

National Braille Association
3 Town Line Circle
Rochester, NY 14623
716-427-8260
http://www.nationalbraille.org

National Council of Private
 Agencies for the Blind
8770 Manchester Road
St. Louis, MO 63069
314-968-9000

National Council of State
 Agencies for the Blind
1213 29th Street, NW
Washington, DC 20007
202-333-5841

National Easter Seals Society
230 West Monroe
Suite 1800
Chicago, IL 60606
312-726-6200 or 800-221-6827;
 TDD 312-726-4258
http://www.easter-seals.org

National Eye Institute
2020 Vision Place
Bethesda, MD 20892
301-496-5248
http://www.nei.nih.gov

National Eye Research Foundation
910 Skokie Boulevard
Northbrook, IL 60062
847-564-6522
http://www.nerf.org

National Federation of the Blind
1800 Johnson Street
Baltimore, MD 21230
410-659-9314
http://www.nfb.org

National Glaucoma Research
 Program of the American Health
 Assistance Foundation

15825 Shady Grove Road
Suite 140
Rockville, MD 20850
301-948-3244
http://www.ahaf.org

National Industries for the Blind
1901 North Beauregard Street
Suite 200
Alexandria, VA 22311
703-998-0770
http://www.nib.org

National Multiple Sclerosis Society
733 Third Avenue
Sixth Floor
New York, NY 10017
212-986-3240
http://www.nmss.org

National Rehabilitation
  Information Center
1010 Wayne Avenue
Suite 800
Silver Spring, MD 20910
1-800-346-2742 or 301-562-2403
http://www.naric.com

National Society to Prevent
  Blindness
4200 California Street
#101
San Francisco, CA 94118-1314
415-387-0934; fax 415-387-1689
http://www.eyeinfo.org

New Eyes for the Needy
P.O. Box 332
549 Millburn Avenue
Short Hills, NJ 07078
201-376-4903

ODPHP (Office of Disease
  Prevention and Health
  Promotion)
Office of Public Health and Science
200 Independence Avenue, SW,
  Room 738G
Washington, DC 20201
202-401-6295; fax 202-205-9478
http://www.odphp.osophs.dhhs.
  gov

Opticians Association of America
7023 Little River Turnpike
Suite 207
Annadale, VA 22003
703-916-8856
http://www.opticians.org

Randolph-Sheppard Vendors of
  America
1808 Faith Place
#B
Terrytown, LA 70056
504-368-7785 or 800-467-5299
http://www.acb.org/rsva

Recording for the Blind
20 Roszel Road
Princeton, NJ 08540
609-452-0606 or 1-800-883-7201
http://www.rfbd.org

Research to Prevent Blindness
645 Madison Avenue
New York, NY 10022
212-752-4333 or 800-621-0026
http://www.rpbusa.org

Smith-Kettlewell Eye Research
  Institute
2318 Fillmore Street
San Francisco, CA 94115
415-345-2000
http://www.ski.org

Taping for the Blind
3935 Essex Lane
Houston, TX 77027
713-622-2767

Telephone Pioneers of America
930 15th Street
Suite 1200
Denver, CO 80202
303-571-1200; fax 303-572-0520
http://www.telephone-pioneers.org

United States Association for Blind
  Athletes
33 North Institute Street
Colorado Springs, CO 80903
719-630-0422
http://www.usaba.org

United States Braille Chess Association
428 West Lima Street
Findlay, OH 45840
419-422-2833
http://www.crisscrosstech.com/
usbca

Vision Council of America: Better
Vision Institute
1700 Diagonal Road
Suite 500
Alexandria, VA 22314
703-548-4560 or 877-642-3253
http://www.visionsite.org

APPENDIX 6
SCHOOLS FOR THE BLIND AND VISUALLY IMPAIRED STUDENTS (BY STATE)

ALABAMA

Alabama Institute for Deaf and
Blind
205 East South Street
Talladega, AL 35160
256-761-3259
http://www.aidb.state.al.us

Southwest Alabama Regional School
for the Deaf and Blind
8901 Airport Boulevard
Mobile, AL 36608-9503
334-633-0241

ARIZONA

Arizona State Schools for the Deaf
and the Blind
1200 West Speedway Boulevard
Tucson, AZ 85745
520-770-3700; TTD/TTY 520-770-
3213
http://www.asdb.org

ARKANSAS

Arkansas School for the Blind
2600 West Markham

Little Rock, AR 72203
1-800-362-1810; TTD/TTY 501-296-
1833

CALIFORNIA

Blind Children's Learning Center
18542-B Vanderlip Avenue
Santa Ana, CA 92705
714-573-8888
http://www.blindkids.org

Blind Children's Center
4120 Marathon Street
Los Angeles, CA 90029
323-664-2153
http://www.blindcntr.org

California School for the Blind
500 Walnut Avenue
Fremont, CA 94536
510-794-3800
http://goldmine.cde.ca.gov/csmt/
apendd.html

Palomar College Adapted Computer
Training Center
1140 Mission Road
Sand Marcos, CA 92069

760-744-1150; TDD/TTY 760-471-
8506
http://www.palomar.edu

COLORADO

Colorado School for the Deaf and
  the Blind
33 North Institute Street
Colorado Springs, CO 80903-3599
719-578-2100; TDD/TTY 719-577-
2101
http://www.csdb.org

CONNECTICUT

Connecticut Institute for the
  Blind/Oak Hill School
120 Holcomb Street
Hartford, CT 06112
860-242-2274
http://www.ciboakhill.org/index.htm

FLORIDA

Florida School for the Deaf and
  Blind
207 North San Marco Avenue
St. Augustine, FL 32084
904-827-2200 or 1-800-344-3732
http://www.fsdb.k12.fl.us

GEORGIA

Georgia Academy for the Blind
2895 Vineville Avenue
Macon, GA 31204
478-751-6083
http://www.gabmacon.org

IDAHO

Idaho School for the Deaf and Blind
1450 Main Street
Gooding, ID 83330
208-934-4457
http://www.isdb.state.id.us

ILLINOIS

Hadley School for the Blind
700 Elm Street
Winnetka, IL 60093
847-446-8111 or 1-800-323-4238;
  TDD/TYY 847-441-8111
http://www.hadley-school.org

Hope School
50 Hazel Lane
Springfield, IL 62705-5810
217-585-5437; TTD/
  TTY 217-529-5766
http://www.thehopeschool.org

Illinois School for the Visually
  Impaired
658 East State Street
Jacksonville, IL 62650
217-479-4400
http://www.il.us/agency/dhs/isvi.
  htm

Philip J. Rock Center and
  School
818 DuPage Boulevard
Glen Ellyn, IL 60137
630-790-2474 or 1-800-771-1158;
  TDD/TTY 630-790-4723
http://www.project-reach-illinois.
  org

INDIANA

Gary Community School
  Corporation
Lew Wallace Building
Suite B122
415 West 45th Avenue
Gary, IN 46408
219-980-6305

Indiana School for the Blind
7725 North College Avenue
Indianapolis, IN 46240
317-253-1481

IOWA

Iowa Braille and Sight-Saving
  School
1002 G Avenue
Vinton, IA 52349
319-472-5221 or 1-800-645-4579
http://www.iowa-braille.k12.ia.us

KANSAS

Kansas State School for the Blind
1100 State Avenue
Kansas City, KS 66102
913-281-3308 or 1-800-572-5463
http://www.kssb.net

KENTUCKY

Kentucky School for the Blind
1867 Frankfort Avenue
Louisville, KY 40206
502-897-1583
http://www.ksb.k12.ky.us

LOUISIANA

Louisiana School for the Visually
   Impaired
1120 Government Street
Baton Rouge, LA 70802-4897
225-342-8694

MARYLAND

Maryland School for the Blind
3501 Taylor Avenue
Baltimore, MD 21236-4499
410-444-5000 or 800-400-4915;
   TDD/TTY 410-319-5703
http://www.mdschblind.org

Ruth Parker Eason School
648 Old Mill Road
Millersville, MD 21108-1373
410-222-3815

MASSACHUSETTS

Perkins School for the Blind
175 North Beacon Street
Watertown, MA 02472
617-924-3434
http://www.perkins.pvt.k12.ma.us

MICHIGAN

Michigan School for the Blind
1667 Miller Road
Flint, MI 48503-5096

810-257-1420 or 1-800-622-6730
   ext. 420
http://www.msdb.k12.mi.us

MINNESOTA

Minnesota State Academy for
   the Blind
P.O. Box 68
Fairbault, MN 55021
507-333-4800 or 1-800-657-3634
http://www.msab.state.mn.us

MISSISSIPPI

Mississippi School for the Blind
1252 Eastover Drive
Jackson, MS 39211
601-984-8200; TTD/TTY
   601-984-8097
http://www2.mde.k12.ms.us/msb

MISSOURI

Blue Springs Special Services
   Center
2103 West Vesper
Blue Springs, MO 64015
816-224-1360

Children's Center for the Visually
   Impaired
3101 Main Street
Kansas City, MO 64111-1921
816-333-3166

Missouri School for the Blind
3815 Magnolia Avenue
St. Louis, MO 63110
314-776-4320 or 1-800-622-5672
http://www.msb.k12.mo.us

MONTANA

Montana School for the Deaf
   and Blind
3911 Central Avenue
Great Falls, MT 59405
406-771-6000
http://www.sdb.mt.us

NEBRASKA

Nebraska Center for the Education
of Children who are Blind or
Visually Impaired
824 Tenth Avenue
Nebraska City, NE 68410
402-873-5513 or 1-800-826-4355
http://www.ncecbvi.org

NEW JERSEY

LIFT
P.O. Box 4264
Warren, NJ 07059
908-707-9840 or 1-800-552-5438
http://www.lift-inc.org

Matheny School and Hospital
Main Street
Peapack, NJ 07977
908-234-0011
http://www.matheny.org

St. Joseph's School for the Blind
253 Baldwin Avenue
Jersey City, NJ 07306
201-653-0578 or 1-800-457-8563
http://school.nj.com/school/sjsb

NEW MEXICO

New Mexico School for the
Visually Handicapped
1900 North White Sands
Boulevard
Alamogordo, NM 88310
505-437-3505 or 1-800-437-3505
http://www.nmsvh.k12.nm.us

NEW YORK

Lavelle School for the Blind
3830 Paulding Avenue
Bronx, NY 10469
718-882-1212

New York Institute for Special
Education
999 Pelham Parkway
Bronx, NY 10469

718-519-7000; TDD/
TTY 718-519-6196
http://www.nyise.org

New York State School for the Blind
2A Richmond Avenue
Batavia, NY 14020
716-343-5384 or (toll-free)
1-877-697-7382
http://web.nysed.gov/vesid/nyssb.
htm

NORTH CAROLINA

Governor Morehead School
2303 Mail Service Center
301 Ashe Avenue
Administration Building
Raleigh, NC 27699-2303
919-733-6381
http://www.governormorehead.net

NORTH DAKOTA

North Dakota Vision Services:
School for the Blind
500 Stanford Road
Grand Forks, ND 58203-2799
701-795-2708 or 1-800-421-1181
http://www.ndsb.k12.nd.us

OHIO

Ohio State School for the Blind
5220 North High Street
Columbus, OH 43214
614-752-1152

OKLAHOMA

Oklahoma School for the Blind
3300 Gibson Street
Muskogee, OK 74403
918-781-8200 or (toll-free)
1-877-229-7136
http://www.osb.k12.ok.us/index/
html

OREGON

Oregon School for the Blind
700 Church Street, SE

Salem, OR 97301
503-378-3820

PENNSYLVANIA

Overbrook School for the Blind
6333 Malvern Avenue
Philadelphia, PA 19151-2597
215-877-0313

Royer-Greaves School for
the Blind
118 South Valley Road
Paoli, PA 19301-1444
610-644-1810
http://royer-greavesschoolforblind.
com

Western Pennsylvania School for
Blind Children
201 North Bellefield Avenue
Pittsburgh, PA 15213-1499
412-621-0100

SOUTH CAROLINA

South Carolina School for the Deaf
and the Blind
355 Cedar Springs Road
Spartanburg, SC 29302
864-585-7711 or (toll-free)
1-888-447-2732; TDD/
TTY 803-798-4936
http://www.scsdb.k12.sc.us

SOUTH DAKOTA

South Dakota School for the Blind
and Visually Impaired
423 17th Avenue SE
Aberdeen, SD 57401
605-626-2580 or (toll-free)
1-888-275-3814; TDD/
TTY 605-626-7829
http://www.sdsbvi.sdbor.edu/

TENNESSEE

Tennessee School for the Blind
115 Stewarts Ferry Pike
Nashville, TN 37214
615-231-7340

http://volweb.utk.edu/Schools/
tsb/

TEXAS

Texas School for the Blind and Visually Impaired
1100 West 45th Street
Austin, TX 78756-3494
512-454-8631 or 1-800-872-5273;
TDD/TTY 512-206-9188
http://www.tsbvi.edu

UTAH

Utah School for the Blind
742 Harrison Boulevard
Ogden, UT 84404
801-629-4700 or 1-800-990-9328;
TDD/TTY 801-629-4701
http://www.usdb.k12.ut.us

VIRGINIA

Virginia School for the Deaf and
Blind at Staunton
P.O. Box 2069
Staunton, VA 24402
540-332-9000 or 1-800-522-8732

Virginia School for the Deaf, Blind
and Multi-Disabled
at Hampton
700 Shell Road
Hampton, VA 23661-2299
757-247-2050
http://www.vsdbh.org

WASHINGTON

Washington State School for
the Blind
2214 East 13th Street
Vancouver, WA 98661-4120
360-696-6321
http://www.wssb.wa.gov

WEST VIRGINIA

West Virginia Schools for the Deaf
and Blind
301 East Main Street

Romney, WV 26757
304-822-4800

WISCONSIN

Wisconsin Center for the Blind and
Visually Impaired

1700 West State Street
Janesville, WI 53546
608-758-6146 or 1-800-832-9784;
TDD/TTY 608-758-6127

APPENDIX 7
PERIODICALS

ABLA Newsletter
American Blind Lawyers Association
P.O. Box 1590
Indianola, MS 38751
662-887-5398

ACB Parents Newsletter
Council of Citizens with Low Vision
5707 Brockton Drive
Suite 302
Indianapolis, IN 46220
317-254-1332 or 800-733-2258

AER Report
Association for Education and
  Rehabilitation of the Blind and
  Visually Impaired
4600 Duke Street
Suite 430
Alexandria, VA 22304
703-823-9690 or 877-492-2708
http://www.aerbvi.com

AFB News
American Foundation for the Blind
11 Penn Plaza
Suite 300
New York, NY 10001
212-502-7660 or 800-232-5463;
  TDD 212-502-7662
http://www.afb.org

American Council of the Blind
  Federal Employees News Council
  of Citizens with Low Vision

5707 Brockton Drive
Suite 302
Indianapolis, IN 46220
317-254-1332 or 800-733-2258

The American Lupus Society
  Quarterly
The American Lupus Society
23751 Madison Street
Torrance, CA 90505
213-373-1335

American Rehabilitation
U.S. Department of Education
Mary Switzer Building
Room 3212
330 C Street, SW
Washington, DC 20202
202-205-5482

Blindness, Visual Impairment,
  Deaf-Blindness, Semiannual
  Listing of Current Literature
Association for Education of the
  Visually Handicapped
Room 700
919 Walnut Street
Philadelphia, PA 19107

The Blind Teacher
American Council of the Blind
1155 15th Street NW
Suite 1004
Washington, DC 20005

202-467-5081 or 800-424-8666; fax
202-467-5085
http://www.acb.org

Braille Book Review
National Library Service for the
Blind and Physically Handicapped
1291 Taylor Street, NW
Washington, DC 20542
202-707-5100
http://www.loc.gov./uls

Braille Forum
American Council of the Blind
1155 15th Street, NW
Suite 1004
Washington, DC 20005
202-467-5081 or 800-424-8666; fax
202-467-5085
http://www.acb.org

The Braille Mirror
Braille Institute of America
741 N. Vermont Avenue
Los Angeles, CA 90029
323-663-1111
http://www/brailleinstitute.com

Braille Memorandum
Braille Revival League
1010 Vermont Avenue, NW
Washington, DC 20005

Braille Monitor
National Federation of the Blind
1800 Johnson Street
Baltimore, MD 21230
410-659-9314
http://www/afb.org

CCB Outlook
Canadian Council of the Blind
396 Cooper Street
Suite 401
Ottawa, Ontario K2P 2H7 Canada
613-567-0311 or 877-304-0968

CCLV Newsletter
Council of Citizens with Low Vision
5707 Brockton Drive
Suite 302
Indianapolis, IN 46220
317-254-1332 or 800-733-2258

Deaf Blind New sSummary
Xavier Society for the Blind
154 East 23rd Street
New York, NY 10010
212-473-7800

Deafblind Weekly
Xavier Society for the Blind
154 East 23rd Street
New York, NY 10010
212-473-7800

Diabetes '90
American Diabetes Association
1701 Beauregard Street
Alexandria, VA 22314
703-549-1500 or 800-342-2383
http://www.diabetes.org

Diabetes Self-Management
R.A. Rapaport Publishing Inc.
150 West 22nd Street
New York, NY 10011

Dialogue
Dialogue Publications Inc.
3100 South Oak Park Avenue
Berwyn, IL 60402

*Education of the Visually
Handicapped*
Heldref Publications
4000 Albemarle Street, NW
Washington, DC 20016

Encore
Division for the Blind and
Visually Handicapped
Library of Congress
1291 Taylor, NW
Washington, DC 20542
202-707-5100
http://www.loc.gov/nls

Exceptional Children
Council for Exceptional Children
1110 North Glebe Road
Suite 300
Arlington, VA 22201
703-620-3660 or 888-221-6830;
TDD 703-264-9446
http://www.cec.sped.org

Free Press
Wisconsin School for the Visually
  Handicapped
American Printing House for
  the Blind
1700 W. State Street
Jamesville, WI 53545
608-755-2977 or 1-800-832-9784

Guide Dog News
Guide Dogs for the Blind
350 Los Ranchitos Road
San Rafael, CA 94903
415-499-4000 or 800-295-4050
http://www.guidedogs.com

Heresay
Association of Radio Reading
  Services
National Office
4200 Wisconsin Avenue, NW
Suite 106-346
Washington, DC 20016
202-347-0955

HKI Report
Helen Keller International
90 Washington Street
15th Floor
New York, NY 10006
212-943-0890
http://www.hki.org

Inside MS
National Multiple Sclerosis
  Society
205 East 42nd Street
New York, NY 10017-5706
212-986-3240

Insight
Prevent Blindness News
National Society for the Prevention
  of Blindness
500 E. Remington Road
Schaumburg, IL 60173
312-843-2020

Insight
John Milton Society for the Blind
  in Canada
40 St. Clair Avenue, E.

#202
Toronto, ON M4T 1M9 Canada
416-960-3953

International Eye Foundation Newsletter
International Eye Foundation
7801 Norfolk Avenue
Bethesda, MD 20814

Jottings
Gospel Association for the Blind
7850 South U.S. Highway 1
Bunnell, FL 32110
904-586-5885

Journal of Visual Impairment and
  Blindness
American Foundation for the Blind
11 Penn Plaza
Suite 300
New York, NY 10001
212-502-7660 or 800-232-5463;
  TDD 212-502-7662
http://www.afb.org

Journal of Visual Rehabilitation
Media Productions and
  Marketing Inc.
2440 O Street
Suite 202
Lincoln, NE 68510
402-474-2676

Log of the Bridgetender
Friends in Art of ACB
Council of Citizens with Low Vision
5707 Brockton Drive
Suite 302
Indianapolis, IN 46220
317-254-1332 or 800-733-2258

Long Cane News Letter
Boston College
140 Commonwealth Avenue
Chestnut Hill, MA 02167

Lutheran Braille Evangelism Bulletin
Lutheran Braille Evangelism
  Association
1740 Eugene Street
White Bear Lake, MN 55110
651-426-0469

Mainstream
Pennsylvania Association for
the Blind
2843 North Front Street
Harrisburg, PA 17110
http://www.pablind.org

MS Quarterly Report
Demos Publications
156 Fifth Avenue
Suite 1018
New York, NY 10010
212-255-8768

NARIC Quarterly
National Rehabilitation
Information Center
8455 Colesville Road
Suite 935
Silver Spring, MD 20910-3319

NBA Bulletin
National Braille Association
3 Townline Circle
Rochester, NY 14623
716-427-8260
http://www.members.aol.com/
nbaoffice/index.htm

*News About Library Services for the
Blind and Physically Handicapped*
SC State Library—DBPH
301 Gervais Street
P.O. Box 821
Columbia, SC 29202
803-737-9970 or 1-800-922-7818

NEWSBITS
Talking Computers Inc.
140 Little Falls Road
Suite 205
Falls Church, VA 22046
1-800-458-6338

Opportunity
National Industries for the Blind
1901 North Beauregard Street
Alexandria, VA 22311
703-998-0770
http://www.nib.org

Paw Tracks
Council of Citizens with
Low Vision

5707 Brockton Drive
Suite 302
Indianapolis, IN 46220
317-254-1332 or 800-733-2258

*Pilot Guide Dog Foundation
Newsletter*
Pilot Guide Dog Alumni
Foundation
1123 Wolfram Street
Chicago, IL 60657
312-671-1336

Recording for the Blind News
20 Roszel Road
Princeton, NJ 08540
609-452-0606 or 1-800-221-4792

Reflections
Council of Citizens with
Low Vision
5707 Brockton Drive
Suite 302
Indianapolis, IN 46220
317-254-1332 or 800-733-2258

Scene
Braille Institute of America
741 N. Vermont Avenue
Los Angeles, CA 90029
323-663-1111
http://brailleinstitute.org

Seeing Eye Guide, The
Seeing Eye Inc.
Washington Valley Road
Morristown, NJ 07960
973-539-4425 or 800-539-4425
http://www.seeingeye.org

Sightsaving
National Society for the
Prevention of Blindness
79 Madison Avenue
New York, NY 10016

Smith-Kettlewell Technical File: A Quarterly Journal for the Blind and Visually Impaired
Smith-Kettlewell Eye Research
Foundation
2318 Fillmore Street
San Francisco, CA 94115

415-345-2000
http://www.ski.org

Standard-Bearer
National Accreditation Council for
   Agencies Serving the Blind
260 Northland Boulevard
Suite 223
Cincinnati, OH 45246
513-772-8449

Student Advocate
National Alliance of Blind
   Students
1010 Vermont Avenue, NW
Suite 1100
Washington, DC 20005
202-393-3666 or 1-800-425-8666

Talking Book Topics
National Library Service for the
   Blind and Physically Handicapped
Library of Congress
1291 Taylor Street, NW
Washington, DC 20542
202-707-5100
http://www.gov.nls

Towers
Overbrook School for the Blind
6333 Malvern Avenue
Philadelphia, PA 19151

Update
National Library Service for the
   Blind and Physically
   Handicapped
Library of Congress
1291 Taylor Street, NW
Washington, DC 20542
202-707-5100
http://www.loc.gov/nls

USABA Newsletter
U.S. Association for Blind Athletes
33 North Institute Street
Colorado Springs, CO 80903
719-630-0422
http://www.usaba.org

Utah Eagle
Utah Schools for the Deaf
   and Blind

Utah State Board of Education
742 Harrison Boulevard
Ogden, UT 84404
801-629-4700 or 800-990-9328;
   TDD 801-629-4701
http://www.usdb.k12.ut.us

VIDPI News
Visually Impaired Data Processors
   International
Council of Citizens with
   Low Vision
5707 Brockton Drive
Suite 302
Indianapolis, IN 46220
317-254-1332 or 800-733-2258

VISTA Newsletter
Council of Citizens with
   Low Vision
5707 Brockton Drive
Suite 302
Indianapolis, IN 46220
317-254-1332 or 800-733-2258

Vendorscope
Council of Citizens with Low
   Vision
5707 Brockton Drive
Suite 302
Indianapolis, IN 46220
317-254-1332 or 800-733-2258

Visionary
Illinois Society for Prevention of
   Blindness
407 South Dearborn Street
Suite 1000
Chicago, IL 60605
312-922-8710 or 800-433-4772
http://eyehealthillinois.org

Washington Weekly Review
(AFB Washington Review)
American Foundation for the
   Blind
11 Penn Plaza
Suite 300
New York, NY 10001
212-502-7660 or 800-232-5463;
   TDD 212-502-7662
http://www.afb.org

Worksight
Mississippi State University
Rehabilitation Research and Train-
    ing Center on Blindness and Low
    Vision

P.O. Box 6189
Mississippi State, MS 39762
601-325-2001 or 1-800-675-7782
www.blind.msstate.edu/irr

APPENDIX 8
RADIO READING SERVICES

Alabama Radio Reading Service
    Network
650 11th Street South
Birmingham, AL 35294
205-934-6576 or 800-444-9246
http://www.wbhm.org

Arkansas Radio Reading for the
    Blind, Inc.
2600 West Markham
Little Rock, AR 72208
510-663-4540
http://pages.prodigy.com/blindnet

Central Indiana Radio Reading, Inc.
1401 North Meridian Street
Indianapolis, IN 46202
317-636-2020
http://www.wfyi.org

Central Ohio Radio Reading Service
2955 W. Broad Street
Columbus, Ohio 43204
614-274-7650
http://www.corrs.org

Central Savannah River Area Radio
    Reading Service Inc.
c/o WACG-FM, Augusta College
2500 Walton Way
Augusta, GA 39010
706-737-1661

Chicagoland Radio Information
    Service, Inc.
77 E. Randolph Pedestrian Walkway

Chicago, IL 60601
312-541-8400
http://www.mcs.net/~cmeans/
    cris.html

Connecticut Radio Information
    Services
589 Jordan Lane
Wethersfield, CT 06109
860-956-3579
http://www.cslib.org/cris

Detroit Radio Information Service
4600 Cass Avenue
Detroit, MI 48201
313-577-4146
http://www.wdetfm.org

Evergreen Radio Reading Service of
    the Washington Library
    for the Blind and Physically
    Handicapped
821 Lenora Street
Seattle, WA 98129
206-615-0400

Georgia Radio Reading Service
260 14th Street, NW
Atlanta, GA 30318
404-685-2820 or 877-937-3378
http://www.galinks.com/garrs

Houston Taping for the Blind Radio
3935 Essex Lane
Houston, TX 77027
713-622-2767

Iowa Radio Reading Information
Service
100 E. Euclid Avenue
Des Moines, IA 50313
515-243-6833 or 877-404-4747

Idaho Radio Reading Service
P.O. Box 83720
Boise, ID 83720
208-334-3220

Illinois Radio Reader
59 East Armory
Champaign, IL 61820
217-333-6503
http://www.will.uiuc.edu

INSIGHT/WYMS
5225 West Vliet Street
Milwaukee, WI 53208
414-475-8488
http://www.wyms.org

In-Sight
43 Jefferson Boulevard
Warwick, RI 02888
401-941-3322

In Touch Networks
15 West 65th Street
New York, NY
212-769-6270 or 800-456-3166

KPBS-FM Radio Reading Service
San Diego State University
San Diego, CA 92182
619-594-8170
http://www.kpbs.org

KUT 90.5 FM
University of Texas at Austin
Communications Building B
Austin, TX 78712
512-471-4683
http://www.kut.org

Montana Radio Reading Service
126 East Broadway, #8
Missoula, MT 59802
406-721-1998 or 800-942-7323

North Eastern Indiana Radio Reading Service Inc.
920 Florence Avenue

Fort Wayne, IN 46808
219-422-8230

Northern Illinois Radio
Information Service
Riverfront Museum Park
711 N. Main Street
Rockford, IL 61103
815-961-8000
http://www.northernpublicradio.
org

Radio Information Center for
the Blind
Division of Associated Services
for the Blind
919 Walnut Street
Philadelphia, PA 19107
215-627-0700
http://www.asb.org

Radio Information Service
Wabash Valley College
2200 College Drive
Mt. Carmel, IL 62963
618-262-8641, ext. 253

Radio Reading Service
4235 Electric Road, SW
Suite 105
Roanoke, VA 24014
540-989-8900

Radio Information Service for Blind
and Handicapped
9541 Church Circle Drive
Belleville, IL 62223
618-394-6221

Radio Information Service for Blind
and Print Handicapped of West
Central Illinois
Western Illinois University
504 Memorial Hall
Macomb, IL 61455
309-298-2403
http://www/wiu.edu/usus/miris/wiv

Radio Reading Network of
Maryland
2901 Liberty Heights Avenue
Baltimore, MD 21215
410-333-5720 or 800-5605

Radio Reading Services of Great
Cincinnati, Inc.
2045 Gilbert Avenue
Cincinnati, OH 45202
513-221-8558

Radio Talking Book Service, Inc.
7101 Newport Avenue
Suite 205
Omaha, NE 68152
402-572-3003 or 800-729-7826

Radio Vision
619 Route 17M
Middletown, NY 10940
845-343-1131 or 800-327-7343
http://www.rcls.org

Reading Radio Service
815 North Walnut
Hutchinson, KS 67501
316-662-6646

READ-OUT Radio Reading
Services
P.O. Box 2400
Syracuse, NY 13220
315-453-2424
http://www.wcny.org

RISE
c/o WMHT-FM
P.O. Box 17
Schenectady, NY 12301
518-356-1700
http://www.wmht.org

Sight Seer
West Michigan Radio Reading Service
213 Sheldon Boulevard, SE
Grand Rapids, MI 49503
616-235-0020
http://www.thesightseer.org

South Carolina Educational Radio
for the Blind
1430 Confederate Avenue
Columbia, SC 29201
803-898-8755 or 1-800-922-2222

Sun Sounds of KJZZ
3124 East Roosevelt Street
Phoenix, AZ 85008

602-231-0500
http://www.sunsounds.org

Talking Information Center
130 Enterprise Drive
P.O. Box 519
Marshfield, MA 02050
781-834-4400 or 1-800-696-9505
http://www.radioview.com

Trade Winds Radio Reading
Service
5901 W. Seventh Street
Gary, IN 46406
219-949-4000 or 800-694-4242;
TDD 219-944-3733
http://www.thetimesonline.com/
org/tradewinds

UPDATE Radio Reading Service
Chautauqua Blind Association
510 W. Fifth Street
Jamestown, NY 14701
716-664-6660

Valley Voice Radio Reading Service
for the Print Handicapped
WMRA-FM
James Madison University
Harrisonburg, VA 22807
703-568-3811
http://www.valleyvoice.org

Virginia Voice for the Print
Handicapped
P.O. Box 15546
401 Azalea Avenue
Richmond, VA 23227
804-266-2477

Washington Ear Inc.
35 University Boulevard East
Silver Spring, MD 20901
301-681-6636
http://www.washear.org

WCBU Radio Information Service
1501 W. Bradley Avenue
Peoria, IL 61625
309-677-3585

WYPL-FM
1850 Peabody Avenue
Memphis, TN 38104

901-725-8833
http://www.memphis.lib.tn.us/
  wypl/wyptop.htm

Radio Reading Service GW
285 Dorset Street
Springfield, MA 01108
413-788-6981

Wichita Radio Reading Service
3317 East 17th Street
Wichita, KS 67208
316-987-6600

WKAR Radio Talking Book
283 Communication Arts and
  Sciences Building
East Lansing, MI 48824
517-353-9124; TDD 517-355-7508
http://www.wkar.org

WLRN-FM School Board of
  Dade County Florida
172 N.E. 15th Street
Miami, FL 33132
305-995-2218 or 1-800-273-6677
http://www.wlrn.org

WPLN Talking Library
700 Second Avenue
Nashville, TN 37210
615-862-5874

WRKC-Radio Home Visitor
Kings College
Wilkes-Barre, PA 18711
520-208-5811

WTSU Radio Reading Service
252 Montgomery Street
Suite 312
Montgomery, AL 36104
334-241-9574

WRBH 88.3 FM Reading Radio
3606 Magazine Street
New Orleans, LA 70115
504-899-1144

WUSF Radio Reading Service
University of South Florida WRB
  209
4202 E. Fowler Avenue
Tampa, FL 33620
813-974-8695 or 800-444-4193
http://www.wusf.usf.edu

York County Blind Center's Radio
  Reading Service
1380 Spahn Avenue
York, PA 17403
717-848-1690
http://www.forsight.org

APPENDIX 9
REHABILITATION SERVICES
(BY STATE)

ALABAMA

Alabama Department of
  Rehabilitation Services
2129 East South Boulevard
Montgomery, AL 36116-2455
334-281-8780 or 1-800-441-7607
http://www.rehab.state.al.us

Workshop and Rehabilitation
  Services for the Blind and
  Disabled
2129 East South Boulevard
Montgomery, AL 36116-2455
334-281-8780 or 1-800441-7607
http://www.rehab.state.al.us

ALASKA

Alaska Center for the Blind
3903 Taft Drive
Anchorage, AK 99517-3069
907-248-7770 or 1-800-770-7517
http://www.alaskablind.com

ARIZONA

Arizona Center for the Blind and
  Visually Impaired
3100 East Roosevelt Street
Phoenix, AZ 85008
602-273-7411
http://www.acbvi.org

Tucson Association for the Blind
  and Visually Impaired
3767 East Grant Road
Tucson, AZ 85716
520-795-1331

ARKANSAS

Arkansas Department of Human
  Services: Division of Services for
  the Blind
522 Main Street
Suite 100
Little Rock, AR 72203-3237
501-682-5463 or 1-800-960-9270;
  TDD/TTY 501-682-0093
http://www.state.ar.us/dhs/dsb

CALIFORNIA

California Department of
  Rehabilitation: Services for
  the Blind
2000 Evergreen Street
Sacramento, CA 95815-3832
916-263-8953; TDD/
  TTY 530-345-3897
http://www.rehab.cahwnet.gov/

Society for the Blind
2750 24th Street
Sacramento, CA 95818
916-452-8271
http://www.societyfortheblind.org

COLORADO

Colorado Department of Human
  Services: Rehabilitation Services
2211 West Evans Street
Building B
Denver, CO 80230
720-884-1234
http://www.state.co.us

CONNECTICUT

Connecticut State Board of Education and Services for the Blind
184 Windsor Avenue
Windsor, CT 06095
860-602-4000 or 1-800-842-4510;
  TDD/TTY 860-602-4002
http://www.besb.state.ct.us

DELAWARE

Delaware Department of Health
  and Social Services: Division for
  the Visually Impaired
1901 North Dupont Highway
Biggs Building
New Castle, DE 19720
302-577-4730; TDD/
  TTY 302-577-4750
http://www.state.de.us/dhss/dvi/
  dvihome.htm

DISTRICT OF COLUMBIA

Columbia Lighthouse for the Blind
1120 20th Street, NW
Washington, DC 20036
202-454-6400 or (toll free)
  877-324-5252
http://www.clb.org

FLORIDA

Center for the Visually Impaired
1187 Dunn Avenue
Daytona Beach, FL 32114
904-253-8879 or 1-800-227-1284
http://www.cfiflorida.org

Florida Department of Education:
  Division of Blind Services
2551 Executive Center Circle
Tallahassee, FL 32399

850-488-1330 or 1-800-342-1828
http://www.state.fl.us/dbs

Independent Living for Adult Blind
c/o Florida Community College at
  Jacksonville
101 West State Street
Jacksonville, FL 32202
904-633-8220

GEORGIA

Georgia Department of Human
  Resources: Division of
  Rehabilitation Services
Two Peachtree Street, NW
Suite 35-412
Atlanta, GA 30303-3142
404-657-3000
http://www.vocrehabga.org

Living Independence for Everyone
17-21 East Travis Street
Savannah, GA 31406
912-920-2414 or 1-800-948-4824;
  TDD/TTY 912-920-2419

HAWAII

Hawaii Department of Human
  Services: Ho'opono Services
  for the Blind, Vocational
  Rehabilitation and Services
  for the Blind Division
1901 Bachelot Street
Honolulu, HI 96817
808-692-7716
http://www.rrhi.com/
  hooponoblindservices

IDAHO

Idaho Commission for the Blind and
  Visually Impaired
341 West Washington Street
Boise, ID 83720-0012
208-334-3220
http://www.icbvi.state.id.us

ILLINOIS

Illinois Department of
  Rehabilitation Services: Bureau
  of Blind Services

623 East Adams Street
Springfield, IL 62794-9429
217-785-3887 or 1-800-275-3677;
  TDD/TTY 630-495-2294
http://www.state.il.us/agency/
  dhs/bsnp.html

Chicago Lighthouse for People
  Who Are Blind or Visually
  Impaired
1850 West Roosevelt Road
Chicago, IL 60608
312-666-1331; TDD/
  TTY 312-666-8874
http://www.thechicagolighthouse.
  org

INDIANA

Indiana Family and Social Services
  Administration: Division of
  Disability, Aging and
  Rehabilitative Services
Indiana Government Center
402 West Washington Street
Room W-453
Indianapolis, IN 46204
317-232-7020 or 1-800-545-7763
http://www.state.in.us/fssa

Trade Winds Rehabilitation Center
5901 West Seventh Avenue
Gary, IN 46406-0308
219-949-4000 or 1-800-694-4242;
  TDD/TTY 219-944-3733
http://www.thetimesonline.com/
  org/tradewinds

IOWA

Iowa Department for the Blind
524 Fourth Street
Des Moines, IA 50309-2364
515-281-1333 or 1-800-362-2587;
  TDD/TTY 515-281-1355
http://www.blind.state.ia.us/

KANSAS

Kansas Department of Social and
  Rehabilitation Services: Division
  of Services for the Blind,

Rehabilitation Center for the Blind
2516 SW Sixth Avenue
Topeka, KS 66606
785-296-3311
http://www.state.ks.us/public/srs

Vision Rehabilitation Center
6100 East Central Avenue
Suite 5
Wichita, KS 67208-4237
316-682-4646

KENTUCKY

Kentucky Department for the Blind
209 St. Clair Street
Frankfort, KY 40602
502-575-7315 or 1-800-334-6920
http://www.state.ky.us/agencies/wfo
rce//dfblind/index.htm

Kentucky Department for the Blind:
Independent Living Services,
Charles McDowell Center
8412 Westport Road
Louisville, KY 40242
502-327-6010 or 1-800-346-2115
http://www.state.ky.us/agencies/
wforce/dfblind/kdfbhome.htm

LOUISIANA

Louisiana Center for the Blind
101 South Trenton Street
Ruston, LA 71270
318-251-2891 or 800-234-4166
http://www.lcb-ruston.com

Louisiana Department of Social
Services: Louisiana
Rehabilitation Services
8225 Florida Boulevard
Baton Rouge, LA 70806
225-925-3594 or 800-737-2958
http://www.dss.state.la.us/offlrs/

MAINE

Maine Department of Labor: Bureau
of Rehabilitation Services, Division for the Blind and Visually
Impaired

3 Anthony Avenue
#150 State House Station
Augusta, ME 04333-0150
207-624-5959; TDD/
TTY 207-624-5955

MARYLAND

Johns Hopkins School of Medicine:
Wilmer Ophthalmological
Institute, Lions Vision Research
and Rehabilitation Center
550 North Broadway
Sixth Floor
Baltimore, MD 21205
410-955-0580
http://www.wilmereyeinstitute.org

Maryland State Department of
Education: Division of
Rehabilitation Services
2301 Argonne Drive
Baltimore, MD 21218-1696
410-767-9100 or (toll-free)
1-888-200-7117; TDD/
TTY 410-554-9411
http://www.dors.state.md.us/

Services for the Visually Impaired
8720 Georgia Avenue
Suite 210
Silver Spring, MD 20910
301-589-0894

MASSACHUSETTS

Massachusetts Association for
the Blind
200 Ivy Street
Brookline, MA 02446
617-738-5110 or 1-800-682-9200
URL: http://www.mablind.org

Massachusetts State Commission
for the Blind
88 Kingston Street
Boston, MA 02111-2227
617-727-5550 or 1-800-392-6450
http://www.magnet.state.ma.us/mcb

MICHIGAN

Michigan Commission for the Blind
Training Center

1541 Oakland Drive
Kalamazoo, MI 49008
616-337-3848
http://www.mfia.state.mi.us/mcb

Visual Rehabilitation and Research
Center of Michigan
15401 East Jefferson Avenue
Grosse Pointe Park, MI 48230
313-824-2401

Visually Impaired Center
725 Mason Street
Flint, MI 48503
810-235-2544

MINNESOTA

Minnesota State Academy for the
Blind
P.O. Box 68
Fairbault, MN 55021
507-333-4800 or 1-800-657-3634
http://www.msab.state.mn.us

Minnesota State Services for the
Blind
2200 University Avenue West
Suite 240
St. Paul, MN 55114-1840
651-642-0500 or 1-800-652-9000
TDD/TTY 651-642-0506
http://www.mnworkforcecenter.org/
ssb/

MISSISSIPPI

Addie McBryde Rehabilitation
Center for the Blind
2550 Peachtree Street
Jackson, MS 39296-5314
601-364-2700 or 1-800-443-1000;
TDD/TTY 601-853-5100

Mississippi Department of
Rehabilitation Services: Office
of Vocational Rehabilitation for
the Blind
1281 Highway 51 North
Madison, MS 39110
601-853-5100 or 1-800-443-1000
http://www.mdrs.state.ms.us

MISSOURI

Missouri Rehabilitation Services for
the Blind
3418 Knipp Drive
Jefferson City, MO 65109
573-751-4249 or 1-800-592-6004
http://www.dss.state.mo.us/dfs/
rehab.htm

Rehabilitation Institute: Center
for Blindness and Low Vision
2801 Wyandotte Street
Third Floor
Kansas City, MO 64108
816-753-6533

MONTANA

Montana Department of Public
Health and Human Services:
Developmental Disabilities
Program/Vocational
Rehabilitation/Blind and
Low Vision Services
111 North Sanders
Room 307
Helena, MT 59604
406-444-2590 or (toll free)
1-877-296-1197

NEBRASKA

Nebraska Commission for the Blind
and Visually Impaired
4600 Valley Road
Suite 100
Lincoln, NE 68510-4844
402-471-8100 or (toll free) 877-
809-2419; TDD/TTY
402-471-2891

NEW HAMPSHIRE

New Hampshire Division of Vocational Rehabilitation: Services for
the Blind and Visually Impaired
78 Regional Drive
Building #2
Concord, NH 03301

603-271-3537 or 800-581-6881
http://216.64.49.52/vrweb/blind.
html

NEW JERSEY

New Jersey Commission for the
Blind and Visually Impaired
153 Halsey Street
6th Floor
Newark, NJ 07101
973-648-3333

New Jersey Foundation for the
Blind
230 Diamond Spring Road
Denville, NJ 07834
201-627-0055

NEW MEXICO

New Mexico Commission for the
Blind
1120 Paseo de Peralta
PERA Building
Room 553
Santa Fe, NM 87504
505-827-4479 or (toll free)
1-888-513-7968
http://www.state.nm.us/cftb

NEW YORK

Helen Keller Worldwide
90 West Street
Second Floor
New York, NY 10006
212-766-5266 or 1-800-535-5374
http://www.hkworld.org

New York State Education Depart-
ment: Office of Vocational and
Educational Services for
Individuals with Disabilities
One Commerce Plaza
Room 1606
Albany, NY 12234
518-474-2714 or 1-800-222-5627
http://web.nysed.gov/vesid

Resource Center for Independent
Living

401-409 Columbia Street
Utica, NY 13503-0210
315-797-4642; TDD/TTY
315-797-5837
http://www.rcil.com

Westchester Independent Living
Center
200 Hamilton Avenue
Second Floor
White Plains, NY 10601
914-682-3926; TDD/TTY
914-682-0926
http://www.wilc.org

NORTH CAROLINA

North Carolina Division of Services
for the Blind
2601 Mail Service Center
309 Ashe Avenue
Raleigh, NC 27699-260
919-733-9822; TDD/TTY
919-733-9700
http://www.dhhs.state.nc.us/dsb/

NORTH DAKOTA

North Dakota Department of
Human Services: Vocational
Rehabilitation
600 South Second Street
Suite 1B
Bismarck, ND 58504
701-328-8950 or 1-800-755-2745;
TDD/TTY 701-328-8968

OHIO

Ohio Rehabilitation Services
Commission: Bureau of Services
for the Visually Impaired
400 East Campus View Boulevard
Columbus, OH 43235-4604
614-438-1255 or 1-800-282-4536;
TTD/TTY 614-995-1161
http://www.state.oh.us/rsc

Ohio State University: College of
Optometry, Vision Rehabilitation
Service

338 West 10th Avenue
Columbus, OH 43210
614-292-1104
http://www.optometry.ohiostate.edu

OKLAHOMA

Oklahoma Department of Rehabilitation Services
3535 N.W. 58th Street, Suite 500
Oklahoma City, OK 73112
405-951-3400 or 1-800-845-8476
http://www.onenet.net/~drspiowm

OREGON

Independent Living Resources
4506 S.E. Belmont, Suite 100
Portland, OR 97215-1658
503-232-7411; TDD/TTY 503-232-
8408
http://www.ilr.org

Oregon Commission for the Blind
535 12th Avenue, SE
Portland, OR 97214
503-731-3221 or (toll-free)
1-888-202-5463; TDD/TTY
503-731-3224
http://www.cfb.state.or.us

PENNSYLVANIA

Associated Services for the Blind
919 Walnut Street
Philadelphia, PA 19107
215-627-0600
http://www.asb.org

Association for the Blind and
Visually Impaired
614 North 13th Street
Allentown, PA 18102-2199
610-433-6018
http://www.abvi.org

Center for Vision Rehabilitation
Allegheny General Hospital
Suite 116
Ophthalmology Department
Pittsburgh, PA 15212
412-359-6300 or 1-800-637-3762

RHODE ISLAND

Rhode Island Department of Human
Services: Services for the Blind
and Visually Impaired
40 Fountain Street
Providence, RI 02903-1898
401-277-2382 or 1-800-752-8088
http://www.ors.state.ri.us

SOUTH CAROLINA

South Carolina Commission for
the Blind
1430 Confederate Avenue
Columbia, SC 29201
803-898-8800 or 1-800-922-2222
http://www.sccb.state.sc.us

SOUTH DAKOTA

South Dakota Department of
Human Services: Division of
Service to the Blind and Visually
Impaired
East Highway 34
500 East Capitol
Pierre, SD 57501-5070
605-773-5990 or 1-800-265-9684
http://www.state.sd.us/dhs/

TENNESSEE

Tennessee Rehabilitation Center
460 Ninth Avenue
Smyrna, TN 37167-2010
615-741-4921

Tennessee Services for the Blind and
Visually Impaired
400 Deaderick Street
11th Floor
Nashville, TN 37248-6200
615-313-4914

TEXAS

Texas Commission for the Blind:
Criss Cole Rehabilitation Center
4800 North Lamar
Austin, TX 78756

512-377-0300 or 1-800-252-5204
http://www.tcb.state.tx.us/
    criss_cole.asp

UTAH

Utah Industries for the Blind
P.O. Box 1258
Salt Lake City, UT 84110-1258
Local Telephone: (801) 485-3847

Utah State Division of Services for
    the Blind and Visually Impaired
250 North 1950 West
Suite B
Salt Lake City, UT 84116-7902
801-323-4343 or 1-800-284-1823;
    TDD/TTY 801-323-4395

VERMONT

Vermont Association for the Blind
    and Visually Impaired
37 Elmwood Avenue
Burlington, VT 05401
802-863-1358 or 1-800-639-5861

VIRGINIA

Virginia Rehabilitation Center for
    the Blind and Vision Impaired
401 Azalea Avenue
Richmond, VA 23227
804-371-3151

WASHINGTON

Washington State Department of
    Services for the Blind
402 Legion Way, SE
Suite 100
Olympia, WA 98504-0933
360-586-1224 or 1-800-552-7103;
    TDD/TTY 206-764-4051
http://www.wa.gov/dsb

WEST VIRGINIA

West Virginia Department of
    Education and the Arts: Division
    of Rehabilitation Services,
    Information and Referral Services
    for the Blind and Visually
    Impaired
P.O. Box 50890
State Capitol Complex
Charleston, WV 25305-0890
304-766-4891 or 1-800-642-3021;
    TDD/TTY 304-766-4970

WISCONSIN

Wisconsin Center for the Blind and
    Visually Impaired
1700 West State Street
Janesville, WI 53546
608-758-6146 or 1-800-832-9784;
    TDD/TTY 608-758-6127

Wisconsin Council of the Blind
354 West Main Street
Madison, WI 53703-3115
608-255-1166 or 1-800-783-5213
http://www.wcblind.org

Wisconsin Department of Health
    and Family Services: Division of
    Supportive Living, Bureau for the
    Blind
1 West Wilson Street
Madison, WI 53707
608-266-3139
http://www.dhfs.state.wi.us/

WYOMING

Wyoming Division of Vocational
    Rehabilitation
1100 Hershler Building
Cheyenne, WY 82002
307-777-7389
http://onestop.state.wy.us/appview/
    ujn-home.asp

APPENDIX 10
SCHOLARSHIPS FOR THE BLIND

American Council on Rural Special
  Education Scholarships
Kansas State University
2323 Anderson Avenue
Suite 226
Manhattan, KS 66501-2912
785-532-2737
http://www.kus.edu

American Council of the Blind
  Scholarships
1155 15th Street, NW
Suite 270
Washington, DC 20005
202-467-5081 or 800-424-8666

American Foundation for the Blind
  Scholarships
11 Penn Plaza
Suite 300
New York, NY 10001
212-502-7600 or 800-232-5463
http://www.afb.org

Amy Reiss Blind Student Scholarship
Fordham University Financial Aid
  Office
140 W. 62nd Street
Room 125
New York, NY 10023
http://www.acenet.edu

Association for Education and Reha-
  bilitation of the Blind and Visually
  Impaired
Ferrell Scholarship Fund
4600 Duke Street
Suite 430
Alexandria, VA 22397
703-823-9690

Barbara Jackman Zuckert
  Scholarship
George Washington University

Disabled Support Services
Marvin Center
Suite 436
Washington, DC 20052
202-994-8250

Blinded Veterans Association
  Scholarships
Blinded Veterans Association
477 H Street, NW
Washington, DC 20001
202-371-8880

Christian Record Braille Foundation
  Scholarships
444 South 52nd Street
Lincoln, NE 68506
402-488-0981

Citizens Scholarship Foundation of
  America
Jenneth Cote
Citizens Scholarship Foundations of
  America
Box 112A
Londonderry Turnpike
RFD #7
Manchester, NH 13104

and

Ingrid LeMarie
New Hampshire Charitable Fund
One South Street
Concord, NH 03301
http://www.csfa.org

Council of Citizens with Low Vision
  International
1155 15th Street, NW
Suite 1004
Washington, DC 20005
800-733-2258
http://www.cclvi.org

Council of Citizens with Low Vision,
Carl E. Foley Scholarship
Pennsylvania College of
Optometry
1200 West Godfrey Street
Philadelphia, PA 19141
215-276-6268

Equal Opportunity Publications
445 Broad Hollow Road
Suite 425
Melville, NY 11747
631-421-9421
http://www.eop.com

The Foundation for Exceptional
Children Scholarships
1920 Association Drive
Reston, VA 20190
703-264-3507

Foundation for Science and the
Handicapped Scholarships
Chairperson of the Science Grant
Committee
Division of Rehabilitation
Education
154 Juliet Court
Clarenden Hills, IL 60514

George Peabody College, Vanderbilt
University Department of Special
Education
Nashville, TN 37203
615-322-2249

Itzhak Perlman Award
Denise Warner
Very Special Arts Education Office
Kennedy Center
Washington, DC 20566
202-662-8899

Jewish Braille Institute of America
Inc. Scholarship
110 East 30th Street
New York, NY 10016
212-889-2525

Lighthouse International
Career Incentive and Achievement
Awards
111 East 59th Street

New York, NY 10022
212-821-9428

National Federation of the Blind
Scholarship Committee
805 Fifth Avenue
Grinnell, LA 50112-1653
641-236-3369
http://www.nfb.org

The New Hampshire Charitable
Foundation
37 Pleasant Street
Concord, NH 03301-4005
603-225-6641

Opportunities for the Blind Ind.,
Scholarships
P.O. Box 510
Leonardtown, MD 20650
800-884-1990
http://www.oppblind.com

Recording for the Blind Scholastic
Achievement Awards
Public Relations Department
Recording for the Blind
20 Roszel Road
Princeton, NJ 08540
609-452-0606, ext. 246

Ronnie Milsap Foundation
600 Renaissance Center
Suite 1300
Detroit, MI 48243

Rotary Ambassadorial Scholarships
Rotary International
Scholarship Dept.
1560 Sherman Avenue
Evanston, IL 60601
847-866-3000
http://www.rotary.org

University of Kansas
Research and Training Center on
Independent Living
BCR/4089 Dole
Lawrence, KS 66045
913-864-4095

Vinland National Center
P.O. Box 308

3675 Ihduhapi Road
Loretto, MN 55357
612-479-3555

Vermont Association for
the Blind
Charles E. Leonard Memorial Schol-
arship Fund
P.O. Box 2000
Champlain Mill
Winooski, VT 05404

VSA (Very Special Arts)
1300 Connecticut Avenue, NW
Suite 700
Washington, DC 20036
800-933-8721

Western Michigan University
Department of Rehabilitation
Western Michigan University
Kalamazoo, MI 49008

APPENDIX 11
SPORTS AND RECREATION ORGANIZATIONS AND PUBLICATIONS

*Access to Art: An Art Resource Directory
for the Blind and
Visually Impaired*
American Foundation for
the Blind
11 Penn Plaza
Suite 300
New York, NY 10001
212-502-7660 or 800-232-5463;
TDD 212-502-7662
http://www.afb.org

American Alliance for Health, Physical Education, Recreation and
Dance
1900 Association Drive
Reston, VA 22091
703-476-3481
http://www.aahperd.org

American Blind Bowling
Association
411 Sheriff Street
Mercer, PA 16137
412-662-5748

American Blind Skiers, Inc.
2325 Wilshire Boulevard
Santa Monica, CA 90403
213-828-5514

American Camping Association
5000 State Road 67 North
Martinsville, IN 46151
765-342-8456
http://www.ACAcamps.org

American Horticulture Therapy
Association
909 York Street
Denver, CO 80206
720-865-3616
http://www.ahta.org

American Red Cross
Program of Swimming for the
Handicapped
431 18th Street, NW
Washington, DC 20006
800-797-8022
http://redcross.org

American Music Therapy Association
8455 Colesville Road
Suite 1000
Silver Spring, MD 20910
301-589-3300
http://www.namt.org

American Printing House for
the Blind
1839 Frankfort Avenue
P.O. Box 6085
Louisville, KY 40206
502-895-2405 or 800-223-1839
http://www.aph.org

Association of Disabled American
Golfers
P.O. Box 280649
Lakewood, CO 80228
303-922-5228
http://www.toski.com/golf/adag

Association of Handicapped Artists
5150 Broadway
Depew, NY 14043
716-683-9316

Association of Radio Reading
Services
Sun Sound Reading Service
3124 East Roosevelt Street
Phoenix, AZ 85008
1-800-255-2777

Bemidji State University
Outdoor Program Center
Hobson Memorial Union
Bemidji, MN 56601
218-755-2999

Bibles and Other Scriptures in
Special Media
National Library Service for the
Blind and Physically Handicapped
Reference Circular
Library of Congress
Washington, DC 20542
212-287-5100

Bible Outdoor Leisure Development
(BOLD)
533 East Main Street

Aspen, CO 81611
303-925-2086

Bradford Woods Outdoor Center
5040 State Road
67 North
Martinsville, IN 46151
765-342-8456

Braille Sports Foundation
4601 Excelsior Avenue South
St. Louis Park, MN 55416
612-920-9363

Breckenridge Outdoor Education
Center
917 Airport Road
P.O. Box 697
Breckenridge, CO 80424
970-453-6422

Challenge Alaska
P.O. Box 110065
Anchorage, AK 99511
907-344-7399
http://www.challenge.ak.org

Choice Magazine
100 Riverview Center
Middletown, CT 06457
860-347-6933

Council for Disabled Sailors
American Sailing Association
60 Padanaram Road
Unit 16
Danbury, CT 06810

Courage Center
Department of Sports, Physical
Education and Recreation
3915 Golden Valley Road
Golden Valley, MN 55422
763-520-0520
http://www.courage.org

Disabled Sports USA
41 Hungerford Drive
Suite 100
Rockville, MD 20850
301-217-0960
http://www.dsusa.org

Discovery Blind Sports International
6811 Aitkem Drive
Oakland, CA 94611
510-399-0777

Evergreen Travel Service
4114 North Avenue, SW
#13
Lynnwood, WA 98036
800-435-2288

Independent Living Aids
200 Robbins Lane
Jericho, NY 11753
800-537-2118
http://www.independentliving.com

Information and Research
Utilization Center
American Alliance for Health,
Physical Education, Recreation
and Dance
1900 Association Drive
Reston, VA 20191
800-213-7193
http://www.aahperd.org

Information Center for
Individuals with Disabilities
P.O. Box 750119
Arlington Heights, MA 02475
781-860-0673
http://www.disability.net

International Bicycle Tours Inc.
12 Mid Place
Chappaqua, NY 10514
914-238-4576

Kirkwood Instruction for Blind Skiers
P.O. Box 138
Kirkwood, CA 95646

Louis Braille Foundation for
Blind Musicians
112 East 19th Street
New York, NY 10003

Matilda Ziegler Magazine for the
Blind
80 Eighth Avenue
Room 1304
New York, NY 10011

212-242-0263
http://zieglermag.org

National Arts and the Handicapped
Information Service
Arts and Special Constituency
Project
National Endowment for the Arts
2401 E Street, NW
Washington, DC 20506

National Association for Sports
for Cerebral Palsy
66 East 34th Street
New York, NY 10016
212-481-6359
http://www.uscpaa.org

National Beep Baseball Association
2231 W. First Avenue
Topeka, KS 66606
785-234-2156
http://www.nbaa.org

National Braille Association
3 Towline Circle
Rochester, NY 14623
716-427-8260
http://www.nationalbraille.org

National Camp Directory for the
Blind and Visually Impaired
American Foundation for the Blind
11 Penn Plaza
Suite 300
New York, NY 10001
212-502-7660 or 800-232-5463;
TDD 212-502-7662
http://www.afb.org

National Committee/Arts for the
Handicapped
1300 Connecticut Avenue
Suite 700
Washington, DC 20036
202-628-2800 or 800-933-8721
http://vsarts.org

National Exhibits by Blind Artists
919 Walnut Street
First Floor
Philadelphia, PA 19107
1-800-222-1764

National Gardening Association
180 Flynn Avenue
Burlington, VT 05401
802-863-1308

National Handicapped Sports and
Recreation Association
5932 Illinois Avenue
Orangevale, CA 95662
916-989-0402

National Therapeutic Recreation
Society
22377 Belmont Ridge Road
Ashburn, VA 20148
703-858-0784
http://www.health.gov/nhic

North American Riding for the
Handicapped Association
P.O. Box 33150
Denver, CO 80233
303-252-4610
http://www.harha.org

Outward Bound
945 Pennsylvania Street
Denver, CO 80203
800-243-8520
http://www.outwardbound.org

People-to-People Committee for the
Handicapped
1111 20th Street, NW
Suite 660
Washington, DC 20036
202-653-5007

Peter Burwash International Ltd.
2203 Timberloch Place
#126
The Woodlands, TX 77380
218-363-4707
http://www.pbi-tennis.com

President's Committee on Employment of People with Disabilities
1331 F Street, NW
Washington, DC 20004
202-376-6200
http://www.health.gov/nhic

Recording for the Blind Inc.
20 Roswell Road

Princeton, NJ 08540
609-452-0606
http://www.rfbdnj.org

Santa Monica Blind Skiers Inc.
2325 Wilshire Boulevard
Santa Monica, CA 90403

Science Products
Box A
Southeastern, PA 19399
1-800-888-7401

SIRE, Inc. (Self Improvement
Through Riding)
Rt. 2, Box 56
Hockley, TX 77447
281-356-7588

Skating for the Blind and
Handicapped
1200 East and West Road
West Seneca, NY 14224
716-675-7222
http://www.sabahinc.org

Ski for Light
1400 Carole Lane
Green Bay, WI 54313
414-494-5572

SOAR
5404 NE Alameda Avenue
Portland, OR 97214

Society for the Advancement of
Travel for the Handicapped
374 Fifth Avenue
Suite 610
New York, NY 10016
212-447-7284
http://www.sath.org

Sports Illustrated
Available through the National
Library Service for the Blind and
Physically Handicapped
1291 Taylor Street, NW
Washington, DC 20542

Telesensory Systems
455 North Bernardo Avenue
P.O. Box 7455
Mountain View, CA 94043-5274
1-800-286-8484

Travel Industry and Disabled
  Exchange (TIDE)
5435 Donna Avenue
Tarzana, CA 91356

Travel Information Center
Moss Rehabilitation Hospital
12th Street and Tabor Road
Philadelphia, PA 19141
215-329-5715

United States Blind Chess Association
30 Snell Street
Brockton, MA 02410

United States Blind Golfers
  Association
3094 Shamrock Street North

Tallhassee, FL 32308
850-893-4511
http://www.usbga.org

Vinland National Center
3675 Ihduhapi Road
P.O. Box 308
Loreetto, MN 55357
615-479-3555

West Chester University Outdoor
  Resource Center
West Chester, PA 19380
215-436-1000

APPENDIX 12
ADDITIONAL RESOURCES

Abel, Robert. *The Eye Care Revolution: Prevent and Reverse Common Vision Problems.* New York: Kensington Publishing Company, 1999.

Alexander, Sally Hobart. *Taking Hold: My Journey Into Blindness.* New York: Simon & Schuster, 1994.

———. *Do You Remember the Color Blue?: And Other Questions Kids Ask About Blindness.* New York: Penguin Putnam Books for Young Readers, 2000.

Cassel, Gary H., Michael D. Billig, and Harry G. Randall. *The Eye Book: A Complete Guide to Eye Disorders and Health.* Baltimore, Md.: Johns Hopkins University Press, 1998.

Chapman, Bill G. *Coping with Vision Loss: Maximizing What You Can See and Do.* Alameda, Calif.: Hunter House Incorporated, 2001.

D'Amato, Robert, and Joan Snyder, *Macular Degeneration: The Latest Scientific Discoveries and Treatments for Preserving Your Sight.* New York: Walker & Company, 2000.

Dobree, John Hatherley, and Eric Boulter. *Blindness and Visual Handicap: The Facts.* New York: Oxford University Press, 1982.

Garfield, James B., and Robert Greiner. *Follow My Leader.* New York: Penguin Putnam Books for Young Readers, 1994.

Hermann, Spring. *The Story of Abigail Carter and America's First School for Blind People.* New York: Henry Holt & Company, 1998.

Holbrook, M. Cay. *Children with Visual Impairments: A Parent's Guide*. Bethesda, Md.: Woodbine House, Inc., 1995.

Hull, John M. *On Sight and Insight: A Journey Into the World of Blindness*. London: Oneworld Publications, 1997.

———. *Touching the Rock: An Experience of Blindness*. New York: Vintage Books, 1992.

Kaplan, Robert Michael. *The Power Behind Your Eyes: Improving Your Eyesight with Integrated Vision Therapy*. Rochester, Vt.: Healing Arts Press, 1995.

Kendrick, Deborah. *Jobs to be Proud of: Profiles of Workers Who Are Blind or Visually Impaired*. New York: American Foundation for the Blind Press, 1993.

Kleege, Georgina. *Sight Unseen*. New Haven, Conn.: Yale University Press, 1999.

Landau, Elaine. *Blindness*. New York: Twenty-first Century Press, 1995.

Marks, Edith, and Rita Montauredes. *Coping with Glaucoma: A Guide to Living with Glaucoma for You and Your Family*. Garden City, N.Y.: Avery Publishing Group, Inc., 1997.

———. *The Two in One: Walking with Smokie, Walking with Blindness*. Philadelphia: Temple University Press, 1998.

Michalko, Rod. *The Mystery of the Eye and the Shadow of Blindness*. Toronto: University of Toronto Press, 1998.

Olson, Myrna R., and Sally S. Mangold. *Guidelines and Games for Teaching Efficient Braille Reading*. New York: American Foundation for the Blind Press, 1997.

Price, Ira Marc, and Linda Comac. *Coping with Macular Degeneration: A Guide for Patients and Families to Understanding and Living with Degenerative Vision Disorder*, New York: The Putnam Publishing Group, 2000.

Roberts, Alvin. *Coping with Blindness: Personal Tales of Blindness Rehabilitation*. Carbondale: Southern Illinois University Press, 1998.

Rosenthal, Bruce P., and Kate Kelly. *Living Well with Macular Degeneration: Practical Tips and Essential Information*. New York: NAL, 2001.

Scott, Eileen P., and James E. Jan, and Roger D. Freeman. *Can't Your Child See?: A Guide for Parents and Professionals About Young Children Who Are Visually Impaired*. Austin, Tex.: PRO-ED, 1995.

Schulman, Arlene. *T.J.'s Story: A Book About a Boy Who Is Blind*. Indianapolis, Ind.: The Lerner Publishing Group, 1997.

Shulman, Julius, and Neil Hardy. *Cataracts: From Diagnosis to Recovery—The Complete Guide for Patients and Families*. New York: St. Martin's Press, Inc., 1995.

Solomon, Yale, and Jonathan D. Solomon. *Overcoming Macular Degeneration: A Guide to Seeing Beyond the Clouds*. New York: William Morrow & Co., 2000.

Stark, Walter J. *Cataracts: A Guide for Patients*. H I N, Incorporated, 1997.

Trope, Graham E., *Glaucoma: A Patient's Guide to the Disease*. Toronto: University of Toronto Press, 1996.

Warren, David H. *Blindness and Children: An Individual Differences Approach*. New York: Cambridge University Press, 1994.

White, Peter. *Being Blind*. Mankato, Minn.: Smart Apple Media, 2000.

Zinn, Walter J., and Herbert Solomon. *The Complete Guide to Eyecare, Eyeglasses and Contact Lenses*. Hollywood, Fla.: Lifetime Books, 1996.

BIBLIOGRAPHY

ABLEDATA. *Braille Telephone Device for the Deaf.* Newington, Conn.: ABLEDATA, 1989.

———. *Electronic Travel Aids Printout.* Newington, Conn.: ABLEDATA, 1989.

———. *Kurzweil Reader Printout.* Newington, Conn.: ABLEDATA, 1989.

———. *Speech Synthesizers Printout.* Newington, Conn.: ABLEDATA, 1989.

———. *Telebraille.* Newington, Conn.: ABLEDATA, 1989.

———. *Voice Output Module.* Newington, Conn.: ABLEDATA, 1989.

Abel, Robert. *The Eye Care Revolution: Prevent and Reverse Common Vision Problems.* Clifton, N.J.: Kensington Publishing Corporation, 1999.

Alexandidis, E. *The Pupil.* New York: Springer-Verlag, 1985.

Alpert, Joseph S. *The Heart Attack Handbook.* Boston: Little, Brown, 1985.

American Academy of Ophthalmology. Medem. "Air Bags May Cause Serious Eye Injuries in Children." Available online. URL: http://www.medem.com/MedLB/article_detaillb.cfm?article_ID=ZZZ14RKP6BC.

———. "American Academy of Ophthalmology Says Newly Approved Drug, Visudyne, is Promising." Available online. URL: http://www.medem.com/MedLB/article_detaillb.cfm?article_ID=ZZZY6EF428C.

———. "Corneal Rings Safe and Effective for Correcting Nearsightedness, Two-Year Study Shows." Available online. URL: http://www.medem.com/MedLB/article_detaillb.cfm?article_ID=ZZZHDXJB8RC. Posted September 2001.

———. "Early Ophthalmic Examination Can Lead to Child Abuse Detection and Prevention." Available online. URL: http://www.medem.com/MedLB/article_detaillb.cfm?article_ID=ZZZASLAS2AC.

———. "90% of Sports-Related Eye Injuries Are Preventable, Eye M.D.s Say." Available online. URL: http://www.medem.com/MedLB/article_detaillb.cfm?article_ID=ZZZVYGPIJ7C. Posted on March 23, 2000.

American Foundation for the Blind. *A Different Way of Seeing.* New York: AFB, 1984.

———. *Aging and Vision.* New York: AFB, 1987.

———. *Career Choice for Blind and Visually Impaired Students: Career Planning and Placement Offices.* New York: AFB, 1987.

———. *Directory of Services for Blind and Visually Impaired Persons in the United States.* 23rd ed. New York: AFB, 1988.

———. *Facts about the American Foundation for the Blind.* New York: AFB, 1986.

———. *A Good Employee Is a Good Employee.* New York: AFB, 1987.

———. *Helen Keller,* New York: AFB, 1987.

———. *How Does a Blind Person Get Around?* New York: AFB, 1988.

———. *Is Your Child Blind?* New York: AFB, 1975.

———. *Louis Braille.* New York: AFB, 1987.

———. *Low Vision Questions and Answers: Definitions, Devices, Services.* New York: AFB, 1987.

———. *The M. C. Migel Memorial Library and Information Center.* New York: AFB, 1986.

———. *Parenting Preschoolers: Suggestions for Raising Young Blind and Visually Impaired Children.* New York: AFB, 1984.

————. *The Preschool Deaf-Blind Child: Suggestions for Parents.* New York: AFB, 1974.

————. *Touch the Baby.* New York: AFB, 1987.

————. *Understanding and Living with Glaucoma.* New York: AFB, 1984.

————. *Understanding Braille.* New York: AFB, 1970.

————. *Visually Impaired Professional Personnel.* New York: AFB, 1986.

————. *What Do You Do When You See A Blind Person?* New York: AFB, 1970.

————. *What To Do When You Meet A Deaf-Blind Person.* New York: AFB, 1985.

American Heart Association. *Recovering From a Stroke.* Dallas: AHA, 1986.

————. *1989 Stroke Facts.* Dallas: AHA, 1988.

————. *Stroke: Why Do They Behave that Way?* Dallas: AHA, 1974.

Anderson, Douglas R. *Testing the Field of Vision.* St. Louis: C. V. Mosby Company, 1982.

Anderson, Harry C. *An Experience: Students with Usher Syndrome and their Parents.* Baltimore: RP Foundation Fighting Blindness, 1977.

Anderson, Julia, "How Technology Brings Blind People into the Workplace." *Harvard Business Review* (March–April 1989): 36–39.

Annala, Linda. *Facing the Future with Usher's Syndrome.* Baltimore: RP Foundation Fighting Blindness, 1976.

Apolloni, Tony. "Effective Advocacy: How to Be a Winner." *Exceptional Parent* (February 1985): 14–19.

Architectural and Transportation Barriers Compliance Board. *Uniform Federal Accessibility Standards.* Washington, D.C.: ATBCB, 1984.

Arkenstone, Inc. *Arkenstone Reader with TrueScan.* Sunnyvale, Calif.: Arkenstone, 1989.

————. *Calera Recognition Systems.* Sunnyvale, Calif.: Arkenstone, 1989.

————. *What Is Arkenstone?* Sunnyvale, Calif.: Arkenstone, 1989.

Arthur, Julietta K. *Employment for the Handicapped.* New York: Abingdon Press, 1967.

Artic Technologies. *ARTIC CRYSTAL.* Troy, Mich.: AT, 1989.

————. *ARTIC D'LIGHT.* Troy, Mich.: AT, 1989.

————. *Artic ENCORE!* Troy, Mich.: AT, 1989.

————. *Artic Navigates the Channel.* Troy, Mich.: AT, 1989.

————. *Artic Turbo-Pedals.* Troy, Mich.: AT, 1989.

————. *Artic Vision.* Troy, Mich.: AT, 1989.

————. *SynPhonix.* Troy, Mich.: AT, 1989.

Bailey, Ian L. "The Aged Blind." *The Australian Journal of Optometry* (January 1975): 31–39.

Bankes, James L. Kennerley. *Clinical Ophthalmology.* New York: Churchill Livingstone, 1987.

Barnes, Broda O., and Lawrence Galton. *Hypothyroidism: The Unsuspected Illness.* New York: Thomas Y. Crowell Company, 1976.

Barraga, Natalie C. *Visual Handicaps and Learning.* Belmont, Calif.: Wadsworth Publishing Company Inc., 1976.

Bath, Patricia E. "Blindness Prevention Through the Programs of Community Ophthalmology in Developing Countries." In *Ophthalmology.* Vol. 2. Edited by K. Shimizu and J. Oosterhuis. Amsterdam: Excerpta Medica, 1979.

Begbie, G. Hugh. *Seeing and the Eye.* New York: Doubleday, 1973.

Berkeley Systems, Inc. *Corporate Background.* Berkeley, Calif.: BSI, 1989.

————. *inLARGE: The Software Magnifying Glass.* Berkeley, Calif.: BSI, 1989.

———. *inTOUCH: The Tactile Macintosh Screen.* Berkeley, Calif.: BSI, 1989.

———. *outSPOKEN: The Talking Macintosh Interface.* Berkeley, Calif.: BSI, 1989.

Berland, Theodore, and Richard A. Perritt, M.D. *Living With Your Eye Operation.* New York: St. Martin's Press, 1974.

Berlinski, Peter. "A Hidden Resource." *Worklife* (Fall 1988): 2.

Biklen, Douglas, and Robert Bogdan. "Media Portrayals of Disabled People: A Study in Stereotypes." *Interracial Books for Children Bulletin* 8, no. 6–7 (1977): 4–9.

"Bill of Rights for People with Disabilities." *Tips and Trends* 1, no. 6 (June–July 1989): 1.

BIT Corporation. *Winter 1989 Catalog, Edition #9.* Boston: BIT, 1989.

Bitter, James A. *Introduction to Rehabilitation.* St. Louis: C. V. Mosby Company, 1979.

Blacker, M. M., and D. R. Wekstein, eds. *Your Health After Sixty.* New York: E. P. Dutton, 1979.

Blau, Sheldon Paul, and Dodi Schultz. *Lupus: The Body Against Itself.* New York: Doubleday and Company, Inc., 1977.

Blinded Veterans Association. *BVA Fact Sheet.* Washington, D.C.: BVA, 1989.

———. *Alternatives for Blind or Visually Impaired Veterans.* Washington, D.C.: BVA, 1989.

Blodi, Frederick C. *Herpes Simplex Infections of the Eye.* New York: Churchill Livingstone, 1984.

Boardman, Louise S. *My Son Has Usher's Syndrome.* Baltimore: RP Foundation Fighting Blindness, 1985.

Bonfanti, Barbara H. "Effects of Training on Nonverbal and Verbal Behaviors of Congenitally Blind Adults." *Journal of Visual Impairment and Blindness* (January 1979): 1–9.

Bowe, Frank. *Jobs for Disabled People.* New York: Public Affairs Committee Inc., 1985.

———. "Recruiting Workers with Disabilities." *Worklife* (Summer 1989): 37–41.

Brady, Frank B. *A Singular View—The Art of Seeing With One Eye.* Annapolis, Md.: Frank B. Brady Publisher, 1985.

Braille Institute. *How to Help a Blind Person.* Los Angeles: BI, 1980.

———. *Track and Field Olympics.* Los Angeles: BI, 1989.

———. *When Glasses No Longer Help.* Los Angeles: BI, 1980.

Braille Sports Foundation. *Feeling Sports: February 1989.* Minneapolis: BSI, 1989.

———. *Feeling Sports: September–October 1989.* Minneapolis: BSI, 1989.

Braverman, Sydell. "The Psychological Roots of Attitudes Toward the Blind." *Attitudes Toward Blindness.* New York: American Foundation for the Blind, 1951.

Brock, Peter. *Love in the Lead.* New York: E. P. Dutton, 1954.

Brockhurst, Robert J. *Controversy in Ophthalmology.* Philadelphia: W. B. Saunders Company, 1977.

Brooks, Dennis L. *Don't Be Afraid of Cataracts.* Secaucus, N.J.: Arthur Henley, Lyle Stuart, 1978.

Brown, Bruce. "Supercharging Your Scanner." *PC Magazine* (March 28, 1989): 5.

Burde, Ronald M., Peter J. Savino and Jonathan D. Trobe. *Clinical Decisions in Neuro-Ophthalmology.* St. Louis: The C. V. Mosby Company, 1985.

Butler, Beverly. *Maggie By My Side.* New York: Dodd, Mead and Company, 1987.

Caird, F. I., and John Williamson, eds. *The Eye and It's Disorders in the Elderly.* Bristol: John Wright and Sons Ltd., 1986.

California State Health and Welfare Agency. *California State Plan for Rehabilitation Facilities Part I 1979–1984*. Sacramento, Calif.: CSHWA, 1984.

California State University, Northridge. *CSUN Assistive Technology Center*. Northridge, Calif.: CSUN, 1989.

———. Personal correspondence between Dr. Harry Murphy, Director of the Office of Disabled Student Services, and the writer. October 24, 1989.

Calne, R. Y. *The Oxford Companion to Medicine Volume II N–Z*. New York: Oxford University Press, 1986.

Carden, Robert G. "Vitamins for Healthier Eyes." *Let's LIVE* (September 1985): 10–11.

Carr, Ronald E., et al. *The Eye and Your Vision*. New York: National Association for Visually Handicapped, 1988.

Carroll Center for the Blind. *The Carroll Center for the Blind*. Newton, Mass.: CCB, 1989.

———. *Services for the Carroll Center for the Blind*. Newton, Mass.: CCB, 1989.

Carroll, Rev. Thomas J. "A Look at Aging." *The New Outlook* (April 1972): 97–103.

———. *Blindness*. Boston: Little, Brown and Company, 1961.

Cassel, Gary H., Michael D. Billig, and Harry G. Randall. *The Eye Book: A Complete Guide to Eye Disorders and Health*. Baltimore: Johns Hopkins University Press, 1998.

Cassie, Dhyan. *So Who's Perfect*. Scottdale, Pa.: Herald Press, 1984.

Cauwels, Janice M. *The Body Shop*. St. Louis: C. V. Mosby Company, 1986.

Cawood, Liz Tilton, ed. *WORDS: Work Oriented Rehabilitation Dictionary and Synonyms*. Seattle: Northwest Association of Rehabilitation Industries Inc., 1976.

The Center for the Partially Sighted. *Myths and Realities of Visual Impairment*. Santa Monica, Calif.: CPS, 1985.

———. *The Center for the Partially Sighted and You*. Santa Monica, Calif.: CPS, 1985.

———. *The CPS at a Glimpse*. Santa Monica, Calif.: CPS, 1987.

Chase, Allan. *The Truth About STD*. New York: William Morrow, 1983.

Chawla, Hector Bryson. *Essential Ophthalmology*. New York: Churchill Livingstone, 1981.

Chong, Curtis. "Speech Output for the IBM Personal Computer." *The Braille Monitor* (January 1986): 37–47.

Clark, Matt, Carl Robinson and Ingrid Wickelgren, "Interchangeable Parts." *Newsweek* (September 12, 1988): 61–63.

Clearinghouse on the Handicapped. *Programs for the Handicapped*. Washington, D.C.: CH, 1983.

———. *Pocket Guide to Federal Help for Individuals with Disabilities*. Washington, D.C.: CH, 1987.

Cohen, Jerome. "The Effects of Blindness on Children's Development." *Children* (January/February 1966): 23–27.

Computerized Books for the Blind. *Computerized Books for the Blind*. Missoula, Mont.: CBB, 1989.

Conte, Luca E. *Sheltered Employment Services and Programs*. Washington, D.C.: National Rehabilitation Information Center, 1983.

Cook, Paul F., Peter R. Dahl and Margaret Ann Gale. *Vocational Opportunities*. Salt Lake City, Utah: Olympus Publishing Company, 1978.

Cooley, Donald G. *After 40 Health and Medical Guide*. Des Moines, Iowa: Better Homes and Gardens Books, 1980.

Coombs, Jan. *Living With the Disabled: You Can Help*. New York: Sterling Publishing Co. Inc., 1984.

Corsaro, Maria, and Carole Korzeniowsky. *STD: A Commonsense Guide*. New York: St. Martin's Press, 1980.

Council for Exceptional Children. *Overview: 1988–89*. Reston, Va.: CEC, 1989.

County of Santa Clara: Social Services Agency. *Social Services Agency Guide*. San Jose, Calif.: SSA, 1989.

Cull, John G., and Richard E. Hardy. *Behavior Modification in Rehabilitation Settings*. Springfield, Ill.: Charles C. Thomas, 1974.

Cupak, K. "The Importance of Eye Camps in Underdeveloped Countries." In *Ophthalmology*. Vol. 2. Edited by K. Shimizu and J. Oosterhuis. Amsterdam: Excerpta Medica, 1979.

Curtis, Patricia. *Greff: The Story of a Guide Dog*. New York: E. P. Dutton, 1982.

Cutsworth, T. *The Blind in School and Society*. New York: American Foundation for the Blind Inc., 1951.

D'Amato, Robert, and Joan Snyder. *Macular Degeneration: The Latest Scientific Discoveries and Treatments for Preserving Your Sight*. New York: Walker & Company, 2000.

Davidoff, Jules B. *Differences in Visual Perception*. New York: Academic Press Inc., 1975.

Davidson, Margaret. *Louis Braille*. New York: Hastings House Publishers, 1971.

Department of Health and Human Services. *Section 504 of the Rehabilitation Act of 1973*. Washington, D.C.: DHHS, 1989.

Deur, Lynne. *Doers and Dreamers: Social Reformers of the Nineteenth Century*. Minneapolis: Lerner Publications Company, 1972.

DeVita, Vincent, et al., eds. *AIDS: Etiology, Diagnosis, Treatment, Prevention*. New York: J. B. Lippincott, 1985.

Dickman, Irving R. *What Can We Do About Limited Vision?* Public Affairs Pamphlet Number 491A, New York: Public Affairs Committee Inc., 1984.

Dickman, Irving R., and Sol Gordon. *Getting Help for a Disabled Child—Advice from Parents*. Public Affairs Pamphlet Number 615, New York: Public Affairs Committee Inc., 1983.

Dickey, Thomas W. "Meeting the Vocational Needs of the Older Blind Person." *The New Outlook* (May 1975): 218–225.

Dietl, Dick. "Operation Job Match Helping Fill the Worker Void." *Worklife* (January/February/March 1988): 10–11.

Discovery Blind Sports International. *Discovery Blind Sports International*. Kirkwood, Calif.: DBSI, 1989.

Dodds, Allan G., David D. Clark-Carter and C. Ian Howarth. "The Sonic Pathfinder: An Evaluation." *Journal of Visual Impairment and Blindness* (May 1984): 203–206.

Dudley, Rosemary, and Wade Rowland. *How to Find Relief from Migraine*. New York: Beaufort Books Inc., 1982.

Duke-Elder, Stewart, and Peter A. MacFaul. *System of Ophthalmology: Volume XIV: Injuries, Part 2 Non-Mechanical Injuries*. St. Louis: C. V. Mosby Company, 1972.

Dukeminier, Jesse. "Organ Donation: Legal Aspects." In *The Encyclopedia of Bioethics*, edited by Warren T. Reich. New York: Macmillan (1978): 1157–1159.

Duncan, John, ed., *Environmental Modifications for the Visually Impaired: A Handbook*. New York: American Foundation for the Blind, 1988.

Dyke, Peter J., Gunter Haase and Mark May. "Diagnosis and Care of Bell's Palsy." *Patient Care* (October 1988): 107–118.

Eden, John. *The Eye Book*. New York: Penguin Books, 1978.

Editors of Prevention Magazine. *Prevention's New Encyclopedia of Common Diseases.* Emmaus, Pa.: Rodale Press, 1984.

Eichel, Valerie J. "A Taxonomy for Mannerisms of Blind Children." *Journal of Visual Impairment and Blindness* (May 1979): 167–177.

Emiliani, P. L., ed. *Development of Electronic Aids for the Visually Impaired.* Boston: Dr. W. Junk Publishers, 1986.

Enabling Technologies Company. *The Marathon Brailler.* Stuart, Fla.: ETC, 1989.

———. *PED-30.* Stuart, Fla.: ETC, 1989.

———. *Romeo Braille Printer.* Stuart, Fla.: ETC, 1989.

———. *The TED-600.* Stuart, Fla.: ETC, 1989.

ERIC Clearinghouse on Handicapped and Gifted Children. *ERIC Digest: Selecting Software for Special Education Instruction.* Reston, Va.: ERIC, 1986.

———. *ERIC Digest: Visual Impairments.* Reston, Va.: ERIC, 1982.

———. *Research and Resources on Special Education: Abstract 13.* Reston, Va.: ERIC, 1987.

———. *Research and Resources on Special Education: Abstract 14.* Reston, Va.: ERIC, 1987.

———. *Research and Resources on Special Education: Abstract 19.* Reston, Va.: ERIC, 1988.

Esche, Jeanne, and Carol Griffin. *A Handbook for Parents of Deaf-Blind Children.* Lansing, Mich.: Michigan School for the Blind, 1980.

Esterman, Ben. *The Eye Book.* Arlington: Great Ocean Publishers, 1977.

Eye Bank Association of America. *Background Information on Eye Bank Association of America.* Washington, D.C.: EBAA, 1988.

———. *Questions Most Frequently Asked About Eye Donation and Corneal Transplantation.* Washington, D.C.: EBAA, 1988.

———. *A Summary of the Programs and Services of the Eye Bank Association of America.* Washington, D.C.: EBAA, 1988.

EyeCare Info.com. "Ocular Pharmacology." Available online. URL: http://www.eyecareinfo.com/professionals/ocular_pharmacology.shtml.

Faye, Eleanor, E. *Clinical Low Vision.* Boston: Little, Brown, 1984.

Featherstone, Helen. *A Difference in the Family.* New York: Basic Books Inc., 1980.

Feman, Stephen S., and Robert D. Reinicke, eds. *Handbook of Pediatric Ophthalmology.* New York: Grune & Stratton, 1978.

Ferguson, Dianne L. "Parent Advocacy Network." *Exceptional Parent* (March 1984): 41–45.

Ferrara, Peter J., ed. *Social Security.* Washington, D.C.: Cato Institute, 1985.

Finkelstein, Daniel. "Blindness and Disorders of the Eye." *The Braille Monitor* (December 1988): 578–579.

"First Lady's Thyroid to be Irradiated." *San Jose Mercury News,* 12 April 1989, pp. 2A.

Foley, Conn, and H. F. Pizer. *The Stroke Fact Book.* New York: Bantam Books, 1985.

Fonda, Gerald E. *Management of Low Vision.* New York: Thieme-Stratton Inc., 1981.

Foundation Fighting Blindness (the). "Clinical Trial Finds Antioxidants and Zinc Beneficial in Reducing Risk of Severe AMD." Available online. URL: http://www.blindness.org/html/science/wzinc.html.

———. "Foundation Hosts Important Stem Cell Meeting." Available online. URL: http://www.blindness.org/html/science/wstemcell.html. Posted November 2000.

———. "Gene Therapy Reverses Blindness in Dogs, Opens Possibility for Human Treatment Trials." Available online. URL: http://www.blindness.org/html/science/wdogcomments.html.

————. "Researchers Restore Vision in an Animal Model of Childhood Blindness." Available online. URL: http://www.blindness.org/html/science/rpe65rev.html.

————. "Usher Syndrome Gene Identified." Available online. URL: http://www.blindness.org/html/science/wusherwork.html.

Foundation for the Junior Blind. *Needs Assessment: California Services for Persons with Visual Impairments.* Los Angeles: FJB, 1987.

Fraiberg, S. *Insights from the Blind.* New York: Basic Books, 1977.

Frames, Robin. "Insight Into Eyesight." *MS Facts and Issues.* New York: National Multiple Sclerosis Society, 1985.

Freeman, Paul B. "Optical and Nonoptical Aids for Patients with Age-Related Macular Degeneration." *Sightsaving* 54, no. 1 (1985): 20–23.

Freese, Arthur S. *Cataracts and Their Treatment.* Public Affairs Pamphlet Number 545, New York: Public Affairs Pamphlets, 1977.

————. *The Bionic People Are Here.* New York: McGraw-Hill Book Company, 1979.

————. *The Miracle of Vision.* New York: Harper & Row, Publishers, 1977.

————. *Stroke: The New Hope and the New Help.* New York: Random House, 1980.

Freid, Jacob. "The Blind Senior Citizen's Needs." *The Braille Monitor* (March/April 1977): 110–112.

Froyd, Helen E. "Counseling Families of Severely Visually Handicapped Children." *The New Outlook* (June 1973): 251–257.

Gallin, John I., and Anthony S. Fauci, eds. *Acquired Immunodeficiency Syndrome (AIDS).* New York: Raven Press, 1985.

Galloway, N. R. *Common Eye Diseases and Their Management.* Berlin: Springer-Verlag, 1985.

Garrett, James F., and Edna S. Levine, eds. *Rehabilitation Practices with the Physically Disabled.* New York: Columbia University Press, 1973.

Geist, Chrisann Schiro, and William A. Calzaretta. *Placement Handbook for Counseling Disabled Persons.* Springfield, Ill.: Charles C. Thomas, 1982.

Gilbard, Jeffrey P. "Can My Eye Irritation Be Related to My Lupus?" *Lupus News* 8, no. 1 (1988): 2.

Gittinger Jr., John W. *Ophthalmology: A Clinical Introduction.* Boston: Little, Brown, 1984.

Gliedman, John, and William Roth. *The Unexpected Minority.* New York: Harcourt, Brace, Jovanovich, 1980.

Goldberg, Maxwell H., and John R. Swinton. *Blindness Research: The Expanding Frontiers.* University Park: Pennsylvania State University Press, 1969.

Goldenson, Robert M., ed. *Disability and Rehabilitation Handbook.* New York: McGraw-Hill Book Company, 1978.

Graedon, Joe, and Teresa Graedon. *The Graedon's People's Pharmacy For Older Adults.* New York: Bantam Books, 1988.

————. *The People's Pharmacy.* New York: St. Martin's Press, 1985.

Green, Charles. "Disabled Rights Bill Endorsed." *San Jose Mercury News.* 8 September 1989, pp. 1A.

Grover, John W. *VD: The ABC's.* Englewood Cliffs, N.J.: Prentice-Hall, 1971.

Guide Dog Foundation for the Blind Inc. *Guide Dog Foundation for the Blind Inc. Puppy Program.* Smithtown, New York: GDFB, 1989.

————. *Guide Dog Foundation for the Blind Inc. Training Program.* Smithtown, N.Y.: GDFB, 1989.

————. *The Guideway.* Smithtown, N.Y.: GDFB, 1989.

Guide Dogs for the Blind Inc. *Legislation Pertaining to Dog Guides in the United States (1970)*. San Rafael, Calif.: GDB, 1970.

———. *Fact Sheet*. San Rafael, Calif.: GDB, 1987.

Guiding Eyes for the Blind Inc. *Guiding Eyes for the Blind*. Yorktown Heights, N.Y.: GEB, 1987.

———. *Guiding Eyes for the Blind: The Pursuit of Independence*. Yorktown Heights, N.Y.: GEB, 1987.

Hadley School for the Blind. *Student Course Catalog 1988–1989*. Winnetka, Ill.: HSB, 1988.

Hagen, Dolores. *Microcomputer Resource Book for Special Education*. Reston, Va.: Reston Publishing Company Inc., 1984.

Hamilton, Helen Klusek, ed. *Professional Guide to Diseases, Second Edition*. Springhouse, Pa.: Springhouse Corporation, 1987.

Hamilton, Richard. *The Herpes Book*. Los Angeles: J. P. Tarcher Inc., 1980.

Harper, Forine Watson. "Gestures of the Blind." *Education of the Visually Handicapped* (Spring 1978): 14–20.

Haskins, James. *Who Are the Handicapped?* New York: Doubleday, 1978.

Havener, William H. *Ocular Pharmacology*. St. Louis: C. V. Mosby Company, 1970.

———. *Synopsis of Ophthalmology: The Ophthalmoscopy Book*. St. Louis: C. V. Mosby Company, 1984.

Keller, Helen. *Midstream*. Westport, Conn.: Greenpress Publishers, 1929.

Helen Keller International. *Facts About Helen Keller International*. New York: HKI, 1988.

———. Personal correspondence between Victoria Sheffield and the writer. August 14, 1989.

Helen Keller National Center for Deaf-Blind Youths and Adults. *Helen Keller National Center for Deaf-Blind Youths and Adults*. Sands Point, N.Y.: HKNC, 1988.

———. *Guidelines for Helping Deaf-Blind Persons*. Sands Point, N.Y.: HKNC, 1988.

Henkind, Paul, Martin Mayers, and Arthur Berger, eds. *Physicians' Desk Reference for Ophthalmology*. Oradell, N.J.: Medical Economics Company Inc., 1987.

Henter-Joyce Inc. *The Experts in Access Technology*. St. Petersburg, Fla.: HJI, 1989.

———. *Forum-Mate*. St. Petersburg, Fla.: HJI, 1989.

———. *JAWS*. St. Petersburg, Fla.: HJI, 1989.

Heppe, Cherie. *Of Dog Guides and White Canes*. Baltimore: National Federation of the Blind, 1986.

Herman, Scott C., ed. *Transportation Research Record 934*, Washington, D.C.: Transportation Research Board, National Research Council, 1983.

Hayes, Anthony D. "The Sonic Pathfinder: A New Electronic Travel Aid." *Journal of Visual Impairment and Blindness* (May 1984): 200–202.

Holleb, Arthur I., ed. *American Cancer Society Cancer Book*. New York: Doubleday and Company Inc., 1986.

Hoshmand, Lisa T. "Blindisms: Some Observations and Propositions." *Education of the Visually Handicapped* (May 1975): 56–59.

Howard, Ian P. *Human Visual Orientation*. New York: John Wiley, 1982.

Howe Press of Perkins School for the Blind. *Newsletter Summer 1987*. Watertown, Mass.: HP, 1987.

———. *Newsletter Summer 1988*. Watertown, Mass.: HP, 1988.

———. *Newsletter Winter 1987*. Watertown, Mass.: HP, 1987.

HumanWare, Inc. *Braille-n-Print*. Loomis, Calif.: HWI, 1989.

————. *ClearView.* Loomis, Calif.: HWI, 1989.

————. *Index Advanced.* Loomis, Calif.: HWI, 1989.

————. *Index Classic.* Loomis, Calif.: HWI, 1989.

————. *Index Domino.* Loomis, Calif.: HWI, 1989.

————. *KeyBraille.* Loomis, Calif.: HWI, 1989.

————. *KeyNote PC.* Loomis, Calif.: HWI, 1989.

————. *Mountbatten Brailler.* Loomis, Calif.: HWI, 1989.

————. *Mowat Sensor.* Loomis, Calif.: HWI, 1989.

————. *Sonicguide.* Loomis, Calif.: HWI, 1989.

————. *Speakwriter 2000.* Loomis, Calif.: HWI, 1989.

————. *Viewpoint.* Loomis, Calif.: HWI, 1989.

IBM Corporation. *Resource Guide for Persons with Vision Impairments.* Atlanta: IBM, 1989.

————. *Technology for Persons with Disabilities.* Atlanta: IBM, 1989.

Independent Living Aids Inc. *Can-Do Products.* Plainview, N.Y.: ILA, 1989.

————. *Portable Electronic Magnifying Viewers for People on the Go.* Plainview, N.Y.: ILA, 1989.

International Association of Lions Clubs. *Glaucoma.* Oak Brook, Ill.: IALC, 1987.

International Conference on the Education of the Deaf. *Deaf-blind Children and Their Education.* Rotterdam: University Press, 1971.

Jackson, Tom, and Paul Krantz. "Removing Everyday Barriers." *Better Homes and Gardens* (September 1988): 37–41.

Jacobbi, Marianne. "Battling Lyme Disease." *Family Circle Magazine* (July 25, 1989): 17–20.

James, John S. "CMV Retinitis—Ganciclovir, Foscarnet, and Other Treatments: Background, History, and Emerging Controversy." *AIDS Treatment News,* no. 71 (December 1988): 1–7.

Jampol, Lee M. "Lasers—Past, Present, and Future." *Sight-saving* 53, no. 4 (1984–85): 10–11.

Jenkins, William M., et al. *Rehabilitation of the Severely Disabled.* Dubuque, Iowa: Kendall/Hunt Publishing Company, 1976.

Jernigan, Kenneth. *Blindness: Is the Public Against Us?* Baltimore: National Federation of the Blind, 1975.

————. *Blindness: Of Visions and Vultures.* Baltimore: National Federation of the Blind, 1976.

————. *Blindness, Simplicity, Complexity, and the Public Mind.* Baltimore: National Federation of the Blind, 1982.

————. *Blindness: The Coming of the Third Generation.* Baltimore: National Federation of the Blind, 1986.

————. *Blindness: The Pattern of Freedom.* Baltimore: National Federation of the Blind, 1985.

————. *Disability and Visibility: Uncle Tom, Blind Tom, and Tiny Tim.* Baltimore: National Federation of the Blind, 1970.

————. "Facts You Should Know Concerning Disability Insurance." *The Braille Monitor* (June 1989): 362–364.

————. *Focus on the Education of Blind Children.* New York: National Federation of the Blind, 1988.

Job Accommodation Network. JAN. Morgantown, W. Va.: JAN, 1989.

————. *JAN Update.* Morgantown, W. Va.: JAN, 1989.

———. *Job Accommodation Network: Typical Questions.* Morgantown, W. Va.: JAN, 1989.

———. *Job Accommodation Network: A System that Works for the Employer.* Morgantown, W. Va.: JAN, 1989.

———. *Job Accommodation Network: A System that Works for the Job-Ready Person with a Disability.* Morgantown, W. Va.: JAN, 1989.

———. *Job Accommodation Network: A System that Works for the Rehabilitation Professional.* Morgantown, W. Va.: JAN, 1989.

Joffee, E. "Role of Electronic Travel Aids: Field Applications of the Russell Pathsounder." *Journal of Visual Impairment and Blindness* (October 1987): 389–390.

John-Hall, Annette. "Blindness Can't Stop These Athletes." *San Jose Mercury News,* 14 July 1989, pp. 1D.

Johnson, Eric W. *V.D.* New York: J.B. Lippincott Company, 1978.

Johnson, Kurt L. *Incentives and Disincentives in the Vocational Rehabilitation Process.* Washington D.C.: National Rehabilitation Information Center, 1983.

Johnson, Patty T. *Helen Keller: Girl From Alabama.* Huntsville, Ala.: Strode Publishers, 1980.

Jose, Randall T. *Understanding Low Vision.* New York: American Foundation for the Blind, 1983.

Kaplan, Elizabeth W., ed., *Transportation Research Record 1098.* Washington D.C.: Transportation Research Board, National Research Council, 1986.

Katz, Alfred H., and Knute Martin. *A Handbook of Services for the Handicapped.* Westport, Conn.: Greenwood Press, 1982.

Katz, Susan. *Empowering the Disabled.* HealthNet Reference Library. Columbus, Ohio: CompuServe, 1987.

Keith, C. Gregory. *Genetics and Ophthalmology.* London: Churchill Livingstone, 1978.

Keller, Helen. "My Dreams." *Century Magazine* 77, no. 1 (1908): 69–74.

———. *The World I Live In.* New York: Century Company, 1908.

Kelman, Charles D. *Cataracts: What You Must Know About Them.* New York: Crown Publishers Inc., 1982.

———. *Through My Eyes.* New York: Crown Publishers, 1985.

Kelley, Jerry D., ed. *Recreation Programming for Visually Impaired Children and Youth.* New York: American Foundation for the Blind, 1981.

Kendrick, Deborah. *Jobs to be Proud of: Profiles of Workers Who are Blind or Visually Impaired.* New York: American Foundation for the Blind Press, 1993.

Kestenbaum, Alfred. *Applied Anatomy of the Eye.* New York: Grune and Stratton, 1963.

Kimmins, Charles W. *Children's Dreams.* London: George Allen & Unwin Ltd., 1937.

Kirchner, Corinne, and Ziva Simon. "Blind and Visually Handicapped College Students—Part I: Estimated Numbers." *Journal of Visual Impairment and Blindness* (February 1984): 78–81.

Kirtley, Donald. *The Psychology of Blindness.* Chicago: Nelson-Hall, 1975.

Kirtley, Donald, and Katherine Cannistraci. "Dreams of the Visually Handicapped: Toward a Normative Approach." *AFB Research Bulletin #27* (April 1974): 111–133.

Kirtley, Donald, and Kenneth Sabo. "Aggression in the Dreams of Blind Women." *Journal of Visual Impairment and Blindness.* 77, no. 6 (June 1983): 269–270.

———. "Symbolism in the Dreams of the Blind." *International Journal of Rehabilitation Research.* 2, no. 2 (1979): 225–232.

Knight, John J. "Mannerisms in the Congenitally Blind Child." *The New Outlook* (November 1972): 297–301.

Koby, Melvin M. *The "Eyes" Have It—The Eyes and Lupus.* San Jose, Calif.: Bay Area Lupus Foundation, 1981.

Koek, Karin E., Susan B. Martin, and Annette Novallo, eds. "American Association of the Deaf-Blind." *Encyclopedia of Associations,* 23rd ed. Detroit: Gale Research Inc., 1989.

Koestler, Frances A. *The Unseen Minority.* New York: David McKay Company Inc., 1976.

Kornzweig, Abraham L. "Progress in the Prevention of Blindness Among the Aged." *The New Outlook* (September 1971): 210–213.

Kozin, Franklin. *General Clinical Overview of Lupus.* San Jose, Calif.: Bay Area Lupus Foundation, 1986.

Krames Communications. *A Guide to Eye Safety.* Daly City: Kans., 1987.

Kraus, Lewis E. "Disability and Work." *Worklife* (Fall 1989): 37–39.

Kreisler, Nancy, and Jack Kreisler. *Catalog of Aids for the Disabled.* New York: McGraw-Hill, 1982.

Kubler-Ross, Elisabeth. *On Death and Dying.* New York: MacMillan Publishing Co. Inc., 1969.

Kugelmass, J. Alvin. *Louis Braille.* New York: Julian Messner, 1951.

Kuklin, Susan. *Mine for a Year.* New York: Coward-McCann Inc., 1984.

Kwitko, Marvin L., and Frank J. Weinstock. *Geriatric Ophthalmology.* New York: Grune & Stratton Inc., 1985.

Lance, James W. *Migraine and Other Headaches.* New York: Scribner's, 1986.

Langston, Deborah P. *Living With Herpes.* New York: Doubleday, 1983.

Lash, Joseph P. *Helen and Teacher.* New York: Dell, 1980.

Lassiter, Robert A., et al., eds. *Vocational Evaluation, Work Adjustment, and Independent Living for Severely Disabled People.* Springfield, Ill.: Charles C. Thomas, 1983.

Lauer, Harvey, and Leonard Mowinski. *Computer Aids for the Visually Impaired.* HealthNet Reference Library. Columbus, Ohio: Compuserve, 1989.

———. *Recommending Computers for the Visually Impaired: A Moving Target or a Losing War?* HealthNet Library. Columbus, Ohio: CompuServe, 1989.

Lavin, John H. *Stroke: From Crisis to Victory.* New York: Franklin Watts, 1985.

Lee, Yvonne, "Lyon Makes Text Bigger Now Without Add-In Card." *InfoWorld* (July 10, 1989): 24.

Leflar, Robert B., and Helen Lillie. *Cataracts.* Washington, D.C.: Public Citizen's Health Research Group, 1981.

"Legal Services Corporation." *The Guide to American Law.* Vol. 7. Washington, D.C.: Legal Services Corporation (1984): 132–133.

Lehrer, Steven. *Alternative Treatments for Cancer.* Chicago: Nelson-Hall, 1979.

Leontief, Wassily, "The New Technology: How Did We Get Here, Where Are We Going?" *The Future of Work for Disabled People: Employment and the New Technology.* New York: American Foundation for the Blind, 1986.

Leslie, G. Robert, ed. *Supportive Personnel in Rehabilitation Centers: Current Practices and Future Needs.* Pittsburg: Association of Rehabilitation Centers Inc., 1967.

Lesnoff-Caravaglia, Gavi, eds. *Aging and the Human Condition.* New York: Human Services Press Inc., 1982.

Lindenberg, Richard, Frank B. Walsh, and Joel G. Sacks. *Neuropathology of Vision.* Philadelphia: Lea and Febiger, 1973.

Lions Clubs International. Fact Sheet. Oak Brook, Ill.: LCI, 1989.

Lions Clubs History. Oak Brook, Ill.: LCI, 1989.

Lions International Helen Keller Day. Oak Brook, Ill.: LCI, 1987.

Lions Dog Guide Schools. Oak Brook, Ill.: LCI, 1988.

Llyod, Judy H. "Use of Telescopic Aids for Vocational Purposes." *Journal of Visual Impairment and Blindness* (May 1984): 216–220.

Lowenfeld, Berthold. "The Social Impact of Blindness upon the Individual." *New Outlook for the Blind* 58, no. 4 (April 1964): 273–277.

Luckiesh, M. *Visual Illusions.* New York: Dover Publications Inc., 1965.

Lukoff, Irving, et al. *Attitudes Toward Blind Persons.* New York: American Foundation for the Blind, 1972.

Lunt, Suzanne. *A Handbook for the Disabled.* New York: Scribner's, 1982.

Lyme Borreliosis Foundation, Inc. *Lyme Disease: A Serious Health Threat.* Tolland, Conn.: LBF, 1989.

Lyon Computer Discourse Limited. *Lyon Large Print Program.* North Vancouver, B.C.: LCD, 1989.

Lyon, John. Personal Correspondence. November 9, 1989.

MacDonald, A. B. "Lyme Disease: A Neuro-ophthalmologic View." *Journal of Clinical Neuro-ophthalmology* 7, no. 4 (1987): 10.

Mainstream Inc. *Putting Disabled People in Your Place: Focus on Blind and Vision-Impaired Individuals.* Washington, D.C.: MI, 1985.

Malcolm, Andrew H. "Is There Too Little Order in the Transplant Business?" *The New York Times,* 13 April 1986.

Malikin, David, and Herbert Rusalem, eds. *Vocational Rehabilitation of the Disabled: An Overview.* New York: University Press, 1969.

Malone, Mary. *Annie Sullivan.* New York: G. P. Putnam's Sons, 1971.

Maloney, William F., Lincoln Grindle and Donald E. Pearcy. *Consumer Guide to Modern Cataract Surgery.* Fallbrook, Calif.: Lasenda Publishers, 1986.

Mangold, Sally. Personal Interview. San Francisco, Calif.: July 13, 1989.

Mann, Richard C. *Diagnosis: Cerebral Palsy.* Oklahoma City: United Cerebral Palsy of Oklahoma, 1986.

Manninen, Diane L., and Roger Evans. "Public Attitudes and Behavior Regarding Organ Donation." *Journal of American Medical Association* 253, no. 21 (June 7, 1985): 3111–3115.

Martin, Paul. "Medicine's New Superstar: The Atom." *The Lion* (February 1989): 14–16.

Massengill, R. K. *Supersight: The Lens Implant Miracle.* Boston: Health Institute Press, 1986.

Maumenee, Irene H. "Discoveries in Genetic Eye Disease." *Sightsaving* 53, no. 4 (1984–85): 14–15.

Maurer, Marc. *Preparation and the Critical Nudge.* Baltimore: National Federation of the Blind, 1988.

May, Michael, and Ronald Salviolo. *Blind Alpine Skiing and Racing.* Kirkwood, Calif.: Kirkwood Instruction of Blind Skiers, 1986.

McGarry, Barbara D. "Legislative Advocacy for the Blind in America: The Historical Involvement of Consumers and Professionals." In *Yearbook of the AERBVI 1983.* Alexandria, Va.: The Association for Education and Rehabilitation of the Blind and Visually Impaired (1983): 31–39.

McGlen, Brian. Pfizer International. Telephone interview. May 5, 1989.

McInnes, J. M., and J. A. Treffry. *Deaf-Blind Infants and Children.* Toronto: University of Toronto Press, 1982.

Meehan, Michaelann. RP Foundation. Telephone interview. May 11, 1989.

Meighan, Thomas. *An Investigation of the Self Concept of Blind and Visually Handicapped Adolescents.* New York: American Foundation for the Blind, 1971.

Mendelsohn, Steven B. *Financing Adaptive Technology.* New York: Smiling Interface, 1987.

Menitove, Jay E., and Jerry Kolins, eds. *AIDS.* Arlington: American Association of Blood Banks, 1986.

Meredith, Travis A. *The Eye: Disease, Diagnosis, Treatment.* Bowie, Md.: Robert J. Brady Company, 1975.

Miller, Barbara S., and William H. Miller. "Extinguishing 'Blindisms': A Paradigm for Intervention." *Education of the Visually Handicapped* (Spring 1976): 7–14.

Miller, David. *Ophthalmology: The Essentials.* Boston: Houghton Mifflin Professional Publishing, 1979.

Miller, Stephen J. H. *Parson's Diseases of the Eye.* New York: Churchill Livingstone, 1978.

Mitchell, Joyce Slayton. *See Me More Clearly.* New York: Harcourt, Brace, Jovanovich, 1980.

Moore, Thomas, Eye Bank Association of America. Telephone interview. March 6, 1989.

Morain, Claudia. "First Lady Slimmer, But Illness Isn't Worth It." *San Jose Mercury News,* 1 April 1989, pp. 3C.

Morris, Ian. "Technology and Disabled People: A Global View." *The Future of Work for Disabled People: Employment and the New Technology.* New York: American Foundation for the Blind, 1986.

Moses, Howard. "Americans with Disabilities Act—1989: Extending Civil Rights Protection." *NARIC Quarterly* 2, no. 2 (Summer 1989): 1–13.

Mueller, Conrad G., and Mae Rudolph. *Light and Vision.* New York: Time-Life Books, 1972.

Mullen, Peggy Boucher. *Consumer Guide to Prescription Drugs.* Lincolnwood, Ill.: Publications, International, 1987.

Munna, Raymond. *As I See It: Radial Keratotomy Before, During, and After Surgery.* Metairie, La.: Granite Publishers, 1985.

Murphy, Jo Anne. *How Does a Blind Person Get Around?* New York: American Foundation for the Blind, 1988.

Myers, Lawrence. *Living with MS.* Healthnet Library. Columbus, Ohio: CompuServe, 1988.

Murray, Thomas H. "The Gift of Life Must Always Remain a Gift." *Discover* (March 1986): 90–92.

Nash, David T. *Coronary! Prediction and Prevention.* New York: Scribner's, 1978.

National Alliance for Eye and Vision Research. "The Demographics of Eye and Vision Disorders." Available online. URL: http://www.eyeresearch.org/naevr/demographics.html.

———. "Age-Related Macular Degeneration: Questions and Answers." Available online. URL: http://www.eyeresearch.org/naevr/amd_qa.html.

———. "Age-Related Macular Degeneration: Facts and Figures." Available online. URL: http://www.eyeresearch.org/naevr/amd_ff.html.

National Association for Parents of the Visually Impaired. *Awareness: First Quarter.* Camden, N.Y.: NAPVI, 1989.

National Association for Visually Handicapped. *Classification of Impaired Vision.* New York: NAVH, 1973.

———. *Every Low Vision Patient Should Know* . . New York: NAVH, 1985.

———. *Fact Sheet.* New York: NAVH, 1985.

———. *Family Guide.* New York: NAVH, 1980.

———. *Guide to Visual Aids and Illumination.* New York: NAVH, 1986.

———. *The Heartbreak of Being "A Little Bit Blind!"* New York: NAVH, 1982.

———. *Problems of the Partially Seeing.* New York: NAVH, 1985.

National Braille Association. *National Braille Association.* HealthNet Reference Library. Columbus, Ohio: Compuserve 1989.

National Eye Institute (The). "Glaucoma Awareness Month Emphasizes Treatments that Reduce Side Effects, Help Save Vision." Available online. URL: http://www.nei.nih.gov/news/121300.htm. Posted December 13, 2001.

———. "New Eye Disease Treatment May Improve Patients' Quality of Life." Available online. URL: http://www.nei.nih.gov/news/6_21_99.htm. Posted June 21, 1999.

———. "Help Now Available for People with Low Vision. New Program Targets 1 in 20 Americans." Available online. URL: http://www.nei.nih.gov/news/1099.htm. Posted October 19, 1999.

———. "Blacks, Whites Benefit from Different Surgical Glaucoma Treatments." Available online. URL: http://www.nei.nih.gov/news/pr798.htm. Posted July 6, 1998.

———. "Antiviral Drug Sharply Reduces Return of Herpes of the Eye." Available online. URL: http://www.nei.nih.gov/news/hedsII.htm. Posted July 29, 1998.

———. "Life With Low Vision: A Report on Qualitative Research Among People With Low Vision and Their Caregivers." Available online. URL: http://www.nei.nih.gov/nehep/execsum.htm. Posted June 1997.

———. "New Treatment for Eye Disease Reduces Need for Strong Drugs." Available online. URL: http://www.nei.nih.gov/news/newtreatment.htm. Posted May 27, 1997.

National Eye Research Foundation. *The National Eye Research Foundation.* Northbrook, Ill.: NERF, 1988.

National Federation of the Blind. *Do You Know a Blind Person?* New York: NFB, 1988.

———. *What Is the National Federation of the Blind?* New York: NFB, 1988.

National Industries for the Blind. *National Industries for the Blind.* Wayne, N.J.: NFB, 1989.

National Information Center for Handicapped Children and Youth. *General Information about Handicaps and People with Handicaps.* Washington, D.C.: NICHCY, 1982.

National Institute on Disability and Rehabilitation Research. *Data on Disability from the National Health Interview Survey, 1983–85.* Washington, D.C.: NIDRR, 1988.

———. *Disability Statistics Bulletin, No. 1, Spring 1988.* Washington, D.C.: NIDRR, 1988.

National Institute of Handicapped Research. *Rehab Brief: Disabled Americans: Self Perceptions.* Washington, D.C.: NIHR, 1987.

———. *Rehab Brief: Sports for Disabled Individuals.* Washington, D.C.: NIHR, 1981.

———. *Rehab Brief: Works Disincentives.* Washington, D.C.: NIHR, 1980.

———. *Rehab Brief: Sensory Aids for Visually Impaired Clients.* Washington, D.C.: NIHR, 1987.

National Multiple Sclerosis Society. *What is Multiple Sclerosis?* New York: NMSS, 1987.

National Rehabilitation Association. *Technology and Employment of Persons with Disabilities.* Alexandria, Va.: NRA, 1989.

National Rehabilitation Information Center. *Consumerism and Advocacy in Vocational Rehabilitation.* Silver Spring, Md.: NARIC, 1983.

———. *NARIC Guide to Disability and Rehabilitation Periodicals.* Silver Spring, Md.: NARIC, 1989.

———. *REHABDATA.* Silver Spring, Md.: NARIC, 1989.

National Society to Prevent Blindness. *AMD.* New York: NSPB, 1985.

———. *Annual Report.* New York: NSPB, 1988.

———. *Cataract.* New York: NSPB, 1986.

———. *Diabetic Retinopathy.* New York: NSPB, 1986.

———. *Facts and Figures: Adult Eye Problems.* New York: NSPB, 1980.

———. *Glaucoma . . . Sneak Thief of Sight.* New York: NSPB, 1985.

———. *The Sight Saving People.* New York: NSPB, 1987.

———. *1987 Sports and Recreational Eye Injuries.* New York: NSPB, 1987.

———. *Vision Problems in the U.S.: Facts and Figures.* New York: NSPB, 1980.

Neal, Helen. *Low Vision.* New York: Simon & Shuster, 1987.

Nelson, Eugene C., and Ellen Roberts, Jeannette Simmons and William A. Tisdale, *Medical and Health Guide for People Over Fifty.* Glenview, Ill.: Scott, Foresman and Company, 1986.

"New Cell-transplant Operation May Eventually Be Able to Treat Blindness." *San Jose Mercury News,* 9 September 1989, pp. 19A.

Newell, Frank W. *Ophthalmology: Principles and Concepts.* St. Louis: C. V. Mosby Company, 1982.

Newington Children's Hospital. *ABLEDATA.* Newington, Conn.: NCH, 1989.

———. *ABLEDATA Printout.* Newington, Conn.: NCH, 1989.

New York State Office of Advocate for the Disabled. *What Makes Disabled People Disabled?* Albany, N.Y.: NYOAD, 1982.

Noir Medical Technologies. *Noir: A Chemical Sunglass.* South Lyon, Mich.: NMT, 1985.

Northern California Society to Prevent Blindness. *Coping with Sight Loss in Northern California.* San Francisco: NCSPB, 1989.

O'Brien, Robert, and Morris Chafetz. *The Encyclopedia of Alcoholism.* New York: Facts On File Publications, 1982.

O'Bryant, Tom. "Facts About Hiring People with Disabilities." *Worklife* (Fall 1988): 8–10.

Oi, Walter Y., and William F. Gallagher. "Attitudes Toward Employment, Technology and Independence: Introductory Remarks." *The Future of Work for Disabled People: Employment and the New Technology.* New York: American Foundation for the Blind, 1986.

Opteq Vision Systems. *Opteq II Typing System.* Brookfield, Wisc.: OVS, 1989.

———. *Opteq IV.* Brookfield, Wisc.: OVS, 1989.

———. *Opteq V.* Brookfield, Wisc.: OVS, 1989.

———. *Opteq VFF.* Brookfield, Wisc.: OVS, 1989.

————. *Opteq Vision Systems*. Brookfield, Wisc.: OVS, 1989.

Orlansky, Michael D. *Mainstreaming the Visually Impaired Child*. Camden, N.Y.: National Association for Parents of the Visually Impaired Inc., 1989.

Ottoson, David, and Semir Zeki. *Central and Peripheral Mechanisms of Color Vision*. London: Macmillan Press Ltd., 1985.

Owen, Mary Jane. "Hammers, Saws and Obligations: The Control of Specialized Tools in a Competitive Marketplace." *Worklife* (Spring 1989): 30–32.

Pagon, Roberta A. "Retinitis Pigmentosa." *Survey of Ophthalmology* 33, no. 3 (November–December 1988): 137–153.

"Parental Leave on Line." *NAPVI Awareness* (Third Quarter 1987): 5.

Parr, John Cuthbert. *Introduction to Ophthalmology*. New York: Oxford University Press, 1978.

Perkins School for the Blind. *1987 Annual Report*. Watertown, Mass.: PSB, 1987.

————. *Perkins' Programs*. Watertown, Mass.: PSB, 1988.

Perry, Lewis C. "Howe, S.G." *McGraw-Hill Encyclopedia of World Biography* 5 (1973): 378–379.

Pfaffenberger, Clarence J., et al. *Guide Dogs for the Blind: Their Selection, Development, and Training*. New York: Elsevier Scientific Publishing Company, 1976.

Phillips, Calbert I. *Basic Clinical Ophthalmology*. London: Pitman Publishers Limited, 1984.

Pimentel, Albert. *Handling the Upper Secondary and College Usher's* Syndrome Student. Baltimore: RP Foundation Fighting Blindness, 1976.

Pinckney, Cathey and Edward R. *The Patient's Guide to Medical Tests*. New York: Facts On File Publications, 1982.

President's Committee on Employment of People With Disabilities. *Annual Work Plan 1989*. Washington, D.C.: PCEPD, 1989.

————. *Disabled Adults in America*. Washington, D.C.: PCEPD, 1985.

————. *People with Disabilities in Our Nation's Job Training Partnership Act Programs*. Washington, D.C.: PCEPD, 1987.

————. *Ready, Willing, and Available*. Washington, D.C.: PCEPD, 1989.

————. *This is the President's Committee*. Washington, D.C.: PCEPD, 1988.

Price, Ira Marc, and Linda Comac. Coping with Macular Degeneration: *A Guide for Patients and Families to Understand and Living With Degenerative Vision Disorder*. New York: Putnam, 2000.

Pritikin, Roland I. "Eyeglasses." *Groliers Academic American On-Line Encyclopedia*. Columbus, Ohio: Grolier Electronic Publishing, 1988.

Raised Dot Computing Inc. *Raised Dot Computing*. Madison, Wisc.: RDC, 1989.

Read, Leah Fowler. "An Examination of the Social Skills of Blind Kindergarten Children." *Education of the Visually Handicapped* (Winter 1989): 142–155.

Recording for the Blind. *Recording for the Blind: A Service to People*. Princeton, N.J.: RB, 1986.

————. *Recording for the Blind: How the Service Works*. Princeton, N.J.: RB, 1986.

————. *What is Recording for the Blind?* Princeton, N.J.: RB, 1986.

Retinitis Pigmentosa Foundation Fighting Blindness. *Answers to Your Questions About Retinitis Pigmentosa*. Baltimore: RPFFB, 1983.

————. *Answers to Your Questions About Usher's Syndrome*. Baltimore: RPFFB, 1988.

————. *Backgrounder: Usher's Syndrome*. Baltimore: RPFFB, 1988.

————. *Explore the Bright Side of Darkness*. Baltimore: RPFFB, 1988.

————. *Night Vision Aid Fact Sheet*. Baltimore: RPFFB, 1987.

————. Personal correspondence between Michaelann R. Meehan. Information and Referral Coordinator, and the winter. 6 July 1989.

Reynolds, James D. *Amblyopia*. HealthNet Reference Library. Columbus, Ohio: CompuServe, 1989.

————. *Cataracts*. HealthNet Reference Library. Columbus, Ohio: CompuServe, 1989.

————. *Cataract Surgery*. HealthNet Reference Library. Columbus, Ohio: CompuServe, 1989.

————. *Color Blindness*. HealthNet Reference Library. Columbus, Ohio: CompuServe, 1989.

————. *Corneal Transplant*. HealthNet Reference Library. Columbus, Ohio: CompuServe, 1989.

————. *Diabetic Retinopathy*. HealthNet Reference Library. Columbus, Ohio: CompuServe, 1989.

————. *Eye Care Professionals*. HealthNet Reference Library. Columbus, Ohio: CompuServe, 1989.

————. *Glaucoma*. HealthNet Reference Library. Columbus, Ohio: CompuServe, 1989.

————. *Glaucoma Surgery*. HealthNet Reference Library. Columbus, Ohio: CompuServe, 1989.

————. *Hypertensive Retinopathy*. HealthNet Reference Library. Columbus, Ohio: CompuServe, 1989.

————. *Lasers in Ophthalmology*. HealthNet Reference Library. Columbus, Ohio: CompuServe, 1989.

————. *Miscellaneous Neurological Disorders*. HealthNet Reference Library. Columbus, Ohio: CompuServe, 1989.

————. *Nasolacrimal System*. HealthNet Reference Library. Columbus, Ohio: CompuServe, 1989.

————. *Ocular Herpes*. HealthNet Reference Library. Columbus, Ohio: CompuServe, 1989.

————. *Ocular Trauma (Eye Injury)*. HealthNet Reference Library. Columbus, Ohio: CompuServe, 1989.

————. *Orbital Cellulitis*. HealthNet Reference Library. Columbus, Ohio: CompuServe, 1989.

————. *Radial Keratotomy*. HealthNet Reference Library. Columbus, Ohio: CompuServe, 1989.

————. *Refractive Errors*. HealthNet Reference Library. Columbus, Ohio: CompuServe, 1989.

————. *Retinal Detachment*. HealthNet Reference Library. Columbus, Ohio: CompuServe, 1989.

————. *Retinal Detachment Surgery*. HealthNet Reference Library. Columbus, Ohio: CompuServe, 1989.

————. *Retinitis Pigmentosa.*HealthNet Reference Library. Columbus, Ohio: CompuServe, 1989.

————. *Strabismus*. HealthNet Reference Library. Columbus, Ohio: CompuServe, 1989.

————. *Strabismus Surgery*. HealthNet Reference Library. Columbus, Ohio: CompuServe, 1989.

————. *Uveitis*. HealthNet Reference Library. Columbus, Ohio: CompuServe, 1989.

Rhode, Stephen J., and Stephen P. Ginsberg, eds. *Ophthalmic Technology*. New York: Raven Press, 1987.

Rice, Mary. *Medications In Lupus Therapy*. San Jose, Calif.: Bay Area Lupus Foundation, 1983.

Rivlin, Barbara Pogul. "Recent Study Compares Employment Trends." *NARIC Quarterly* 2, no. 2 (Fall 1989): 1, 8–10.

Roehrig, Arthur. *Living with Usher's Syndrome*. Baltimore: RP Foundation Fighting Blindness, 1985.

Roth, Wendy Carol. "Let Us Work!" *Parade Magazine*, 17 September 1989, p. 16.

Rudrud, Eric H., et al. *Proactive Vocational Habilitation*. Baltimore: Paul H. Brookes Publishing Company, 1984.

Sabo, Kenneth, and Donald Kirtley. "Objects and Activities in the Dreams of the Blind." *International Journal of Rehabilitation Research* 5, no. 2 (1982): 241–242.

Sachsenweger, Rudolf. *The Illustrated Handbook of Ophthalmology*. London: Wright PSG, 1984.

San Francisco Lighthouse for the Blind. *At Ease!* San Francisco: SFLB, 1982.

Saper, Joel R., and Kenneth R. Magee. *Freedom from Headaches*. New York: Simon & Shuster, 1981.

Sargent, Jean Vieth. *An Easier Way*. New York: Walker & Company, 1981.

Sarno, John E., and Martha Taylor Sarno. *Stroke: A Guide for Patients and Their Families*. New York: McGraw-Hill Book Company, 1969.

Scadden, Lawrence. "The Changing Workplace: View from a Disabled Technologist." *The Future of Work for Disabled People: Employment and the New Technology*. New York: American Foundation for the Blind, 1986.

Scholl, Geraldine T. *Foundations of Education for Blind and Visually Handicapped Children and Youth*. New York: American Foundation for the Blind Inc., 1986.

Schweitzer, N. M. J., ed. *Ophthalmology*. Amsterdam: Excerpta Medica, 1982.

Scoblionkov, Deborah. "Blindness Isn't a Handicap—It's a Nuisance." *McCall's* (October 1989): 49–52.

Scott, Eileen P. *Your Visually Impaired Student*. Baltimore: University Park Press, 1982.

Scott, Neil. Personal interview. Northridge, Calif.: March 10, 1989.

Seeing Eye Inc. A Digest of Legislation Relating to Travel with Dog Guides in the United States and Canada. Morristown, N.J.: SEI, 1988.

———. *Can a Seeing Eye Dog Help You or Someone You Know?* Morristown, N.J.: SEI, 1989.

———. *Q and A: Facts About the Seeing Eye*. Morristown, N.J.: SEI, 1980.

———. *The Seeing Eye*. Morristown, N.J.: SEI, 1980.

———. *The Seeing Eye Has a Scientific Breeding Station*. Morristown, N.J.: SEI, 1989.

———. *The Seeing Eye, How It Started*. Morristown, N.J.: SEI, 1989.

Seeing Technologies Inc. *The SEETEC Systems*. Minneapolis: STI, 1989.

Sensory Aids Foundation. *Annual Program Report, 1988*. Palo Alto, Calif.: SAF, 1988.

———. *Doing the Job is Easy. The Hard Part is Getting It!* Palo Alto, Calif.: SAF, 1989.

———. *SAF Fact Sheet*. Palo Alto, Calif.: SAF, 1989.

Shafto, Marjorie, and Gerald L. Hunt. *Every Woman's Guide to the Body at 40*. New York: Perigee Books, 1987.

Sherman, Spencer E. *A Consumer's Guide to Contact Lenses*. New York: The Dial Press, 1982.

Shields, M. Bruce. "Major Advances in Glaucoma Therapy." *Sightsaving* 53, no. 4 (1984–85): 6–11.

Shimizu, Koichi, and Jendo A. Oosterhuis. *Ophthalmology*. Vol. 1. Amsterdam: Excerpta Medica, 1979.

Sholton, David B. *The Dry Eye Syndrome*. San Jose, Calif.: Bay Area Lupus Foundation, 1981.

"Shopping Bag." *NAPVI Awareness* (First Quarter 1989): 2–7.

Shulman, Julius. *Cataracts*. New York: Simon & Shuster, New York 1984.

———. *No More Glasses*. New York: Simon & Shuster, 1987.

Sickle Cell Anemia Research and Education, Inc. *Facts About Sickle Cell Anemia*. Oakland, Calif.: SCARE, 1977.

Silverman, Harold M., and Gilbert I. Simon. *The Pill Book*. New York: Bantam Books, 1979.

Skurzynski, Gloria. *Bionic Parts for People*. New York: Four Winds Press, 1978.

Smith, Eleanor. *Earning Power*. HealthNet Reference Library. Columbus, CompuServe, 1989.

Smith, Elizabeth Simpson. *A Guide Dog Goes to School*. New York: William Morrow, 1987.

Smith-Kettlewell Eye Research Institute. *The Smith-Kettlewell Eye Research Institute*. San Francisco: SKERI, 1989.

———. *The Smith-Kettlewell Rehabilitation Engineering Center: Annual Report of Progress*. San Francisco: SKERI, 1987.

———. *The Smith-Kettlewell Rehabilitation Engineering Center: Annual Report of Progress*. San Francisco: SKERI, 1988.

Sobel, David S., and Tom Ferguson. *The People's Book of Medical Tests*. New York: Summit Books, 1985.

Sommer, A. *Field Guide to the Detection and Control of Xerophthalmia*. Geneva: World Health Organization, 1982.

Sperber, Al. *Out of Sight*. Boston: Little, Brown and Company, 1976.

Staff of Ready Reference Press. *Directory of Information Resources for the Handicapped*. Santa Monica, Calif.: Ready Reference Press, 1980.

Staff of Peninsula Center for the Blind. *The First Steps*. Palo Alto, Calif.: Peninsula Center for the Blind, 1980.

Stark, Walter J. *Cataracts: A Guide for Patients*. Wall Township, N.J.: H I N, Inc., 1997.

State of California Department of Rehabilitation. *Business Enterprise Training Program*. Sacramento, Calif.: CDR, 1983.

———. *Regulations: Business Enterprise Program for the Blind*. Sacramento, Calif.: CDR, 1983.

Stephens, John W. *Understanding Diabetes*. Beaverton, Oreg.: The Touchstone Press, 1987.

Summers, Laureen. "Reimbursing Adaptive Technology." *NARIC Quarterly* 2, no. 4 (Winter 1989): 1, 7–11, 17.

Swail, J., and E. L. Bryenton. "Sensory 6: An Electronic Travel Aid for Blind Persons." *Journal of Visual Impairment and Blindness* (May 1987): 217–219.

Tait, Perla. "Play and the Intellectual Development of Blind Children." *The New Outlook* (December 1972): 361–369.

Talal, Norman, and Dan Lechay. *Are You Aware of Lupus?* San Jose, Calif.: Bay Area Lupus Foundation, 1989.

Talking Computers Inc. *NEWSBITS*. Falls Church, Va.: TCI, 1989.

———. *NEWSBITS Auditory Magazine: February 1989*. Falls Church, Va.: TCI, 1989.

———. *NEWSBITS Auditory Magazine: June 1989*. Falls Church, Va.: TCI, 1989.

————. *News From Talking Computers, Inc.* Falls Church, Va.: TCI, 1989.

————. *Talk-To-Me Tutorials.* Falls Church, Va.: TCI, 1989.

Taylor, Robert B. *Feeling Alive After 65.* New York: Arlington House Publishers, 1973.

Telephone Pioneers of America. *Pioneering: The Service Connection.* New York: TPA, 1986.

Telesensory Systems, Inc. *Focus on Technology.* Mountain View, Calif.: TSI, 1989.

————. *LapVert.* Mountain View, Calif.: TSI, 1989.

————. *Navigator.* Mountain View, Calif.: TSI, 1989.

————. *Optacon II.* Mountain View, Calif.: TSI, 1989.

————. *See What You've Been Missing.* Mountain View, Calif.: TSI, 1989.

————. *Voyager.* Mountain View, Calif.: TSI, 1989.

Thackray, John. "The High Cost of Workplace Eye Trauma." *Sightsaving* 51, no. 1 (1982): 19–22.

Thijssen, J. M., and A. M. Verbeek, eds. *Ultrasonography in Ophthalmology.* Boston: Dr. W. Junk Publishers, 1981.

Transceptor Technologies, Inc. *Introducing the Personal Companion.* Ann Arbor, Mich.: TTI, 1989.

Transcript of Phil Donahue Show. *"What They Did for Love."* 13 February 1989, Mutimedia Entertainment, New York.

Trevor-Roper, P. D. and P. V. Curran. *The Eye and Its Disorders.* Oxford, U.K.: Blackwell Scientific Publications, 1984.

Turriff, Tod W. National Society to Prevent Blindness. Telephone interview. 16 November 1989.

"UCLA Finds Gene Tied to Blindness in Mice." *San Jose Mercury News,* 15 December 1989, pp. 17A.

United Cerebral Palsy Association. *Cerebral Palsy—Facts and Figures.* New York: UCPA, 1986.

————. *What Is Cerebral Palsy.* New York: UCPA, 1978.

United States Association for Blind Athletes. *SportsScoop: July and August 1989.* Colorado Springs, Colo.: USABA, 1989.

————. *Sports Summaries: Alpine Skiing.* Colorado Springs, Colo.: USABA, 1989.

————. *Sports Summaries: Goal Ball.* Colorado Springs, Colo.: USABA, 1989.

————. *Sports Summaries: Gymnastics.* Colorado Springs, Colo.: USABA, 1989.

————. *Sports Summaries: Judo.* Colorado Springs, Colo.: USABA, 1989.

————. *Sports Summaries: Nordic Skiing.* Colorado Springs, Colo.: USABA, 1989.

————. *Sports Summaries: Powerlifting.* Colorado Springs, Colo.: USABA, 1989.

————. *Sports Summaries: Speed Skating.* Colorado Springs, Colo.: USABA, 1989.

————. *Sports Summaries: Swimming.* Colorado Springs, Colo.: USABA, 1989.

————. *Sports Summaries: Tandem Cycling.* Colorado Springs, Colo.: USABA, 1989.

————. *Sports Summaries: Track and Field.* Colorado Springs, Colo.: USABA, 1989.

————. *Sports Summaries: Wrestling.* Colorado Springs, Colo.: USABA, 1989.

————. *United States Association for Blind Athletes.* Colorado Springs, Colo.: USABA, 1989.

University of Maryland Medicine. "Refractive Errors." Available online. URL: http://www.umm.edu/eyecare/visprobs.htm.

————. "Age-Related Macular Degeneration (AMD)." Available online. URL: http://www.umm.edu/eyecare/macular.htm.

U.S. Bureau of the Census. *Disability, Functional Limitation, and Health Insurance Coverage: 1984/85.* Washington, D.C.: USBC, 1986.

U.S. Department of Health and Human Services. *Diabetic Retinopathy.* NIH Publication No. 85–2171. Washington, D.C.: Government Printing Office, 1987.

———. *Vision Research: A National Plan, 1983–1987 Volume Two/Part One.* NIH Publication No. 83–2471. Washington, D.C.: Government Printing Office, 1987.

———. *Vision Research: A National Plan, 1983–1987 Volume Two/Part Two.* NIH Publication No. 83–2472. Washington, D.C.: Government Printing Office, 1987.

———. *Vision Research: A National Plan, 1983–1987 Volume Two/Part Four.* NIH Publication No. 83–2472. Washington, D.C.: Government Printing Office, 1987.

———. *Vision Research: A National Plan, 1983–1987 Volume Two/Part Five.* NIH Publication No. 83–2475. Washington, D.C.: Government Printing Office, 1987.

U.S. Department of Labor. *Interviewing Guides for Specific Disabilities.* Washington, D.C.: DOL, 1977.

U.S. Postal Service. *Mailing Free Matter for Blind and Visually Handicapped Persons.* Washington, D.C.: USPS, 1985.

Vander, James F., and Janice A. Gault. *Ophthalmology Secrets.* Philadelphia: Hanley & Belfus, Inc., 1998.

Vaughn, Daniel, and Taylor Asbury. *General Ophthalmology.* Los Altos, Calif.: Lange Medical Publications, 1977.

Vaughn, Lewis, ed. *The Complete Book of Vitamins and Minerals for Health.* Emmaus, Pa.: Rodale Press, 1988.

Vernon, McCay, Joann A. Boughman and Linda Annala. *Considerations in Diagnosing Usher's Syndrome: RP and Hearing Loss.* Baltimore: RP Foundation Fighting Blindness, 1982.

Veterans Administration. *Federal Benefits for Veterans and Dependents.* Washington, D.C.: VA, 1988.

Vision Place (The). "Treating Glaucoma with Eye Drops." Available online. URL: http://www.thevisionplace.com/VisionPlaceIII/discover/treatglcdrops.htm.

———. "Laser Treatment for Glaucoma." Available online. URL: http://www.thevisionplace.com/VisionPlaceIII/discover/treatglclaser.htm.

Wall, M., and D. R. May. "Threshold Amsler Grid Testing in Maulopathies." *Ophthalmology* (September 1987): 1126–33.

Walsh, Sara R., and Robert Holzberg, eds. *Understanding and Educating the Deaf-Blind/Severely and Profoundly Handicapped.* Springfield, Ill.: Charles C. Thomas Publisher, 1981.

Ware, Mary A., and Lois O. Schwab. "Child Rearing by Blind Parents." *The New Outlook* (June 1971): 169–174.

Waring, A. O. "Results of the Prospective Evaluation of Radial Keratotomy (PERK) Study on Year After Surgery." *Ophthalmology* 92, no. 2 (February 1985): 177–198.

Warren, David H. *Blindness and Early Childhood Development.* New York: American Foundation for the Blind, 1977.

———. "Blindness and Early Development: Issues in Research Methodology." *The New Outlook* (February 1976): 53–60.

Weale, R. A. *Focus on Vision.* Cambridge, Mass.: Harvard University Press, 1982.

Weinberg, Nancy, and Rosina Santana. "Comic Books: Champions of the Disabled Stereotype." *Rehabilitation Literature* 39, nos. 11–12 (November–December 1978): 327–331.

Weiner, Florence. *No Apologies.* New York: St. Martin's Press, 1986.

Weisgerber, Robert A., et al., eds. *Training the Handicapped for Productive Employment.* Rockville, Md.: Aspen Publications, 1980.

Western Blind Rehabilitation Center. *WBRC Clinical Summary.* Palo Alto, Calif.: WBRC, 1987.

———. *Western Blind Rehabilitation Center.* Palo Alto, Calif.: WBRC, 1987.

Wilensky, Jacob T., and John E. Read, eds. *Primary Ophthalmology.* New York: Grune and Stratton Inc., 1984.

World Health Organization. *Available Data On Blindness (Update 1987).* New York: WHO, 1987.

———. *Control of Vitamin A Deficiency and Xerophthalmia.* Geneva: WHO, 1982.

———. *Guidelines for Programmes for the Prevention of Blindness.* Geneva: WHO, 1979.

———. *The Use of Residual Vision by Visually Disabled Persons.* Copenhagen: WHO, 1981.

Woods, Virgil L. *Update in Lupus Research.* San Jose, Calif.: Bay Area Lupus Foundation, 1984.

Woodworth, Robert S., and Harold Schlosberg. *Experimental Psychology.* New York: Henry Holt and Company, 1958.

Worden, Helen W. "Aging and Blindness." *The New Outlook* (December 1976): 433–437.

Yanoff, Myron. "Magnetic Views of the Eye and Brain." *Sightsaving* 53, no. 4 (1984–85): 16–17.

Yudkin, John. *The Penguin Encyclopedia of Nutrition.* New York: Viking Press, 1985.

Ziegler, Martha. "Strength in Numbers: The National Network of Parent Coalitions." *Exceptional Parent* (June 1983): 57–58.

Zimmerman, Phillip. "HealthWatch: Nutritional Approaches to Degenerative Eye Diseases." *Townsend Letter for Doctors* (February/March 1988): 2.

Zinn, Walter J., and Herbert Solomon. *The Complete Guide to Eye Care, Eyeglasses, and Contact Lens.* Hollywood, Fla.: Frederick Fell Publishers Inc., 1986.

INDEX

Page numbers in **boldface** indicate extensive treatment of a topic.